NCLEX-RN®
Content Review Guide

FIFTH EDITION

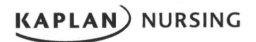
KAPLAN) NURSING

© 2017 by Kaplan, Inc.

Published by Kaplan Publishing, a division of Kaplan, Inc.
750 Third Avenue,
New York, NY 10017

ISBN Course: 978-1-5062-1462-7

ISBN Retail: 978-1-5062-1460-3

10 9 8 7 6 5 4 3 2 1

Judy Hyland, M.S.N., R.N.

Executive Director of Nursing

Barbara Arnoldussen, M.B.A., R.N.

Judith A. Burckhardt, Ph.D., R.N.

Barbara Dobish, M.S.N., R.N.

Cindy Finesilver, M.S.N., R.N.

Pamela Gardner, M.S.N., R.N.

Barbara J. Irwin, M.S.N., R.N.

Ellen Mahoney, C.S., D.N.S., R.N.

Marlene Redemske, M.S.N., M.A., R.N.

Table Of Contents

Introduction

Welcome! By using Kaplan Nursing resources, you've taken an important step toward passing the National Council Licensure Examination for Registered Nurses (NCLEX-RN®* examination).

Our many years of experience indicate that your success on the NCLEX-RN® examination is keyed to two specific factors: your educational background and your preparation for the exam. It is the amount and intensity of study you devote that will earn you the greatest benefit from the resources. The best results come to those who actively participate in exam preparation. We will show you how the NCLEX-RN® examination works, what you do and don't need to know, and the smartest way to take the NCLEX-RN® examination. We provide you with data to help you analyze your practice performance and determine where you need to make improvements. We will give you all the help, advice, and encouragement we can, but only you can do the work. Get to know all the benefits that Kaplan Nursing has to offer so you can make the most of your study time.

After you complete your resources and take the NCLEX-RN® examination, please tell us how you did. Kaplan's Research and Curriculum Development Team works hard to ensure that our course materials employ the most effective and innovative teaching methods. In order to evolve and improve, we need your help. Please take a few moments to share your thoughts on how the materials helped you. Thank you in advance for choosing Kaplan for your studies.

KAPLAN
750 Third Avenue,
New York, NY 10017
Attn: NCLEX Curriculum

customer.care@kaplan.com (kaptest.com)
integrated.support@kaplan.com (nursing.kaplan.com)

Our best wishes for an interesting and satisfying nursing career.

*NCLEX is a trademark of N.C.S.B.N., Inc.

Please note: All Kaplan lectures, web content, and printed and electronic media are the property of Kaplan Nursing and are copyrighted under law.

Chapter 1

THE NCLEX–RN® EXAMINATION

Units

1. **The NCLEX–RN® Examination**

Have you talked to graduate nurses about their experiences taking the NCLEX-RN® exam? They probably told you that the test wasn't like any nursing test they had ever taken. How can that be? The NCLEX-RN® exam is primarily multiple-choice test questions, and as a nursing student you are used to taking multiple-choice tests. In fact, you've taken so many tests by the time you graduate from nursing school that you probably believe there can't be any surprises on a nursing test. Yet there is one more surprise waiting for you, and it is called the NCLEX-RN® exam.

The NCLEX-RN® exam is similar to other standardized exams in some ways, yet different in others:

- The NCLEX-RN® exam is written by nurse specialists who are experts in a content area of nursing.
- All content is selected to allow the beginning practitioner to prove minimum competency on all areas of the test plan.
- NCLEX-RN® questions are written at 4 different levels based on Bloom's Taxonomy for the Cognitive Domain: knowledge, understanding, application, and analysis.
- Minimum competency questions are the passing level questions. They are asked at the application level, not the knowledge level. All the responses to a question are similar in length and subject matter and are grammatically correct.
- All test items have been extensively tested. National Council knows that the questions are valid; all correct responses are documented in two different sources.

What does this mean for you?

- National Council defines what is minimum-competency, entry-level nursing.
- Questions and answers are written in such a way that you will not be able to predict or recognize the correct answer.
- National Council is knowledgeable about the strategies regarding length of answers, grammar, etc. They make sure you can't use these strategies to select correct answers. English majors have no advantage!
- The answer choices have been extensively tested. The people who write the test questions make the incorrect answer choices look attractive to the unwary test-taker.

▶ WHAT BEHAVIORS DOES THE NCLEX-RN® EXAMINATION TEST?

The NCLEX-RN® exam does not want to test your body of nursing knowledge; it assumes you have a body of knowledge because you have graduated from nursing school. Likewise, it does not want to test your understanding of the material; it assumes you understand the nursing knowledge you learned in nursing school. So what does this exam test?

<u>The NCLEX-RN® exam primarily tests your nursing judgment and discretion.</u> It tests your ability to think critically and solve problems. The test writers recognize that as a beginning practitioner you will be managing LPNs/LVNs and nursing assistants to provide care to a group of clients. As the leader of the nursing team, you are expected to make safe and competent judgments about client care.

▶ CRITICAL THINKING AND CLINICAL JUDGMENT

What does the term critical thinking mean? Critical thinking is problem solving that involves thinking creatively.

Using clinical judgment, you successfully solve problems every day in the clinical area. You are probably comfortable with this concept when actually caring for clients. Although you've had lots of practice critically thinking in the clinical area, you may have had less practice thinking critically and using clinical judgment on test questions. Why is that?

During nursing school, you take exams developed by nursing faculty to test a specific body of content. Many of these questions are at the knowledge level. This involves recognition and recall of ideas or material that you read in your nursing textbooks and discussed in class. This is the most basic level of testing.

In nursing school, you are also given test questions written at the comprehension level. These questions require you to understand the meaning of the material. If you are answering minimum competency questions on the NCLEX-RN® exam, you will not see many comprehension-level questions. The test writers assume you know and understand the facts you learned in nursing school.

Minimum competency questions on the NCLEX-RN® exam are written at the application and/or analysis level. Remember, the exam tests your ability to make safe judgments about client care. Your ability to solve problems is not tested with knowledge- or comprehension-level questions. Application involves taking the facts that you know and using them to make a nursing judgment. You must be able to answer questions at the application level to prove your competence on the NCLEX-RN® exam.

▶ STRATEGIES THAT DON'T WORK ON THE NCLEX-RN® EXAMINATION

Whether you realize it or not, you developed a set of strategies in nursing school to answer teacher-generated test questions that are written at the knowledge/comprehension level. These strategies include:

- "Cramming" hundreds of facts about disease processes and nursing care
- Recognizing and recalling facts, rather than understanding the pathophysiology and the needs of a client with an illness
- Knowing who wrote the question and what is important to that faculty
- Predicting answers based on what you remember
- Selecting the response that is a different length compared with the other choices
- Selecting the answer choice that is grammatically correct
- When in doubt, choosing answer choice C

▶ CRITICAL THINKING AND CLINICAL JUDGMENT ON THE NCLEX-RN® EXAMINATION

- The NCLEX-RN® exam is not a test about recognizing facts.
- You must be able to correctly identify what the question is asking.
- Only focus on background information that is necessary to answer the question.

Remember, the NCLEX-RN® exam tests your ability to think critically. Critical thinking for the nurse involves:

- Observation
- Deciding what is important
- Looking for patterns and relationships
- Identifying the problem
- Transferring knowledge from one situation to another
- Applying knowledge
- Discriminating between possible choices and/or courses of action
- Evaluating according to established criteria

▶ FACTS ABOUT THE NCLEX-RN® EXAMINATION

The Purpose of the Exam

- To determine if you are a safe and competent nurse
- To safeguard the public
- To test for minimum competency to practice nursing

Test Content
- Based on the knowledge and activities of an entry-level nurse
- Written by nursing faculty and clinical specialists
- Majority of questions are self-contained, multiple-choice questions with four possible answer choices
- Some questions may ask you to select all answers that apply, fill in the blank, listen to an audio item, or answer questions that include graphics
- Some questions may ask you to use the mouse to identify a location on a graphic, drag and drop answers from an unordered answer column to an ordered answer column, or click on an exhibit tab
- Based on integrated nursing content—not on the medical model of medical, surgical, obstetrics, pediatrics, and psychiatric nursing
- Includes 15 experimental questions being tested for future exams; these questions do not count

Administration of the CAT
- The CAT (Computer Adaptive Test) is adapted to your knowledge, skills, and ability level.
- The question sequence is determined interactively.
- The computer selects questions based on the item difficulty and the test plan.
- You individually schedule a date and time to take the exam at a testing center.
- You sit at an individual computer station.

Taking the Exam
- Computer knowledge is not required to take this exam.
- You use a mouse to highlight and lock in your answer.
- You receive instructions and a practice exercise before beginning the exam.
- Any necessary background information appears on the screen with the question.
- The computer selects a first question on or around the passing level.
- The next question is selected by the computer on the basis of your response to the first question. If you receive a question that is similar to a question already answered, do not assume that you answered the first question incorrectly. Select the BEST answer to every question.
- If your answer is correct, the next question requires a higher level of critical thinking.
- If your answer is incorrect, the next question requires a lower level of critical thinking.
- Questions are selected to precisely measure your ability in each area of the test plan.

Timing

- There is no time limit for each individual question.
- You will answer a minimum of 75 questions to a maximum of 265 questions.
- The maximum time for the exam is 6 hours, including the practice exercise and all breaks.
- A pop-up window appears reminding you to take a break after 2 hours and 3.5 hours of testing. The time continues to run during all breaks.

The exam will end:

- When the computer has determined your ability, or
- When a maximum of 6 hours of testing is reached, or
- When a maximum of 265 questions have been answered.

Scoring

- It is a pass/fail exam.
- You are required to choose an answer before the computer will provide your next question. Take your best educated guess if you have to.
- The 15 experimental questions are not counted.

Concerns

- You can't change answers once you select NEXT. Questions are selected by the computer according to the accuracy of your previous responses.
- You can't scroll back.
- You can't skip a question. You must answer the question to go on.

Advantages

- Testing is available year-round, 15 hours a day, 6 days a week, in 6-hour time slots.
- Results are released by the individual State (Province or Territory) Board; length of time before you receive results will vary by State (Province or Territory) Board.
- If you fail, your state will determine when you can re-test.

▶ WHAT THE NCLEX-RN® EXAMINATION TESTS: CLIENT NEEDS

- Safe and Effective Care
    - Management of Care (17–23%)
    - Safety and Infection Control (9–15%)
- Health Promotion and Maintenance (6–12%)
- Psychosocial Integrity (6–12%)
- Physiological Integrity
    - Basic Care and Comfort (6–12%)
    - Pharmacological and Parenteral Therapies (12–18%)
    - Reduction of Risk Potential (9–15%)
    - Physiological Adaptation (11–17%)

▶ REGISTRATION

Registration information is available from your State (Province or Territory) Board of Nursing or your nursing school senior advisor. To obtain the address and phone number of an individual State Board of Nursing, contact:

National Council of State Boards of Nursing

111 E. Wacker Drive

Suite 2900

Chicago, IL 60601-4277

www.ncsbn.org

Chapter 2

KAPLAN'S REVIEW FOR THE NCLEX-RN® EXAMINATION

Units

1. **Kaplan's NCLEX-RN® Course Materials**

2. **How to Use Kaplan's NCLEX-RN® Online Study Center Resources**

3. **Kaplan's RN Decision Tree**

4. **Guide for Test-Takers Repeating the NCLEX-RN® Examination**

This chapter is for students enrolled in a Kaplan NCLEX-RN® Review Course.

If you are interested in the Kaplan NCLEX-RN® Course, start at kaptest.com

You have chosen the best course to prepare for the NCLEX-RN® exam. It is important that you take advantage of all the resources found in Kaplan's Review Course to ensure your success on the exam.

Familiarize yourself with all of the material so you can prepare a study plan that fits into your schedule. Students will have access to online study center resources after payment has been received and for 3 months after the class begins. Since most students test within 8 weeks of graduation, Kaplan has designed a schedule that continues for 8 weeks after class ends.

▶ MATERIALS FOR KAPLAN'S NCLEX-RN® REVIEW COURSE

(Available 24 hours a day, 7 days a week during your enrollment period)

Phase One: Content Review

Orientation to Kaplan's NCLEX-RN® Review Course
- Learn about Kaplan's NCLEX-RN® Review Course
- Explains how to use online assets

Pathway to Success Videos
- Learn how to think your way through the types of questions you will see on the NCLEX-RN® exam
- Establish a way to approach application- and analysis-level questions

Kaplan's Strategy Seminar for the NCLEX-RN® Examination
- Learn what you need to know about the NCLEX-RN® exam

Diagnostic Exam
- 180-question online exam that evaluates your strengths and weaknesses
- Indicates areas of the NCLEX-RN® test plan in which you will need concentrated study

NCLEX-RN® Content Review Guide
- Review frequently tested, minimum-competency nursing content
- Read content sections before class or study session

Video Review of Content
- Guided review of essential nursing content for success on the NCLEX-RN® exam
- Review the content as often as required

Phase Two: Learn How to Answer High-Level Critical Thinking Questions

RN Decision Tree
- Kaplan's critical thinking framework based on clinical nursing judgment
- Enables candidates to correctly answer application/analysis questions utilizing critical thinking

Class Lessons

- Learn how to apply your nursing knowledge to answer questions similar to those on the actual exam
- Discuss critical thinking and clinical judgment specific to the NCLEX-RN® exam
- Review exam-style questions using Kaplan's RN Decision Tree to ensure success on the NCLEX-RN® examination

Review of Questions

- Guided review of questions using Kaplan's RN Decision Tree; includes explanations of correct and incorrect responses
- Master critical thinking by repeating and/or reviewing the questions at your own pace

NCLEX-RN® Practice Test

- 60-Question Test (60 questions is the minimum for a computer decision. Remember: 15 of the first 75 are pretest, non-scored items.)
- Designed using the NCSBN test plan

Roadmap to Success

- Understand the importance of self regulation
- Review selected questions from the RN Practice Test
- Develop your study plan

Phase Three: Practice

The Question Trainers

- 1,000+ practice questions divided into 7 tests
- Provides practice with exam-style questions
- Review the explanations for correct and incorrect answers
- Includes alternate question types

Qbank

- 1500 exam-style questions
- Create customized practice tests
- 4 sample tests (one with all alternate format style questions)
- Receive immediate on-screen feedback
- Review detailed explanations of correct and incorrect answers

Readiness Test

- 180 Application and Analysis Level Question Test
- Complete 1 week before your scheduled NCLEX Examination
- Review and remediate every question

HOW TO USE KAPLAN'S NCLEX-RN®
ONLINE STUDY CENTER RESOURCES

Whether you take the Kaplan NCLEX-RN® Review In-Person, Live Online, or Self-Paced, Kaplan's NCLEX-RN® course offers many resources to ensure your success on the exam. These resources include the *NCLEX-RN® Content Review Guide*, review of exam-style questions, and the online study center. To make the best use of your NCLEX-RN® course, follow these steps and keep track of what you have accomplished.

This is the recommended study plan for utilizing the Kaplan NCLEX-RN® Prep resources. These resources are designed to give you plenty of realistic practice for success on test day. As you begin your preparation, please keep in mind that preparing for the NCLEX-RN® is a marathon, not a sprint! It is important to not rush your studies, but also not to procrastinate.

While you are utilizing the Kaplan NCLEX-RN® Prep resources, it is important that you follow these steps: analyze, review/remediate, think, study, and then continue practicing. Thoughtful review is the key to your NCLEX-RN® success.

▶ PHASE ONE: PRIOR TO YOUR KAPLAN NCLEX REVIEW COURSE

Phase one of the course is designed to help the student establish and review the essential nursing knowledge content. This content provides the base for the student to move to the higher-level critical thinking questions.

As you are completing tests, look at your **Analysis** page to see how you performed on each test. Aim for a score of 65 percent or higher *(Institutional students: your school may require higher.)* Use the test analyses to identify the client need categories where you scored the lowest. Use the **Test Reflection Worksheet** as you ask yourself the following, and assess how you are thinking:

1. Did I change any answers? Which way: correct to incorrect, or incorrect to correct?
2. Did I take enough time on each question or did I take too much time on each question?
3. Did I lose concentration, and if so, is there a pattern? Did I need to take a break?

Review/remediate all questions. Ask yourself the following:

1. Did I not know the content of the question?
2. For questions I answered incorrectly, why did the author of this question choose one answer, and why did I choose another?

Use the **Essential Nursing Content/Review of Content Videos** and your *NCLEX-RN® Content Review Guide* eBook to fill in any knowledge gaps, working from your content need area of greatest weakness toward your area of greatest strength.

Remember the goal of this phase: build and review <u>essential</u> nursing content.

▶ PHASE TWO: DECISION TREE, KAPLAN NCLEX REVIEW COURSE

Kaplan's review course consists of 7 three-hour sessions led by one of our expert nurse educators. Your review will concentrate on helping you answer passing-level NCLEX questions utilizing the Decision Tree and your clinical judgment skills in order to ensure success on test day.

While the structure of the lectures is not content focused, you will receive high-yield content tips while reviewing NCLEX-style questions in class.

In the second to last session (7/8) you will complete the **RN Practice Test.** Part of Session Eight is designed to review some of these questions with you.

Remember the goal of this phase: learn and review the Decision Tree process to answer high-level critical thinking questions. These questions are the passing-level questions of the NCLEX-RN® examination.

▶ PHASE THREE: AFTER ATTENDING THE KAPLAN NCLEX REVIEW COURSE

The goal of phase three is practice, practice, practice. The key to your practice is to take the time to review, remediate, and think about how you performed on the test you completed. Identify patterns that you need to change to become more successful on the next test.

Continue to look at your **Analysis** page to see how you performed on each of these tests and **continue to review/remediate** <u>all</u> questions. For Question Trainers 4 and 5, aim for scores of 65 percent or higher. For Question Trainers 6, 7, and the Qbank, aim for scores of 60 percent or higher *(Institutional students: your school may require higher on any of these resources.)*

Use the **Test Reflection Worksheet** and ask yourself:

1. Did I use the Decision Tree?
2. Am I seeing improvement as I progress from test to test?
3. Am I assessing <u>how I am thinking</u>?
4. Did I take a break at the best time for me?

Continue to use the **Online Content Lectures/***Review of Content Videos* and your *NCLEX-RN ® Content Review Guide* eBook to fill in any knowledge gaps, working from your content need area of greatest weakness toward your area of greatest strength.

You should complete all Question Trainers, Qbank questions, and review/remediate all questions before you take the NCLEX.

The day before your test, rest your mind and exercise your body. You are embarking upon the final step towards beginning your exciting new career as a nurse!

Additional Resources

The **Orientation, Decision Tree,** and **Review Class Questions/***Review of Questions* videos revisit information covered in the Review Course. Additional guidance on formulating your study plan leading up to your NCLEX test date can be found in Chapter 2 of the *NCLEX-RN® Content Review Guide* eBook. You can email NCLEX-Expert@kaplan.com for specific questions on the Decision Tree or using critical thinking to answer the question correctly.

▶ STUDY SCHEDULE

Designing your study schedule is a process that only you can do. Consideration for your work, family, and personal time mixed with your study time can only be determined by you. We provide you with a process of creating the schedule, but you have to prioritize your time and fill in the calendar.

Plan a test date that allows you adequate time to complete all of Kaplan's questions prior to testing. Stick closely to your schedule. Delaying test dates can negatively affect your outcome on the NCLEX-RN® exam. (See research at **https://www.ncsbn.org/delaystudy2006.pdf**)

Not completing all the recommended requirements also may affect your outcome.

How to create your study plan: (This process is also in session eight of the class videos)

Timing for Kaplan NCLEX-RN® Resources

RESOURCE	APPROXIMATE TIME TO COMPLETE	APPROXIMATE TIME TO REVIEW
Phase 1		
Diagnostic Test	3 hours	9 hours
Trainer 1	1.5 hours	4.5 hours
Trainer 2	1.5 hours	4.5 hours
Trainer 3	2 hours	6 hours
Content Videos		30 hours
RN Content Review Guide		Determine how long will it take you to read this resource
Phase 2		
Sessions 1–6 and 8	21 hours	
Session 7 NCLEX-RN® Practice Test	1.2 hours	3.6 hours
Phase 3		
Trainer 4	3 hours	9 hours
Trainer 5	3 hours	9 hours
Trainer 6	4 hours	12 hours
Trainer 7	6 hours	18 hours
16–75q Qbank tests	1.5 hrs each (24 hrs)	4.5 hrs each (72 hrs)
Readiness Test	3 hours	9 hours
Total		approximately: 260 hours
Do NOT study the 24 hours before your test. Let your mind rest!		

FIRST METHOD: Use this to choose your date based on how much time you require to prepare. This is the method we recommend.

1. How many days a week can you study? *Example: 5 days a week*
2. How many hours a day can you focus on studying? *Example: 6 hours a day*
3. Multiply your answer from #1 by #2. *Example: 5 x 6 = 30 hours/ week*
4. Divide the total number of hours from the study guide by the numbers of hours you have a week. *Example: 260/30 = 8.7 weeks needed to prepare*
5. Set your date that many weeks from now. *Example: 8 weeks from now*

SECOND METHOD: If you have a date picked out, use this method to determine how many hours a week you have to prepare.

1. How many weeks from today until your test date?
   ◦ *Example: My test is in 5 weeks.*
2. Divide the total hours needed for preparation by the number of weeks you have until your test date.
   ◦ *Example: 260/5 weeks = 52 hours/week*

- ◦ Ask yourself, can you study 52 hours a week?
- ◦ If not, consider moving your test date.

3. Divide the hours per week you got in step 2 by the number of days a week you have available to study.
   - ◦ *Example: I can study 5 days a week.*
   - ◦ 52 hours a week/ 5 days = 10.4 hours a day
   - ◦ Ask yourself, can you study 10.4 hours a day?
   - ◦ If not, consider moving your test date.

4. Calendar Example: Put in your time just like a class.
   Example: studying 6 hours a day for 6 days a week.

Sun	Mon	Tues	Wed	Thur	Fri	Sat
Off	9–12 1–4	9–12 1–4	9–12 1–5	9–12 1–4	9–12 1–4	10–1 2–5

5. Your study plan will look different from everyone else's because you have different work and family needs and study preferences. Use your critical thinking to achieve the best study plan for you.

▶ REVIEWING QUESTIONS

Use the **Test Reflection Worksheet to help you review and remediate each test and every question.** Make sure to review the rationales to all the questions answered. Review the questions you answered correctly to reinforce successful critical thinking. Review the questions you missed to learn from your mistakes. To identify why you missed questions, ask yourself these questions:

1. **Did you miss the question because you did not know the content?**

   If so, look up the content immediately. Focus on understanding the concepts and principles rather than trying to memorize content.

2. **Did you miss the question because you did not correctly identify the topic of the question?**

   You know you have misidentified the topic if you are reading the rationale and it is about a topic you did not consider. Look carefully at the stem of the question and the answers to determine the topic. Refer to the Decision Tree.

3. **Did you miss the question even though you correctly identified the topic?**

   Use all the steps of the Decision Tree. Many times students will choose the second best answer because they did not recognize the patterns found in the answer choices. Another reason students answer questions incorrectly is because they do not thoughtfully consider each answer choice. Slow down and THINK!

▶ MONEY-BACK GUARANTEE

If you are a kaptest.com student and graduate of an NLN or CCNE-accredited nursing program taking the exam for the first time within 6 months of graduation, and you do not pass the NCLEX-RN® exam, you are entitled to either a 100% tuition refund or a free 3-month continuation of your enrollment. If you are an Institutional Program student, check the school policy.

You must meet the following eligibility criteria:

- Take the Kaplan Diagnostic and Readiness Tests from your online account.
- Attend all class sessions: In Person, Live Online, or Self-Paced. Up to 2 live Classroom sessions can be made up online.
- Answer all questions on the 7 Question Trainer tests.

To qualify for the 100% tuition refund, you must not access the Online Study Center resources after the date of your NCLEX-RN® exam. The money-back guarantee applies ONLY to the original 3-month enrollment, and does not apply to any enrollment renewal. You must call 1-800-KAP-TEST within 20 days of the date of your NCLEX-RN® exam for instructions.

The RN Decision Tree is Kaplan Nursing's critical thinking framework to answer application/analysis nursing test questions. Your Kaplan instructor will teach you how to use the Decision Tree and will use it when reviewing test questions. Open your book to these pages when you practice answering questions. Consistently use the Decision Tree to be successful on the NCLEX-RN® exam.

Step 1: Can you identify the topic of the question?

No

Yes

Trap: NCLEX-RN® "hides" the topic of the question.

Read answer choices for clues.
Identify the topic of the question.
Proceed to **Step 2.**

Proceed to **Step 2.**

Step 2: Are the answers assessments or implementations?

A mix of assessments and implementations?

Trap: Is validation required?

Are answers all assessment or implementation?

Read stem to determine if you should assess or implement.

Proceed to **Step 3.**

Select correct answer.

Step 3: Does Maslow apply?

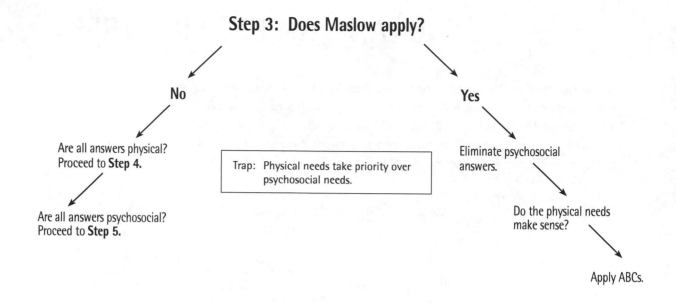

No

Are all answers physical?
Proceed to **Step 4.**

Are all answers psychosocial?
Proceed to **Step 5.**

Trap: Physical needs take priority over psychosocial needs.

Yes

Eliminate psychosocial answers.

Do the physical needs make sense?

Apply ABCs.

Step 4: Are all answers physical?

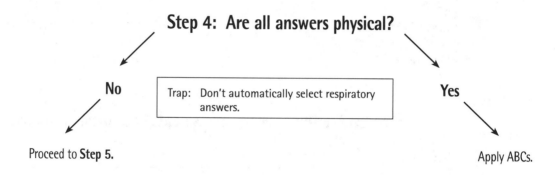

No

Trap: Don't automatically select respiratory answers.

Yes

Proceed to **Step 5.**

Apply ABCs.

Step 5: What is the outcome of each of the remaining answers?

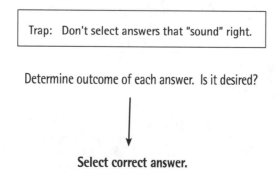

Trap: Don't select answers that "sound" right.

Determine outcome of each answer. Is it desired?

Select correct answer.

GUIDE FOR TEST-TAKERS REPEATING THE NCLEX-RN® EXAMINATION

Some people may never have to read this section, but it's a certainty that others will. The most important advice we can give to repeat test-takers is: don't despair. There is hope. We can get you through the NCLEX-RN® exam. Contact nclex-expert@kaplan.com to assist you if you purchased the Kaplan Review Course to begin the next path to success.

You Are Not Alone

Think about that awful day when your envelope arrived. You just couldn't believe it. You had to tell family, friends, your supervisor, and coworkers that you didn't pass. When this happens, each unsuccessful candidate feels like he or she is the only person that has failed the exam.

Should You Test Again?

Absolutely! You completed your nursing education to become an RN. The initial response of many unsuccessful candidates is to declare, "I'm never going back! That was the worst experience of my life! What do I do now?" When you first received your results, you went through a period of grieving—the same stages that you learned about in nursing school. Three to four weeks later, you find that you want to begin preparing to retake the exam.

How to Interpret Unsuccessful Test Results

Most unsuccessful candidates on the NCLEX-RN® exam will usually say, "I almost passed." Some of you did almost pass, and some of you weren't very close. If you fail the exam, you will receive a Candidate Performance Report from National Council. In this report, you will be told how many questions you answered on the exam. The more questions you answered, the closer you came to passing. The only way you will continue to get questions after you answer the first 75 is if you are answering questions close to the level of difficulty needed to pass the exam. If you answered questions far below the level needed to pass, your exam will end.

Figure 1 shows a representation of what happens when a candidate fails in 75 questions. This student does not come close to passing. In 75 questions, this student demonstrates an inability to consistently answer questions correctly at or above the level of difficulty needed to pass the exam. This usually indicates a lack of nursing knowledge, considerable difficulties with taking a standardized test, or a deficiency in critical thinking skills.

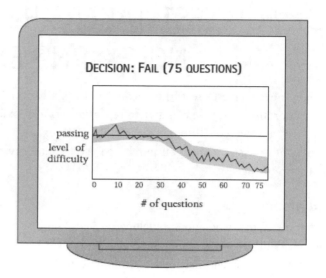

Figure 1

Figure 2 shows what happens when a candidate takes all 265 questions and fails. This candidate "almost passed." If the last question is below the level of difficulty needed to pass, the candidate fails.

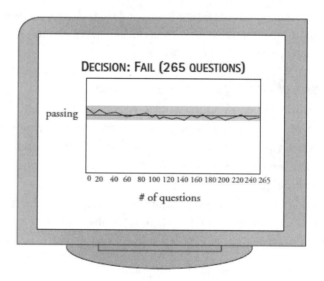

Figure 2

If the last question is above the level of difficulty needed to pass, the candidate passes. If you took a test longer than 75 questions and failed, you were probably familiar with most of the content you saw on the exam, but you may have had difficulty using critical thinking skills or taking a standardized test.

The information contained on the Candidate Performance Report helps you identify your strengths and weaknesses on this particular NCLEX-RN® exam. This knowledge will help you identify where to concentrate your study when you prepare to retake the exam.

▶ COMMON PROBLEMS WITH THE NCLEX-RN®

I saw nursing topics that were not familiar to me.

Review the Candidate Performance Report and identify the client need areas where you were "below passing." Review your Kaplan test results and identify client need areas where your scores were below the benchmark score. If you purchased the Kaplan Preparation Course, review content using the content videos and review your *NCLEX-RN® Content Review Guide,* beginning with your weakest content areas and progressing to your stronger areas.

I saw medications that were not familiar to me.

It is difficult to memorize individual medications. Organize your study of medications based on the classification system. The pharmacology section in your *NCLEX-RN® Content Review Guide* is organized according to medication classifications. You will need to know the generic names of medications in each classification. As you read topics in your guide, if a medication is mentioned, look it up so you understand the context in which it is being used.

I prepared for the exam just like I prepared for tests in nursing school.

The purpose of the NCLEX-RN® exam is to test critical thinking and clinical judgment needed to safely care for clients in all health care settings. Passing-level questions on NCLEX-RN® are written at the application and analysis level. If you prepare for NCLEX-RN® by answering knowledge and comprehension questions, you are not using the type of thinking required. The Decision Tree, taught in the Kaplan Course, has been designed to act as a framework or guide to approach application and analysis level questions.

I memorized facts without understanding the principles of client care.

If you memorize facts about a disease process, that may not help you answer the questions on NCLEX-RN®. NCLEX-RN® tests the candidate's ability to prioritize, provide safe and effective nursing care, and evaluate the client's response to care. Understanding, not memorization, allows you to approach, analyze, and determine the best clinical judgment for each question.

I was not sure about the type of questions I would see on NCLEX-RN®.

Go to www.ncsbn.org and review the candidate information about the alternate-format item questions and the test plan for the exam. When you take Kaplan nursing tests, the questions are written at the level of difficulty needed to pass NCLEX-RN®. The NCLEX-RN® exam is testing your ability to critically think in complex client care situations.

I did not understand Computer Adaptive Testing (CAT).

Review the candidate information on www.ncsbn.org about Computer Adaptive Testing. When taking the NCLEX-RN® exam, the next question depends on only 2 things: first, whether you answered the previous question correctly or incorrectly, and second, the area of the test plan from which the next question must come to maintain the percentages in each area.

I thought I would complete the exam with the minimum amount of questions.

It is possible to pass or fail the test with the minimum or maximum amount of questions or anywhere in between the minimum or maximum number. The computer will continue to give you questions as long as you are around the passing line. You need to prepare to take the maximum number of questions. It's better to be prepared for longer and end up short, than the reverse. If you are getting questions, you are still in the game—stay focused!

I began to lose my concentration when the computer continued to give me questions.

If you lose your concentration, you need to recognize what's happening and regain your ability to concentrate. Take a mental break while sitting at the computer or leave the computer station for a short time. The Kaplan Course uses longer tests that allow you to get in mental shape. Follow the guidelines given for each test.

I had difficulty identifying what the questions were asking.

Take your time and read the question and answers. Do not try to answer a question without identifying the topic. Remember, you cannot answer the question until you are clear about what you are being asked.

I did not carefully consider each answer choice.

NCLEX questions are written so that you may like more than one answer. It is important to consider each answer choice before selecting an answer.

I did not eliminate answers when I considered the answer choices.

Eliminate answers you know are incorrect. If you are not sure about an answer, keep it in for consideration.

I am not good at selecting answers that require me to establish priorities of care.

When you are answering questions, think about answers that provide for client safety or reduce the risk of injury. Is gathering more data or implementation the best and most important action for the nurse to take? Do Maslow's hierarchy or the ABCs apply?

I answered the questions based on my "real world" experiences.

The NCLEX-RN® exam is based on "ivory-tower nursing." When you answer a question, think about what the author of a nursing text book would do. Do not consider what you do at work or what you see others doing.

When I thought 2 answer choices seemed correct, I did not know how to choose the correct one.

Read the question and then each answer choice. Think about priorities: client safety, Maslow, and the ABCs. There is only one best answer. If you can do only one thing and walk away, what will the outcome be for your client?

I began to believe I would not pass.

When you feel this coming on, you need to take a break and do some positive thinking. As long as the computer is still asking you questions, you are still in the running. Tell yourself you are doing okay. Repeat positive thinking statements. Refocus your brain on each question.

Evaluate Your CAT Experience

Some students attribute their failure to the CAT experience. Comments we have heard include:

"I didn't like answering questions on the computer."

"I found the background noise distracting."

"I looked up every time the door opened."

"I should have taken a snack. I got so hungry!"

"After two and a half hours I didn't care what I answered. I just wanted the computer to shut off!"

"I didn't expect to be there for four hours!"

"I should have rescheduled my test, but I just wanted to get it over with!"

Do any of these comments sound familiar? It is important for you to take charge of your CAT experience. Here's how:

- Choose a familiar testing site.
- Select the time of day that you test your best. (Are you a morning or afternoon person?)
- Accept the earplugs when offered.
- Take a snack and a drink for your break.
- Take a break if you become distracted or fatigued during the test.
- Contact the proctors at the test site if something bothers you during the test.
- Plan on testing for six hours. If you get out early, it's a pleasant surprise.
- Say to yourself every day, "I will be successful."

After determining why you failed, the next step is to establish a plan of action for your next test. Remember, you should prepare differently this time.

Consider the following when setting up your new plan of study:

You've Seen the Test

You may wish that you didn't have to walk back into the testing center again, but if you want to be a registered professional nurse, you must go back. But this time you have an advantage over a first time test taker: you've seen the test! You know exactly what you are preparing for, so there are no unknowns. The computer will remember what questions you took before, and you will not be given any of the same questions. But the content of the question, the style of the question, and the kinds of answer choices will not change. You will not be surprised this time.

Study Both Content and Test Questions

By the time you retest, you will be out of nursing school for 3–6 months or longer. Remember that old saying, "What you are not learning, you are forgetting"? Because this exam is based on nursing as it is practiced in the United States and Canada, you must remember all you can about nursing theory and use sound clinical judgment to select the correct answers. You must study content that is integrated and organized like the NCLEX–RN® exam.

You must also master exam-style test questions. It is essential that you be able to correctly identify what each question is asking. You will not predict answers. You will think about each and every answer choice to decide if it answers the reworded question. To master test questions, you must practice answering them. We recommend you answer and review hundreds of exam-style test questions, especially at the application level of difficulty. The Kaplan Course provides all the high-level critical thinking question you will need to prepare.

Know All of the Words and their Meanings

Some students who have to learn a great deal of material in a short period of time have trouble learning the extensive vocabulary of the discipline. For example, difficulty with terminology is a problem for even strong students who study history. They enjoy the concepts, but find it hard to memorize all of the names and dates that allow them to do well on history tests. If you are a student who has trouble memorizing terms, you may find it useful to review a list of the terminology you must know to pass the NCLEX–RN® exam.

Practice Test-Taking Strategies

There is no substitute for mastering the nursing content. But combining this knowledge with test-taking strategies, will help you select a greater number of correct answers. For many students, the strategies mean the difference between a passing test and a failing test. Using strategies effectively can also determine whether you take a short test (75 questions) or a longer test (up to 265 questions).

Test-Taking Strategies That Don't Work on the NCLEX-RN® Examination

Whether you realize it or not, you developed a set of test-taking strategies in nursing school to answer teacher-generated test questions that are written at the knowledge/comprehension level of difficulty. These strategies include:

- "Cramming" hundreds of facts about disease processes and nursing care
- Recognizing and recalling facts rather than understanding the pathophysiology and the needs of a client with an illness
- Knowing who wrote the question and what is important to that instructor
- Predicting answers based on what you remember or who wrote the test question
- Selecting the response that is a different length compared to the other choices
- Selecting the answer choice that is grammatically correct
- When in doubt, choosing answer choice C

These strategies will not work because the NCLEX-RN® exam tests your ability to make safe, competent decisions.

Successful Test-Takers of the NCLEX-RN® Examination:

- Have a good understanding of nursing content
- Have the ability to tackle each test question with a lot of confidence because they assume that they can figure out the right answer
- Don't give up if they are unsure of the answer; they are not afraid to think about the question and the possible choices in order to select the correct answer
- Possess the know-how to correctly identify the question
- Stay focused on the question
- Can pace themselves for a long test, and take a break when they need one

Unsuccessful Test-Takers of the NCLEX-RN® Examination:

- Assume that they either know or don't know the answer to the question
- Memorize facts to answer questions by recall or recognition
- Read the question, read the answers, read the question, and pick an answer
- Choose answer choices based on a hunch or a feeling instead of thinking critically
- Answer questions based on personal experience rather than nursing theory
- Give up too soon because they aren't willing to think hard about questions and answers
- Don't stay focused on the question
- Push through questions without taking a break when they need one

Work to become a successful test-taker!

▶ PREPARE TO RETAKE THE NCLEX-RN® EXAMINATION

(Some resources are only available in the Kaplan NCLEX-RN® Review Course)

1. **Evaluate your content knowledge.**

   Compare your individualized results from the Kaplan Diagnostic Test (course only) with the Candidate Performance Report you received from the National Council of State Boards of Nursing. What similarities are there in the two results? What differences are there? In which areas did you do well? In which areas do you need more study?

2. **Think about your strong and weak areas.**

   You will note that both the Kaplan Diagnostic Test (course only) results and the National Council's Diagnostic Profile are organized according to the Categories of Client Needs. It is important that you have a comprehensive understanding of the concept of Client Needs.

3. **Plan a study schedule.**

   Plan your study time to include all nursing content, but emphasize areas identified as weaknesses on the Kaplan Diagnostic exam (course only) and on your Candidate Performance Report from the National Council. Preparation for retaking the NCLEX-RN® exam should include a minimum of 4–6 weeks of concentrated study. Establish specific daily goals and reward yourself when you accomplish them. Don't let yourself fall behind.

4. **Begin studying.**

   At first you may find it difficult to review the nursing content. You may find yourself saying, "I know this already." You may find yourself remembering the questions that were on your NCLEX-RN® exam. Forget them! You will not see any of the same questions when you retest. Focus your energy on understanding the nursing content.

5. **Read the *NCLEX-RN® Content Review Guide*.**

   Begin with your areas of weakness and work toward your areas of strength. If you don't understand a word or have a question about a topic, look it up in your nursing school textbooks. Include these notes in your *NCLEX-RN® Content Review Guide*.

6. **Watch the Essential Nursing Content Videos (course only).**

   Watch the essential nursing content video in the areas identified as weaknesses on your Candidate Performance Report. Take notes in the *NCLEX-RN® Content Review Guide* as you watch the content videos.

7. **Review the Decision Tree. (Interested in the course? Start at kaptest.com.)**

   Kaplan developed the Decision Tree (course only) to provide you with the critical thinking framework and clinical judgment required to successfully answer passing level questions on the NCLEX-RN® exam. Make the commitment to use the Decision Tree when practicing questions in preparation for the NCLEX-RN® exam and when taking the actual exam.

8. **Review Kaplan's Path to Success Videos. (course only)**

These ideas/practices are not a substitute for knowledge of nursing content, but will provide you with tools to utilize your nursing knowledge and answer application/analysis-level questions correctly.

9. **Review the recorded class lessons.** (course only; for some students this will be available after your in-class course)

The questions reviewed in these lessons are exam-style and of varying levels of difficulty. The discussion of the explanations to the questions does three things: first, it gives you the correct answer; second, it reviews the knowledge and thought processes that lead to the correct answer; third, it points out the wrong thinking behind the incorrect answer choices. If you have difficulty with a question, stop the recording and ask yourself why you missed the question. Did the question concern nursing knowledge you didn't know? Did you misread the question? Did you make an assumption or base your answer on what you have seen in the "real world" instead of "ivory tower nursing"? Was it a test-taking problem?

If there is content that you don't understand or don't remember, look it up.

10. **After you finish, go back and review your notes.**

Do you have a complete understanding of the content areas? If not, more study is needed.

11. **Practice with the Question Trainers.** (course only)

If your evaluation of your previous testing experience identified problems with the computer format of the exam, now is the time to work out any difficulties you experienced when taking the "real thing." Use these 7 practice tests to evaluate your knowledge of nursing content, practice your critical thinking skills, and become comfortable with the testing format.

12. **Practice with the Qbank.** (course only)

Build your confidence by using the Decision Tree to answer Qbank questions. You determine the content and select the number of questions contained in each test (at least 75 questions). Build your Qbank test from all 8 client need areas. This will enable you to consistently review essential nursing content. To make the most of your Qbank experience, only answer questions using "testing mode." Typically, students who use "tutor mode" answer more questions correctly because they view explanations prior to selecting answers. This does not, however, give you accurate feedback about how you are answering questions.

13. **Be Confident!**

Don't schedule to retake the NCLEX-RN® exam until you have allowed yourself sufficient time to prepare. Then, walk into the exam knowing that you are prepared and ready to pass. Take charge of your environment. Arrange the computer keyboard and light for comfort. Approach the exam like a marathon and ration your energy and effort. Be prepared to answer all 265 questions. If you lose your concentration, raise your hand and take a short break. Comprehensive preparation and a positive attitude are the ingredients for success on the NCLEX-RN® exam.

Chapter 3

PHYSIOLOGICAL INTEGRITY: PHARMACOLOGICAL AND PARENTERAL THERAPIES

Units

1. **Blood Component Therapy**

2. **Intravenous Therapy**

3. **Medications**

4. **Adverse Effects of Medications**

BLOOD COMPONENT THERAPY

A. Procedure

    1. Equipment

        a. Blood or blood products (see Table 1)

        b. Tubing with filter

        c. 19-gauge needle for venous access

Table 1 BLOOD COMPONENTS		
PRODUCT	**ADVERSE REACTIONS**	**NURSING CONSIDERATIONS**
Packed red blood cells	Reactions less common than with whole blood	Companion solution–0.9% NaCl Monitor client during transfusion Give over 2–4 h Use standard blood filter Mix cells every 20–30 minutes (squeeze bag) Give over 2–4 h
Platelets	Some febrile reactions	Companion solution–0.9% NaCl Nonwettable filter Give as quickly as possible, 4 units/hour
Plasma	Circulatory overload risk	Administer with straight line set Give as quickly as possible (coagulation factors become unstable)
Albumin	Possible circulatory overload	Use administration set provided 25% albumin–give at 1 mL/min Give as quickly as possible if client in shock
Prothrombin	Hepatitis risk greater than with whole blood Allergic/febrile reactions	Use straight line set
Factor VIII	Allergic and febrile reactions	Use component drip set or syringe

    2. Ask client about allergies or previous blood reactions

3. Type and cross-match blood—ensures that the donor's blood and recipient's blood are compatible (see Table 2)

Table 2 BLOOD GROUP COMPATIBILITY		
BLOOD GROUP	CAN ACT AS DONOR	CAN RECEIVE BLOOD FROM
O	O, A, B, AB	O
A	A, AB	O, A
B	B, AB	O, B
AB	AB	O, A, B, AB

4. Check blood for bubbles, dark color, or cloudiness
5. Check by two nurses
   a. Health care provider's order
   b. Client's identity
   c. Hospital ID band name and number
   d. Blood component tag name and number
   e. Blood type and Rh
6. Check baseline vital signs, including temperature
7. Start with normal saline (0.9% NaCl)
8. Run blood slowly for first 15 minutes
9. Stay with client for first 15–30 minutes after blood starts into the client
10. Recheck vital signs 15 minutes after infusion started
11. If no untoward effects, increase rate; should be infused in 2 hours for each unit (depending on client's cardiovascular status) (see Table 3)
12. Obtain vital signs every hour until completed, then hourly for 3 hours
13. For elderly check vital signs every 15 minutes throughout transfusion
14. For elderly infuse each unit over 3–4 hours
15. Ask client to report itching or flank pain over kidneys
16. Change entire IV line for each unit of blood
17. If transfusion reaction suspected
    a. Stop blood or blood product
    b. Restart normal saline
    c. Save blood container and tubing and return to blood bank
    d. Draw blood sample for plasma, hemoglobin, culture, retyping
    e. Collect urine sample and send to lab for hemoglobin determination
    f. Monitor voiding for hematuria

B. Autologous transfusion
1. Preoperative donation collected 4–6 weeks before surgery
2. Iron supplements may be ordered

3. Benefits
    a. Prevention of viral infection from donated blood
    b. Used for clients with history of transfusion reactions
    c. Rare blood type
4. Contraindications
    a. Acute infection
    b. Chronic disease
    c. Hemoglobin less than 11 g/L, hematocrit less than 33%
    d. Cerebrovascular disease
    e. Cardiovascular disease

Table 3 BLOOD TRANSFUSION REACTIONS			
TYPE OF REACTION	CAUSE	SYMPTOMS	NURSING CONSIDERATIONS
Allergic reaction Hypersensitivity	Hypersensitivity to antibodies in donor's blood	Occurs immediately or within 24 hours Mild—urticaria, itching, flushing Anaphylaxis— hypotension, dyspnea, decreased oxygen saturation, flushing	Prevention—premedicate with antihistamines Stop the blood Restart the 0.9% NaCl Notify the health care provider Supportive care: diphenhydramine, oxygen, corticosteroids
Acute intravascular hemolytic reaction	Incompatibility	Occurs within minutes to 24 hours Nausea, chills, vomiting, pain in lower back, hypotension, increase in pulse rate, decrease in urinary output, hematuria	Stop the blood Supportive care: oxygen, diphenhydramine, airway management
Febrile nonhemolytic reaction (most common)	Antibodies to donor platelets or leukocytes	Occurs in minutes to hours Fever, chills, nausea, headache, flushing, tachycardia, palpitations	Stop the blood Supportive care Antipyretics (avoid aspirin in thrombocytopenic clients) Seen with clients after multiple transfusions
Sepsis	Contaminated blood products	Occurs within minutes to less than 24 hours Tachycardia, hypotension, high fever, chills, shock	Stop the blood Obtain blood culture Antibiotics, IV fluids, vasopressors, steroids
Circulatory overload	Large volume over short time	Occurs within minutes to hours—dyspnea, crackles, increased respiratory rate, tachycardia	Monitor clients at high-risk (elderly, heart disease, children) Slow or discontinue transfusion

▶ PARENTERAL FLUIDS

A. Definition of terms

1. Tonicity—concentration of a substance dissolved in water

2. ECF—extracellular fluid

3. Isotonic fluids—same concentration as ECF

4. Hypertonic solution—solute concentration greater than that of ECF

5. Hypotonic solution—solute concentration less than that of ECF

6. Intake refers to all possible avenues of intake, e.g., oral fluids, food, IV fluids, gavage feedings, irrigations

7. Output refers to all possible avenues of output, e.g., insensible losses, urine, diarrhea, vomitus, sweat, blood, and any drainage

B. Types (see Table 1)

Table 1 INTRAVENOUS FLUIDS		
TYPE OF FLUID	**IV FLUID**	**NURSING CONSIDERATIONS FOR IVS**
Isotonic	0.9% NaCl Lactated Ringer's 5% dextrose in water (is isotonic but becomes hypotonic when glucose metabolized)	Main purpose—to maintain or restore fluid and electrolyte balance Secondary purpose—to provide a route for medication, nutrition, and blood components 　Type, amount, and sterility of fluid must be carefully checked Macrodrip—delivers 10, 12, or 15 drops per milliliter; should be used if rapid administration is needed
Hypotonic	0.45% NaCl	Microdrip—delivers 60 drops per milliliter; should be used when fluid volume needs to be smaller or more controlled, e.g., clients with compromised renal or cardiac status, clients on "keep-open" rates, pediatric clients
Hypertonic	10-15% dextrose in water 3% NaCl Sodium bicarbonate 5%	Maintain sterile technique Monitor rate of flow Assess for infiltration—cool skin, swelling, pain Assess for phlebitis—redness, pain, heat, swelling Change tubing every 72 hours, bag every 24 hours or according to agency policy

C. Administration

1. Calculate IV flow rate (see Table 2)

Table 2 CALCULATIONS FOR IV RATE
1) Milliliters per hour:

$$\frac{\text{Total solution}}{\text{hours to run}} = \text{ml/h}$$

Example: 1,000 ml in 8 hours

$$\frac{1,000}{8} = 125\text{ml/h}$$

2) Drops per minute:

$$\frac{\text{Total volume} \times \text{drop factor}}{\text{time in minutes}} = \text{gtts/min}$$

Example: 1,000 ml in 8 hours, with a drop factor of 15

$$\frac{1,000 \times 15}{8 \times 60} =$$

$$\frac{1,000 \times 1}{8 \times 4} =$$

$$\frac{250}{8} =$$

31.25 or 31 gtts/min

2. Nursing care

   a. Change continuous use standard tubing every 96 hours unless contaminated—if contaminated change immediately

   b. Intermittent use tubing is changed every 24 hours unless contaminated—if contaminated change immediately

   c. Change fluid container every 24 hours

▶ PERIPHERAL IV

A. Location

1. Condition of vein

2. Type of fluid/med to be infused

3. Duration of therapy

4. Client's age, size, status

5. Skill of nurse

6. Non-dominant side for client

7. Type of catheter

B. Insertion of catheter

1. Explain procedure, check ID

2. Have all equipment at the bedside and prepared

3. Apply appropriate PPE

4. Distend veins by applying tourniquet 4–6" above site, apply warmth or have client open and close fist, or hang arm over side of bed to help dilate vein

5. Clean site with alcohol swab; start at center and work outward

6. Repeat cleaning with povidone-iodine

7. Hold skin taut to stabilize vein

8. Insert catheter bevel up at 10–30°, (direct method—thrust catheter through skin and vein in one smooth motion: (indirect method—first pierce skin, then vessel)

9. Lessen the angle and advance catheter; watch for flashback of blood

10. Once you see blood return, advance catheter 1/4" and then remove tourniquet

11. Withdraw needle from catheter, advance catheter up to hub

12. Secure catheter

13. Attach IV tubing

14. Begin IV infusion

15. Check for infiltration or hematoma

C. Complications

  1. Circulatory overload

    a. Assessment

      1) Crackles

      2) Dyspnea

      3) Confusion

      4) Seizures

    b. Nursing care

      1) Reduce IV rate

      2) Assess VS

      3) Assess lab values

      4) Notify HCP

  2. Infiltration (extravasation if tissue-damaging medication is used)

    a. Assessment

      1) Edema

      2) Pain

      3) Coolness in area

      4) Significant decrease in flow rate

      5) Apply tourniquet above infusion site; if infusion continues to drip, it is infiltrated

    b. Nursing care

      1) Discontinue IV

      2) Apply warm compresses to infiltrated site

      3) Apply sterile dressing

      4) Elevate arm

      5) Start IV at new site proximal to infiltrated site if same extremity used; may use different vein distal to infiltrated site (basilic or cephalic)

3. Phlebitis
   a. Assessment
      1) Reddened, warm area around insertion site or on path of vein
      2) Tenderness
      3) Swelling
   b. Nursing care
      1) Discontinue IV
      2) Apply warm, moist compresses
      3) Restart IV at new site
4. Thrombophlebitis (inflammation of the vein with clot formation)
   a. Assessment
      1) Pain
      2) Swelling
      3) Redness and warmth around insertion site or along path of vein
      4) Fever
      5) Leukocytosis
   b. Nursing care
      1) Discontinue IV
      2) Apply warm compress
      3) Elevate the extremity
      4) Restart the IV in the opposite extremity
5. Hematoma
   a. Assessment
      1) Ecchymosis
      2) Immediate swelling at site
      3) Leakage of blood at site
   b. Nursing care
      1) Discontinue IV
      2) Apply pressure with sterile dressing
      3) Apply cool compresses (or ice bag) intermittently for 24 h to site, followed by warm compresses
      4) Restart IV in opposite extremity
6. Clotting
   a. Assessment
      1) Decreased IV flow rate
      2) Back flow of blood into IV tubing
   b. Nursing care
      1) Discontinue IV
      2) Do *not* irrigate or milk the tubing
      3) Do *not* increase the IV flow rate or hang the solution higher
      4) Do *not* aspirate clot from the cannula

▶ **CENTRAL VENOUS ACCESS DEVICES**

Four types: peripherally inserted central catheter (PICC), tunneled central catheter, non-tunneled (percutaneous) central catheter, implanted port

A. Peripherally inserted central catheter (PICC)

1. Venipuncture performed above or below anticubital fossa into basilic, cephalic, or axillary veins of dominant arm (encourages blood flow and reduces risk of dependent edema)

2. Tip of catheter is in superior vena cava or brachiocephelic veins

3. May stay in place several days to months

4. Potential complications

   a. Malposition

   b. Pneumothorax

   c. Dysrhythmias

   d. Nerve or tendon damage

   e. Respiratory distress

   f. Catheter embolism

   g. Thrombophlebitis

5. Nursing care

   a. Change dressing 2–3 times a week and when wet or nonocclusive

   b. Flush with normal saline alone or with normal saline followed by heparinized saline according to agency policy

   c. Do not take blood pressure or draw blood from extremity with PICC line

B. Tunneled central catheter

1. Increases in size (2 gauges, 2.5 cm in length) 2 hours after insertion, becomes softer

2. Long-term use—can remain in place for years

3. Catheter is cuffed and can be single- to double-lumen

4. Venipuncture 2–3 finger breadths above antecubital fossa or 1 finger breadth below anticubital fossa into cephalic, basilic, or median cubital vein

5. Inserted surgically in subclavian vein, advanced to superior vena cava

6. Examples: Hickman, Groshong, Permacath

7. Complications

   a. Thrombosis

   b. Phlebitis

   c. Air embolism

   d. Infection

   e. Bleeding

   f. Vascular perforation

8. Nursing care
   a. Change dressing 2–3 times a week and when wet or nonocclusive
   b. Flush with normal saline alone or with normal saline followed by heparinized saline according to agency policy
   c. Anchor catheter securely
   d. Avoid chemotherapy or parenteral nutrition

C. Non-tunneled percutaneous central catheters
   1. Inserted through subclavian vein
   2. Triple-lumen central catheter–distal lumen (16-gauge) used to infuse or draw blood samples, middle lumen (18-gauge) used for PN infusion, proximal port (18-gauge) used to infuse or draw blood and administer medications
   3. Used for short term IV therapy
   4. Insertion
      a. Placed supine in head-low position (dilates vessel and prevents air embolism)
      b. Client turns head away from site during procedure
      c. While catheter is being inserted, client performs Valsalva maneuver
      d. Antibiotic ointment and transparent dressing applied using sterile technique
      e. Verify position of tip catheter by x-ray
      f. Each lumen secured with Leur-Lok cap and labeled to indicate location (proximal, middle, distal)
   5. Nursing care
      a. Site of catheter is used for less than 6 weeks
      b. Flush each lumen with normal saline alone or with normal saline followed by heparinized saline according to agency policy; flush after insertion, after infusions, after specimen withdrawal, or when disconnected
      c. Never use force to flush catheter; if resistance met, notify health care provider
      d. Dressing changes 2–3 times a week and PRN; place in low- Fowler's position; nurse and client wear masks; alcohol and then iodine swabs used to clean site
      e. Change IV tubing every 72 to 96 hours according to agency policy.

D. Implanted ports

1. Used for long-term therapy

2. Examples: Port-a-Cath, Hickman

3. Surgically placed

4. Allows client increased movement and decreased care

5. Tip of the catheter is under the skin

6. Access requires non-coring needle through the skin into the port

7. Complications:

   a. Embolism

   b. Clotted access

   c. Sepsis

8. Nursing Care:

   a. Cleanse skin prior to access

   b. Never use force to flush the port

▶ ORGANIZATION OF MEDICATIONS

The best way to learn medication information is to use the classification and subclassification systems which group and organize the medications.

Step 1: The *Content Review Guide* is organized by the most common classifications and subclassifications of medications.

Step 2: Identify the medications included in the classification and subclassification. NCLEX-RN® will identify the generic name of the medication.

Step 3: Identify the action or effect of the classification or subclassification.

Step 4: Based on the action of the classification or subclassification, identify the therapeutic use for the medications.

Step 5: Based on the action of the classification or subclassification, identify precautions or contraindications for use of that classification.

Step 6: Adverse effects are more intense effects of the action of the medications included in the classification or subclassification. Knowledge about management of adverse effects is critical when answering questions on NCLEX-RN®.

Step 7: Adverse reactions include potentially dangerous consequences related to the action of the medications in the classification or subclassification. The health care provider should be notified when adverse reactions occur.

Step 8: How do you evaluate the effect of the medications in the classification or subclassification? Is it a therapeutic or desired effect? Is it a nontherapeutic or undesired effect?

Step 9: Identify what the client needs to know to take the medication safely.

EMERGENCY MEDICATION FOR SHOCK, CARDIAC ARREST, AND ANAPHYLAXIS		
MEDICATION	ADVERSE EFFECTS	NURSING CONSIDERATIONS
Norepinephrine	Headache Palpitations Nervousness Epigastric distress Angina, hypertension **tissue necrosis with extravasation**	Vasoconstrictor to increase blood pressure and cardiac output Reflex bradycardia may occur with rise in BP Client should be attended at all times Monitor urinary output Infuse with dextrose solution, not saline Monitor blood pressure Protect medication from light
Dopamine	Increased ocular pressure Ectopic beats Nausea Tachycardia, chest pain, dysrhythmias	Low-dose–dilates renal and coronary arteries High-dose–vasoconstrictor, increases myocardial oxygen consumption Headache is an early symptom of drug excess Monitor blood pressure, peripheral pulses, urinary output Use infusion pump
Epinephrine	Nervousness Restlessness Dizziness Local necrosis of skin	Stimulates alpha and beta adrenergic receptors Monitor BP Carefully aspirate syringe before IM and subcutaneous doses; inadvertent IV administration can be harmful Always check strength: 1:100 only for inhalation, 1:1,000 for parenteral administration (SC or IM) Ensure adequate hydration
Isoproterenol	Headache Palpitations Tachycardia Changes in BP Angina, bronchial asthma Pulmonary edema	Stimulates beta 1 and beta 2 adrenergic receptors Used for heart block, ventricular arrhythmias, and bradycardia Bronchodilator used for asthma and bronchospasms Don't give at hs–interrupts sleep patterns Monitor BP, pulse

EMERGENCY MEDICATION FOR SHOCK, CARDIAC ARREST, AND ANAPHYLAXIS (CONTINUED)		
MEDICATION	**ADVERSE EFFECTS**	**NURSING CONSIDERATIONS**
Phenylephrine	Palpations Tachycardia Hypertension Dysrhythmia Angina Tissue necrosis with extravasation	Potent alpha 1 agonist Used to treat hypotension
Dobutamine hydrocholoride	Hypertension PVCs Asthmatic episodes Headache	Stimulates beta 1 receptors Incompatible with alkaline solutions (sodium bicarbonate) Administer through central venous catheter or large peripheral vein using an infusion pump Don't infuse through line with other meds (incompatible) Monitor EKG, BP, I and O, serum potassium
Milrinone	Dysrhythmia Thrombocytopenia Jaundice	Positive inotropic agent Smooth muscle relaxant used to treat severe heart failure
Sodium nitroprusside	Hypotension Increased intracranial pressure	Dilates cardiac veins and arteries Decreases preload and afterload Increases myocardial perfusion Keep medication in dark after fixed Use infusion pump
Diphenhydramine HCl	Drowsiness Confusion Insomnia Headache Vertigo Photosensitivity	Blocks effects of histamine on bronchioles, GI tract, and blood vessels
Actions	Varies with med	
Indications	Hypovolemic shock Cardiac arrest Anaphylaxis	
Adverse effects	Serious rebound effect may occur Balance between underdosing and overdosing	
Nursing considerations	Monitor vital signs Measure urine output Assess for extravasation Observe extremities for color and perfusion	

ADRENOCORTICAL MEDICATIONS: GLUCOCORTICOID		
MEDICATION	**ADVERSE EFFECTS**	**NURSING CONSIDERATIONS**
Cortisone acetate Hydrocortisone Dexamethasone Methylprednisolone Prednisone Beclomethasone Betamethasone Budesonide	Increases susceptibility to infection May mask symptoms of infection Edema, changes in appetite Euphoria, insomnia Delayed wound healing Hypokalemia, hypocalcemia Hyperglycemia Osteoporosis, fractures Peptic ulcer, gastric hemorrhage Psychosis	Prevents/suppresses cell-mediated immune reactors Used for adrenal insufficiency Overdosage produces Cushing's syndrome Abrupt withdrawal of drug may cause headache, nausea and vomiting, and papilledema (Addisonian crisis) Give single dose before 9 A.M. Give multiple doses at evenly spaced intervals Infection may produce few symptoms due to anti-inflammatory action Stress (surgery, illness, psychic) may lead to increased need for steroids Nightmares are often the first indication of the onset of steroid psychosis Check weight, BP, electrolytes, I and O Used cautiously with history of TB (may reactivate disease) May decrease effects of oral hypoglycemics, insulin, diuretics, K^+ supplements Assess children for growth retardation Protect from pathological fractures Administer with antacids. Do not stop abruptly Methylprednisolone also used for arthritis, asthma, allergic reactions, cerebral edema Dexamethasone also used for allergic disorders, cerebral edema, asthma attack, shock
Action	Stimulates formation of glucose (gluconeogenesis) and decreases use of glucose by body cells; increases formation and storage of fat in muscle tissue; alters normal immune response	
Indications	Addison's disease, Crohn's disease, COPD, lupus erythematosus, leukemias, lymphomas, myelomas, head trauma, tumors to prevent/treat cerebral edema	
Adverse effects	Psychoses, depression, weight gain, hypokalemia, hypocalcemia, stunted growth in children, petechiae, buffalo hump	

ADRENOCORTICAL MEDICATIONS: GLUCOCORTICOID *(CONTINUED)*		
MEDICATION	ADVERSE EFFECTS	NURSING CONSIDERATIONS
Nursing considerations	Monitor fluid and electrolyte balance Don't discontinue abruptly Monitor for signs of infection	
Herbal interactions	Cascara, senna, celery seed, juniper may decrease serum potassium; when taken with corticosteroids may increase hypoglycemia Ginseng taken with corticosteroids may cause insomnia Echinacea may counteract effects of corticosteroids Licorice potentiates effect of corticosteroids	

ADRENOCORTICAL MEDICATIONS: MINERALOCORTICOID		
MEDICATION	ADVERSE EFFECTS	NURSING CONSIDERATIONS
Fludrocortisone acetate	Hypertension, edema due to sodium retention Muscle weakness and dysrhythmia due to hypokalemia	Give PO dose with food Check BP, electrolytes, I and O, weight Give low-sodium, high-protein, high-potassium diet May decrease effects of oral hypoglycemics, insulin, diuretics, K+ supplements
Action	Increases sodium reabsorption, potassium and hydrogen excretion in the distal convoluted tubules of the nephron	
Indications	Adrenal insufficiency	
Adverse effects	Sodium and water retention Hypokalemia	
Nursing considerations	Monitor BP and serum electrolytes Daily weight, report sudden weight gain to health care provider Used with cortisone or hydrocortisone in adrenal insufficiency	

ANTACID MEDICATIONS		
MEDICATION	ADVERSE EFFECTS	NURSING CONSIDERATIONS
Aluminum hydroxide gel Calcium carbonate Aluminum hydroxide and magnesium trisilicate	Constipation that may lead to impaction, phosphate depletion	Monitor bowel pattern Compounds contains sodium; check if client is on sodium-restricted diet Aluminum and magnesium antacid compounds interfere with tetracycline absorption Encourage fluids Monitor for signs of phosphate deficiency—malaise, weakness, tremors, bone pain Shake well Careful use advised for kidney dysfunction
Magnesium hydroxide	Excessive dose can produce nausea, vomiting, and diarrhea	Store at room temperature with tight lid to prevent absorption of CO_2 Prolonged and frequent use of cathartic dose can lead to dependence Administer with caution to clients with renal disease
Aluminum hydroxide and magnesium hydroxide	Slight laxative effect	Encourage fluid intake Administer with caution to clients with renal disease
Action	Neutralizes gastric acids; raises gastric pH; inactivates pepsin	
Indications	Peptic ulcer Indigestion Reflux esophagitis Prevent stress ulcers	
Adverse effects	Constipation, diarrhea Acid rebound between doses Metabolic acidosis	
Nursing considerations	Use medications with sodium content cautiously for clients with cardiac and renal disease Absorption of tetracyclines, quinolones, phenothiazides, iron preparations, isoniazid reduced when given with antacids Effectiveness of oral contraceptives and salicylates may decrease when given with antacids	

ANTIANXIETY MEDICATIONS		
MEDICATION	ADVERSE EFFECTS	NURSING CONSIDERATIONS
Benzodiazepine Derivatives		
Chlordiazepoxide Diazepam	Lethargy, hangover Respiratory depression Hypotension	CNS depressant Use–anxiety, sedation, alcohol withdrawal, seizures May result in toxic build-up in the elderly Potential for physiological addiction/overdose Can develop tolerance and cross-tolerance Cigarette smoking increases clearance of drug Alcohol increases CNS depression
Alprazolam Lorazepam Oxazepam	Drowsiness, light-headedness, hypotension, hepatic dysfunction Increased salivation Orthostatic hypotension Memory impairment and confusion	CNS depressant Safer for elderly Don't combine with alcohol or other depressants Check renal and hepatic function Don't discontinue abruptly (true for all antianxiety medications) Teach addictive potential
Midazolam	Retrograde amnesia Euphoria Hypotension Dysrhythmia Cardiac arrest Respiratory depression	CNS depressant Use–preoperative sedation, conscious sedation for endoscopic procedures and diagnostic tests
Anxiolytics: Nonbenzodiazepine		
Buspirone	Light-headedness Confusion Hypotension, palpitations	Little sedation Requires approximately 3 weeks to be effective Cannot be given as a PRN medication Particularly useful for generalized anxiety disorder (GAD) No abuse potential Used for clients with previous addiction Avoid alcohol and grapefruit juice Monitor for worsening depression or suicidal tendencies
Hydroxyzine	Drowsiness, ataxia Leukopenia, hypotension	Produces no dependence, tolerance, or intoxication Can be used for anxiety relief for indefinite periods

ANTIANXIETY MEDICATIONS *(CONTINUED)*		
MEDICATION	ADVERSE EFFECTS	NURSING CONSIDERATIONS
Herbals		
Kava	Impaired thinking, judgment, motor reflexes, vision, decreased plasma proteins, thrombocytopenia, leukocytopenia, dyspnea, and pulmonary hypertension	Similar activity to benzodiazepines Suppresses emotional excitability and produces mild euphoria Do not take with CNS depressants Should not be taken by women who are pregnant or lactating or by children under the age of 12
Melatonin	Sedation, confusion, headache, and tachycardia	Influences sleep-wake cycles (levels are high during sleep) Used for prevention and treatment of "jet lag" and insomnia Use cautiously if given with benzodiazepines and CNS depressants Contraindicated in hepatic insufficiency, history of cerebrovascular disease, depression, and neurologic disorders
Action	Affects neurotransmitters	
Indications	Anxiety disorders, insomnia, petit mal seizures, panic attacks, acute manic episodes	
Adverse effects	Sedation Depression, confusion Anger, hostility Headache Dry mouth, constipation Bradycardia Elevations in LDH, AST, ALT Urinary retention	
Nursing considerations	Monitor liver function Monitor for therapeutic blood levels Avoid alcohol Caution when performing tasks requiring alertness (e.g., driving car) Benzodiazepines are also used as muscles relaxants, sedatives, hypnotics, anticonvulsants	

ANTICHOLINERGIC MEDICATIONS		
MEDICATION	ADVERSE EFFECTS	NURSING CONSIDERATIONS
Propantheline bromide	Decreased gastric motility Decreased effect of vagus nerve	Used for urinary incontinence and peptic ulcer disease Give 30 minutes ac Give hs dose at least 2 h after last meal Monitor vital signs, I and O
Belladonna	Dry mouth, vertigo	Action peaks in 2 hours
Atropine sulfate	Tachycardia Headache, blurred vision Insomnia, dry mouth Dizziness Urinary retention Angina, mydriasis	Used for bradycardia When given PO give 30 minutes before meals Check for history of glaucoma, asthma, hypertension Monitor I and O, orientation When given in non-emergency situations make certain client voids before taking drug Educate client to expect dry mouth, increased respiration and heart rate Client should avoid heat (perspiration is decreased) Antidote-physostigmine salicylate
Iproproprium Tiotropium Iprotropium plus albuterol	Dry mouth Irritation of pharynx	Used for bronchospasm and long-term treatment of asthma Iproproprium administered as aerosol or in nebulizer Tiotropium administered in powder form by HandiHaler
Benztropine Trihexyphenydil	Urinary retention Blurred vision Dry mouth Constipation	Used for Parkinson's Disease Increase fluids, bulk foods and exercise Taper before discontinuation Orthostatic hypotension precautions
Scopolamine	Urinary retention Blurred vision Dry mouth Constipation Confusion and sedation	Used for motion sickness Contraindicated in acute angle glaucoma
Actions	Competes with acetylcholine at receptor sites in autonomic nervous system; causes relaxation of ciliary muscles (cycloplegia) and dilation of pupil (mydriasis); causes bronchodilation and decreases bronchial secretions; decreases mobility and GI secretions	
Indications	Atropine—bradycardia, mydriasis for ophthalmic exam, preoperatively to dry secretions Scopolamine—motion sickness, vertigo, mydriasis for ophthalmic exam, preoperative to dry secretions	

ANTICHOLINERGIC MEDICATIONS *(CONTINUED)*		
MEDICATION	ADVERSE EFFECTS	NURSING CONSIDERATIONS
Adverse effects	Blurred vision Dry mouth Urinary retention Changes in heart rate	
Nursing considerations	Monitor for urinary retention Contraindicated for clients with glaucoma	

ANTICOAGULANT MEDICATIONS		
MEDICATION	ADVERSE EFFECTS	NURSING CONSIDERATIONS
Action: Inhibits synthesis of clotting factors		
Heparin	Can produce hemorrhage from any body site (10%) Tissue irritation/pain at injection site Anemia Thrombocytopenia Fever Dose dependant on aPTT	Monitor therapeutic partial thromboplastin time (PTT) at 1.5–2.5 times the control without signs of hemorrhage Lower limit of normal 20–25 sec; upper limit of normal 32–39 sec For IV administration: use infusion pump, peak 5 minutes, duration 2–6 hours For injection: give deep SQ; never IM (danger of hematoma), onset 20–60 minutes, duration 8–12 hours **Antidote: protamine sulfate within 30 minutes** Can be allergenic

Low-molecular weight heparin
Enoxaparin
	Bleeding
	  Minimal widespread affect
	  Fixed dose
		Less allergenic than heparin
		Must be given deep SQ, never IV or IM
		Does not require lab test monitoring

Warfarin	Hemorrhage Diarrhea Rash Fever	Monitor therapeutic prothombin time (PT) at 1.5–2.5 times the control, or monitor international normalized ratio (INR) Normal PT 9.5–12 sec; normal INR 2.0–3.5 Onset: 12–24 hours, peak 1.5–3 days, duration: 3–5 days **Antidotes: vitamin K, whole blood, plasma** Teach measures to avoid venous stasis Emphasize importance of regular lab testing Client should avoid foods high in vitamin K: many green vegetables, pork, rice, yogurt, cheeses, fish, milk
Dabigatran	Directly inhibits thrombin	thrombin Used to treat atrial fibrillation Increased risk bleeding age greater than 75, kidney disease, gastrointestinal bleeding, use of NSAIDs
Action: inhibits activity of clotting		
Action	Heparin blocks conversion of fibrinogen to fibrin Warfarin interferes with liver synthesis of vitamin K–dependent clotting factors	

ANTICOAGULANT MEDICATIONS *(CONTINUED)*		
MEDICATION	**ADVERSE EFFECTS**	**NURSING CONSIDERATIONS**
Indications	For heparin: prophylaxis and treatment of thromboembolic disorders; in very low doses (10–100 units) to maintain patency of IV catheters (heparin flush) For warfarin: management of pulmonary emboli, venous thromboembolism, MI, atrial dysrhythmias, post cardiac valve replacement For dipyridamole: as an adjunct to warfarin in postop cardiac valve replacement, as an adjunct to aspirin to reduce the risk of repeat stroke or TIAs	
Adverse effects	Nausea Alopecia Urticaria Hemorrhage Bleeding/heparin-induced thrombocytopetria (HIT)	
Nursing considerations	Check for signs of hemorrhage: bleeding gums, nosebleed, unusual bleeding, black/tarry stools, hematuria, fall in hematocrit or blood pressure, guaiac-positive stools Client should avoid IM injections, ASA-containing products, and NSAIDs Client should wear medical information tag Instruct client to use soft toothbrush, electric razor, to report bleeding gums, petechiae or bruising, epistaxis, black tarry stools Monitor platelet counts and signs and symptoms of thrombosis during heparin therapy; if HIT suspected, heparin discontinued and non-heparin anticoagulant given	
Herbal interactions	Garlic, ginger, ginkgo may increase bleeding when taken with warfarin Large doses of anise may interfere with anticoagulants Ginseng and alfalfa my decrease anticoagulant activity Black haw increases action of anticoagulant Chamomile may interfere with anticoagulants	
Vitamin interaction	Vitamin C may slightly prolong PT Vitamin E will increase warfarin's effect	

ANTICONVULSANT MEDICATIONS		
MEDICATION	**ADVERSE EFFECTS**	**NURSING CONSIDERATIONS**
Clonazepam	Drowsiness Dizziness Confusion Respiratory depression	Benzodiazepine Do not discontinue suddenly Avoid activities that require alertness
Diazepam	Drowsiness, ataxia Hypotension Tachycardia Respiratory depression	IV push doses shouldn't exceed 2 mg/minute Monitor vital signs–resuscitation equipment available if given IV Alcohol increases CNS depression After long-term use, withdrawal leads to symptoms such as vomiting, sweating, cramps, tremors, and possibly convulsions

ANTICONVULSANT MEDICATIONS *(CONTINUED)*		
MEDICATION	**ADVERSE EFFECTS**	**NURSING CONSIDERATIONS**
Fosphenytoin	Drowsiness Dizziness Confusion Leukopenia Anemia	Used for tonic–clonic seizures, status epilepticus Highly protein-bound Contact healthcare provider if rash develops
Levetiracetam	Dizziness Suicidal ideation	Avoid alcohol Avoid driving and activities that require alertness
Phenytoin sodium	Drowsiness, ataxia Nystagmus Blurred vision Hirsutism Lethargy GI upset Gingival hypertrophy	Give oral medication with at least 1/2 glass of water, or with meals to minimize GI irritation Inform client that red-brown or pink discoloration of sweat and urine may occur IV administration may lead to cardiac arrest—have resuscitation equipment at hand Never mix with any other drug or dextrose IV Instruct in oral hygiene Increase vitamin D intake and exposure to sunlight may be necessary with long-term use Alcohol increases serum levels Increased risk toxicity older adults
Phenobarbital	Drowsiness, rash GI upset Initially constricts pupils Respiratory depression Ataxia	Monitor vital signs—resuscitation equipment should be available if given IV Drowsiness diminishes after initial weeks of therapy Don't take alcohol or perform hazardous activities Nystagmus may indicate early toxicity Sudden discontinuation may lead to withdrawal Tolerance and dependence result from long-term use Folic acid supplements are indicated for long-term use Decreased cognitive function older adults

ANTICONVULSANT MEDICATIONS *(CONTINUED)*		
MEDICATION	**ADVERSE EFFECTS**	**NURSING CONSIDERATIONS**
Primidone	Drowsiness Ataxia, diplopia Nausea and vomiting	Don't discontinue use abruptly Full therapeutic response may take 2 weeks Shake liquid suspension well Take with food if experiencing GI distress Decreased cognitive function older adults
Magnesium sulfate	Flushing Sweating Extreme thirst Hypotension Sedation, confusion	Monitor intake and output Before each dose, knee jerks should be tested Vital signs should be monitored often during parenteral administration Used for pregnancy-induced hypertension
Valproic acid	Sedation Tremor, ataxia Nausea, vomiting Prolonged bleeding time	Agent of choice in many seizure disorders of young children Do not take with carbonated beverage Take with food Monitor platelets, bleeding time, and liver function tests
Carbamazepine	Myelosuppression Dizziness, drowsiness Ataxia Diplopia, rash	Monitor intake and output Supervise ambulation Monitor CBC Take with meals Wear protective clothing due to photosensitivity Multiple drug interactions
Ethosuximide	GI symptoms Drowsiness Ataxia, dizziness	Monitor for behavioral changes Monitor weight weekly
Gabapentin	Increased appetite Ataxia Irritability Dizziness Fatigue	Monitor weight and behavioral changes. Can also be used to treat postherpetic neuralgia
Lamotrigine	Diplopia Headaches Dizziness Drowsiness Ataxia Nausea, vomiting Life-threatening rash when given with valproic acid	Take divided doses with meals or just afterward to decrease adverse effects

ANTICONVULSANT MEDICATIONS *(CONTINUED)*		
MEDICATION	ADVERSE EFFECTS	NURSING CONSIDERATIONS
Topiramate	Ataxia Confusion Dizziness Fatigue Vision problems	Adjunct therapy for intractable partial seizures Increased risk for renal calculi Stop drug immediately if eye problems—could lead to permanent damage
Action	Decreases flow of calcium and sodium across neuronal membranes	
Indications	Partial seizures: phenobarbitol, carbamazepine, gabapentin Generalized tonic-clonic seizures: phenobarbitol, carbamazepine Absence seizures: ethosuximide Status epilepticus: diazepam, phenytoin	
Adverse effects	Cardiovascular depression Respiratory depression Agranulocytosis Aplastic anemia	
Nursing considerations	Tolerance develops with long-term use Don't discontinue abruptly Caution with use of medications that lower seizure threshold (MAO inhibitors) Barbiturates and benzodiazepines also used as anticonvulsants Increased risk adverse reactions older adults	

ANTIDEPRESSANT MEDICATIONS: HETEROCYCLICS	
Examples	Bupropion Trazodone
Actions	Does not inhibit MAO; has some anticholinergic and sedative effects; alters effects of serotonin on CNS
Indications	Treatment of depression and smoking cessation
Adverse effects	Dry mouth Nausea Bupropion–insomnia and agitation Trazodone–sedation, orthostatic hypotension
Nursing considerations	May require gradual reduction before stopping Avoid use with alcohol, other CNS depressants for up to 1 week after end of therapy

ANTIDEPRESSANT MEDICATION: MONOAMINE OXIDASE (MAO) INHIBITORS	
Examples	Phenelzine sulfate, isocarboxazid, tranylcypromine
Actions	Interferes with monoamine oxidase, allowing for increased concentration of neurotransmitters (epinephrine, norepinephrine, serotonin) in synaptic space, causing stabilization of mood
Indications	Depression Chronic pain syndromes
Adverse effects	Hypertensive crisis when taken with foods containing tyramine (aged cheese, bologna, pepperoni, salami, figs, bananas, raisins, beer, Chianti red wine) or OTC meds containing ephedrine, pseudoephedrine Photosensitivity Weight gain Sexual dysfunction Orthostatic hypotension
Nursing considerations	Not first-line drugs for depression Should not be taken with SSRIs Administer antihypertensive medications with caution Avoid use of other CNS depressants, including alcohol Discontinue 10 days before general anesthesia Medications lower seizure threshold Monitor for urinary retention

ANTIDEPRESSANT MEDICIATION: SELECTIVE SEROTONIN REUPTAKE INHIBITORS	
Example	SSRIs: fluoxetine, paroxetine, sertraline hydrochloride, citalopram SNRIs: venlafaxine, duloxetine
Actions	Inhibits CNS neuronal uptake of serotonin; acts as stimulant counter-acting depression and increasing motivation
Indications	Depression Obsessive-compulsive disorders Obesity Bulimia
Adverse effects	Headache, dizziness Nervousness Insomnia, drowsiness Anxiety Tremor Dry mouth GI upset Taste changes Sweating Rash URI Painful menstruation Sexual dysfunction Weight gain
Nursing considerations	Take in A.M. Takes 4 weeks for full effect Monitor weight Good mouth care Do not administer with MAOIs–risk of serotonin syndrome Monitor for thrombocytopenia, leukopenia, and anemia

ANTIDEPRESSANT MEDICATIONS: TRICYCLICS	
Examples	Amitriptyline Imipramine
Actions	Inhibits presynaptic reuptake of neurotransmitters norepinephrine and serotonin; anticholinergic action at CNS and peripheral receptors
Indications	Depression Obstructive sleep apnea

ANTIDEPRESSANT MEDICATIONS: TRICYCLICS *(CONTINUED)*	
Adverse effects	Sedation
	Anticholinergic effects (dry mouth, blurred vision)
	Confusion (especially in elderly)
	Photosensitivity
	Disturbed concentration
	Orthostatic hypotension
	Bone marrow depression
	Urinary retention
Nursing considerations	Therapeutic effect in 1–3 weeks; maximum response in 6–9 weeks
	May be administered in daily dose at night to promote sleep and decrease adverse effects during the day
	Orthostatic hypotension precautions
	Instruct client that adverse effects will decrease over time
	Sugarless lozenges for dry mouth
	Do not abruptly stop taking medication (headache, vertigo, nightmares, malaise, weight change)
	Avoid alcohol, sleep-inducing drugs, OTC drugs
	Avoid exposure to sunlight, wear sunscreen
	Older adults: strong anticholinergic and sedation effects

ANTIDEPRESSANT MEDICATION OVERVIEW		
MEDICATION	ADVERSE EFFECTS	NURSING CONSIDERATIONS
Monoamine oxidase inhibitors (MAOIs) Isocarboxazid Tranylcypromine sulfate Phenelzine sulfate	Postural hypotension If foods with tyramine ingested, can have hypertensive crisis: headache, sweating, palpitations, stiff neck, intracranial hemorrhage Potentiates alcohol and other medications	Inhibits monoamine oxidase enzyme, preventing destruction of norepinephrine, epinephrine, and serotonin Avoid foods with tyramine—aged cheese, liver, yogurt, herring, yeast, beer, wine, sour cream, pickled products Avoid caffeine, antihistamines, amphetamines Takes 3-4 weeks to work Avoid tricyclics until 3 weeks after stopping MAO inhibitors Monitor vital signs Sunblock required
Tricyclics Amitriptyline hydrochloride Imipramine Desipramine hydrochloride Doxepin Nortriptyline	Sedation/drowsiness, especially with Elavil Blurred vision, dry mouth, diaphoresis Postural hypotension, palpitations Nausea, vomiting Constipation, urinary retention Increased appetite	Increases brain amine levels Suicide risk high after 10-14 days because of increased energy Monitor vital signs Sunblock required Increase fluid intake Take dose at bedtime (sedative effect) Use sugarless candy or gum for dry mouth Delay of 2-6 weeks before noticeable effects

ANTIDEPRESSANT MEDICATION OVERVIEW (CONTINUED)

MEDICATION	ADVERSE EFFECTS	NURSING CONSIDERATIONS
Selective serotonin reuptake inhibitors Fluoxetine Paroxetine Sertraline hydrochloride Citalopram **Serotonin-norepinephrine reuptake inhibitors** Venlafaxine Duloxetine	Palpitations, bradycardia Nausea, vomiting, diarrhea or constipation, increased or constipation, increased or decreased appetite Urinary retention Nervousness, insomnia	Decreases neuronal uptake of serotonin Take in AM to avoid insomnia Takes at least 4 weeks to work Can potentiate effect of digoxin, warfarin, and diazepam Used for anorexia
Heterocyclics/Atypical Bupropion Trazodone	Dry mouth Nausea	May require gradual reduction before stopping Avoid use with alcohol, other CNS depressants for up to 1 week after end of therapy
Herbals St. John's Wort	Dizziness, hypertension, allergic skin reaction, phototoxicity	Avoid use of St. John's wort and MAOI within 2 weeks of each other Do not use alcohol Contraindicated in pregnancy Avoid exposure to sun and use sunscreen Discontinue 1 to 2 weeks before surgery
Herbal interactions	St. John's wort—interacts with SSRIs; do not take within 2 weeks of MAOI Ginseng may potentiate MAOIs Avoid Ma huang or ephedra with MAOIs Kava kava should not be combined with benzodiazepines or opioids due to increased sedation Increase use of Brewer's yeast with MAOIs can increase blood pressure	

ANTIDIABETIC MEDICATIONS: INSULIN

INSULIN TYPES	ONSET OF ACTION	PEAK ACTION	DURATION OF ACTION	TIME OF ADVERSE REACTION	CHARACTERISTICS
Rapid-acting					
Lispro	15–30 min	0.5–2.5 h	3–6 h	Mid-morning: trembling, weakness	Client should eat within 5–15 min after injection; also used in insulin pumps
Aspart	15–30 min	1–3 h	3–5 h		
Glulisine	10–15 min	1–1.5 h	3–5 h		
Short-acting Regular	30–60 min	1–5 h	6–10 h	Mid-morning, midafternoon: weakness, fatigue	Clear solution; given 20–30 min before meal; can be alone or with other insulins
Intermediate-acting Isophane (NPH) Insulin detemir	1–2 h	6–14 h 12–24 h	16 h varies	Early evening: weakness, fatigue	White and cloudy solution; can be given after meals

ANTIDIABETIC MEDICATIONS: INSULIN *(CONTINUED)*					
INSULIN TYPES	ONSET OF ACTION	PEAK ACTION	DURATION OF ACTION	TIME OF ADVERSE REACTION	CHARACTERISTICS
Very long-acting Glargine (Lantus)	3–4 h	Continuous (no peak)	24 h		Maintains blood glucose levels regardless of meals; cannot be mixed with other insulins; given at bedtime
Action	Reduces blood glucose levels by increasing glucose transport across cell membranes; enhances conversion of glucose to glycogen				
Indications	Type 1 diabetes; type 2 diabetes not responding to oral hypoglycemic medications; gestational diabetes not responding to diet				
Adverse effects	Hypoglycemia				
Nursing considerations	Teach client to rotate sites to prevent lipohypertrophy, fibrofatty masses at injection sites; do not inject into these masses				
	Only regular insulin can be given IV; all can be given SQ				
Herbal interactions	Bee pollen, ginkgo biloba, glucosamine may increase blood glucose				
	Basil, bay leaf, chromium, echinacea, garlic, ginseng may decrease blood glucose				

ANTIDIABETIC MEDICATIONS: ORAL HYPERGLYCEMIC MEDICATIONS		
MEDICATION	ADVERSE EFFECTS	NURSING CONSIDERATIONS
Sulfonylureas Glimepiride Glipizide Glyburide	GI symptoms and dermatologic reactions	Only used if some pancreas beta-cell function Stimulates release of insulin from pancreas Many drugs can potentiate or interfere with actions Take with food if GI upset occurs
Biguanides Metformin	Nausea Diarrhea Abdominal discomfort	No effect on pancreatic beta cells; decreases glucose production by liver Not given if renal impairment Can cause lactic acidosis Avoid alcohol Do not give with alpha-glucodiase inhibitors
Alpha glucosidase inhibitors Acarbose Miglitol	Abdominal discomfort Diarrhea Flatulence	Delays digestion of carbohydrates Must be taken immediately before a meal Can be taken alone or with other medications

ANTIDIABETIC MEDICATIONS: ORAL HYPERGLYCEMIC MEDICATIONS *(CONTINUED)*		
MEDICATION	**ADVERSE EFFECTS**	**NURSING CONSIDERATIONS**
Thiazolidinediones Rosiglitazone Pioglitazone	Infection Headache Pain Rare cases of liver failure	Decreases insulin resistance and inhibits gluconeogenesis Regularly scheduled liver-function studies Can cause resumption of ovulation in perimenopause
Meglitinides Repaglinide	Hypoglycemia GI disturbances URIs Back pain Headache	Increases pancreatic insulin release Medication should not be taken if meal skipped
Gliptins Sitagliptin	Upper respiratory infections Hypoglycemia	Enhances action of incretin hormones
Incretin mimetics Exanatide	GI upset Hypoglycemia Pancreatitis	Interacts with many medications Administer 1 hour before meals
Indications	Type 2 diabetes	
Nursing considerations	Monitor serum glucose levels Avoid alcohol Teaching for disease: dietary control, symptoms of hypoglycemia and hyperglycemia Good skin care	
Herbal interactions	Bee pollen, ginkgo biloba, glucosamine may increase blood glucose Basil, bay leaf, chromium, echinacea, garlic, ginseng may decrease blood glucose	

HYPOGLYCEMIA REVERSAL MEDICATION		
MEDICATION	**ADVERSE EFFECTS**	**NURSING CONSIDERATIONS**
Glucagon	Nausea, vomiting	Given SQ or IM, onset is 8–10 min with duration of 12–27 min Should be part of emergency supplies for diabetics May repeat in 15 min if needed
Action	Hormone produced by alpha cells of the pancreas to simulate the liver to change glycogen to glucose	
Indications	Acute management of severe hypoglycemia	

HYPOGLYCEMIA REVERSAL MEDICATION *(CONTINUED)*		
MEDICATION	**ADVERSE EFFECTS**	**NURSING CONSIDERATIONS**
Adverse effects	Hypotension Bronchospasm Dizziness	
Nursing considerations	May repeat in 15 minutes if needed IV glucose must be given if client fails to respond Arouse clients from coma as quickly as possible and give carbohydrates orally to prevent secondary hypoglycemic reactions	

ANTIDIARRHEAL MEDICATIONS		
MEDICATION	**ADVERSE EFFECTS**	**NURSING CONSIDERATIONS**
Bismuth subsalicylate	Darkening of stools and tongue Constipation	Give 2 h before or 3 h after other medications to prevent impaired absorption Encourage fluids Take after each loose stool until diarrhea controlled Notify health care provider if diarrhea not controlled in 48 h Absorbs irritants and soothes intestinal muscle Do not administer for more than 2 days in presence of fever or in clients less than 3 years of age Monitor for salicylate toxicity Use cautiously if already taking aspirin Avoid use before x-rays (is radiopaque)
Diphenoxylate hydrochloride and atropine sulfate	Sedation Dizziness Tachycardia Dry mouth Paralytic ileus	Onset 45-60 min Monitor fluid and electrolytes Increases intestinal tone and decreases peristalsis May potentiate action of barbiturates, depressants
Loperamide	Drowsiness Constipation	Monitor children closely for CNS effects
Opium alkaloids	Narcotic dependence, nausea	Acts on smooth muscle to increase tone Administer with glass of water Discontinue as soon as stools are controlled
Action	Absorbs water, gas, toxins, irritants, and nutrients in bowel; slows peristalsis; increases tone of smooth muscles and sphincters	
Indications	Diarrhea	
Adverse effects	Constipation, fecal impaction Anticholinergic effects	
Nursing considerations	Not used with abdominal pain of unknown origin Monitor for urinary retention	

ANTIDYSRHYTHMIC MEDICATIONS		
MEDICATION	ADVERSE EFFECTS	NURSING CONSIDERATIONS
CLASS IA Procainamide Quinidine	Hypotension Heart failure	Monitor blood pressure Monitor for widening of the PR, QRS or QT intervals Toxic adverse effects have limited use
CLASS IB Lidocaine	CNS: slurred speech, confusion, drowsiness, confusion, seizures Hypotension and bradycardia	Monitor for CNS adverse effects Monitor BP and heart rate and cardiac rhythm
CLASS IC Flecainide Propafenone HCL		
CLASS II **(Beta-blockers)** Propranolol Esmolol hydrochloride	Bradycardia and hypotension Bronchospasm Increase in heart failure Fatigue and sleep disturbances	Monitor apical heart rate, cardiac rhythm and blood pressure Assess for shortness of breath and wheezing Assess for fatigue, sleep disturbances Assess apical heart rate for 1 minute before administration
CLASS III Amiodarone hydrochloride Ibutilide fumarate	Hypotension Bradycardia and atrioventricular block Muscle weakness, tremors Photosensitivity and photophobia Liver toxicity	Continuous monitoring of cardiac rhythm during IV administration Monitor QT interval during IV administration Monitor heart rate, blood pressure during initiation of therapy Instruct client to wear sunglasses and sunscreen
CLASS IV **(Calcium channel blocker)** Verapamil Diltiazem hydrochloride	Bradycardia Hypotension Dizziness and orthostatic hypotension Heart failure	Monitor apical heart rate and blood pressure Instruct clients about orthostatic precautions Instruct clients to report signs of heart failure to health care provider

ANTIEMETIC MEDICATIONS		
MEDICATION	ADVERSE EFFECTS	NURSING CONSIDERATIONS
Trimethobenzamide HCl	Drowsiness Headache	Give IM deep into upper outer quadrant of gluteal muscle to reduce pain and irritation
Prochlorperazine dimaleate	Drowsiness Orthostatic hypotension Diplopia, photosensitivity	Check CBC and liver function with prolonged use Wear protective clothing when exposed to sunlight

ANTIEMETIC MEDICATIONS (CONTINUED)		
MEDICATION	**ADVERSE EFFECTS**	**NURSING CONSIDERATIONS**
Ondansetron	Headache, sedation Diarrhea, constipation Transient elevations in liver enzymes	New class of antiemetics—serotonin receptor antagonist Administer 30 min prior to chemotherapy
Metoclopramide	Restlessness, anxiety, drowsiness Extrapyramidal symptoms Dystonic reactions	Monitor BP Avoid activities requiring mental alertness Take before meals Used with tube feeding to decrease residual and risk of aspiration Administer 30 min prior to chemotherapy
Meclizine	Drowsiness, dry mouth Blurred vision Excitation, restlessness	Contraindicated with glaucoma Avoid activities requiring mental alertness
Dimenhydrinate	Drowsiness Palpitations, hypotension Blurred vision	Avoid activities requiring mental alertness
Promethazine	Drowsiness Dizziness Constipation Urinary retention Dry mouth	If used for motion sickness, take 1/2 to 1 hour before traveling; avoid activities requiring alertness; avoid alcohol, other CNS depressants
Droperidol	Seizures Arrhythmias Hypotension Tachycardia	Often used either IV or IM in ambulatory care settings; observe for extrapyramidal symptoms (dystonia, extended neck, flexed arms, tremor, restlessness, hyperactivity, anxiety), which can be reversed with anticholinergics
Action	Blocks effect of dopamine in chemoreceptor trigger zone; increases GI motility	
Indications	Nausea and vomiting caused by surgery, chemotherapy, radiation sickness, uremia	
Adverse effects	Drowsiness, sedation Anticholinergic effects	
Nursing considerations	When used for viral infections may cause Reye's syndrome in clients less than 21 years old Phenothiazine medications are also used as antiemetics	
Herbals	Ginger—used to treat minor heartburn, nausea, vomiting; may increase risk of bleeding if take with anticoagulants, antiplatelets, thrombolytic medication; instruct to stop medication if easily bruised or other signs of bleeding noted, report to health care provider; not approved for morning sickness during pregnancy	

ANTIFUNGAL MEDICATIONS		
MEDICATION	ADVERSE EFFECTS	NURSING CONSIDERATIONS
Amphotericin B	IV: nicknamed "amphoterrible" GI upset Hypokalemia-induced muscle pain CNS disturbances in vision, hearing Peripheral neuritis Seizures Hematological, renal, cardiac, hepatic abnormalities Skin irritation and thrombosis if IV infiltrates	Refrigerate medication and protect from sunlight Monitor vital signs; report febrile reaction or any change in function, especially nervous system dysfunction Check for hypokalemia Meticulous care and observation of injection site
Nystatin	Mild GI distress Hypersensitivity	Discontinue if redness, swelling, irritation occurs Instruct client in good oral, vaginal, skin hygiene
Flucanozal	Nausea, vomiting Diarrhea Elevated liver enzymes	Drug excreted unchanged by kidneys; dosage reduced if creatine clearance is altered due to renal failure Administer after hemodialysis
Metronidazole	Headaches, vaginitis, nausea, flu-like symptoms (systemic use)	Reduce dosage hepatic disease Monitor CBC, LFTs, cultures Give tablet with food or milk
Action	Impairs cell membrane of fungus, causing increased permeability	
Indications	Systemic fungal infections (e.g., candidiasis, oral thrush, histoplasmosis)	
Adverse effects	Hepatotoxicity Thrombocytopenia Leukopenia Pruritus	
Nursing considerations	Administer with food to decrease GI upset Small, frequent meals Check hepatic function Teach client to take full course of medication, may be prescribed for prolonged period	

ANTIGOUT MEDICATIONS		
MEDICATION	ADVERSE EFFECTS	NURSING CONSIDERATIONS
Colchicine	GI upset Agranulocytosis Peripheral neuritis	Anti-inflammatory Give with meals Check CBC, I and O For acute gout in combination with NSAIDs
Probenecid	Nausea, constipation Skin rash	For chronic gout Reduces uric acid Check BUN, renal function tests Encourage fluids Give with milk, food, antacids Alkaline urine helps prevent renal stones
Allopurinol	GI upset Headache, dizziness, drowsiness	Blocks formation of uric acid Encourage fluids Check I and O Check CBC and renal function tests Give with meals Alkaline urine helps prevent renal stones Avoid ASA because it inactivates drug
Action	Decreases production and reabsorption of uric acid	
Indications	Gout Uric acid stone formation	
Adverse effects	Aplastic anemia Agranulocytosis Renal calculi GI irritation	
Nursing considerations	Monitor for renal calculi	

ANTIHISTAMINE MEDICATIONS		
MEDICATION	ADVERSE EFFECTS	NURSING CONSIDERATIONS
Chlorpheniramine maleate	Drowsiness, dry mouth	Most effective if taken before onset of symptoms
Diphenhydramine HCl	Drowsiness Nausea, dry mouth Photosensitivity	Don't combine with alcoholic beverages Give with food Use sunscreen Older adults: greater risk of confusion and sedation
Promethazine HCl	Agranulocytosis Drowsiness, dry mouth Photosensitivity	Give with food Use sunscreen
Loratadine Cetirizine Fexofenadine	Drowsiness	Reduce dose or give every other day for clients with renal or hepatic dysfunction
Action	Blocks the effects of histamine at peripheral H_1 receptor sites; anticholinergic, antipruritic effects	
Indications	Allergic rhinitis Allergic reactions Chronic idiopathic urticaria	
Adverse effects	Depression Nightmares Sedation Dry mouth GI upset Bronchospasm Alopecia	
Nursing considerations	Administer with food Good mouth care, sugarless lozenges for dry mouth Good skin care Use caution when performing tasks requiring alertness (e.g., driving car) Avoid alcohol	

ANTI-INFECTIVE: AMINOGLYCOSIDES MEDICATIONS	
Examples	Gentamicin Tobramycin Amikacin
Actions	Bacteriocidal Inhibits protein synthesis of many Gram-negative bacteria
Indications	Treatment of severe systemic infections of CNS, respiratory, GI, urinary tract, bone, skin, soft tissues, acute pelvic inflammatory disease (PID), tuberculosis (streptomycin)
Adverse effects	Ototoxicity, Nephrotoxicity Anorexia, nausea, vomiting, diarrhea
Nursing considerations	Check eighth cranial nerve function (hearing) Check renal function (BUN, creatinine) Usually prescribed for 7–10 days Encourage fluids Small, frequent meals

ANTI-INFECTIVE: CEPHALOSPORIN MEDICATIONS	
Example	Multiple preparations: 1st generation example: cephalexin 2nd generation example: cefoxitin sodium 3rd generation example: ceftriaxone sodium 4th generation example: cefepime HCL 5th generation example: fosamil
Actions	Bacteriocidal Inhibits synthesis of bacterial cell wall
Indications	Pharyngitis Tonsillitis Otitis media Upper and lower respiratory tract infections Dermatological infections Gonorrhea Septicemia Meningitis Perioperative prophylaxis Urinary tract infections

ANTI-INFECTIVE: CEPHALOSPORIN MEDICATIONS *(CONTINUED)*	
Adverse effects	Abdominal pain, nausea, vomiting, diarrhea
	Increased risk bleeding
	Hypoprothrombinemia
	Rash
	Superinfections
	Thrombophlebitis (IV), abscess formation (IM, IV)
Nursing considerations	Take with food
	Administer liquid form to children, don't crush tablets
	Have vitamin K available for hypoprothrombinemia
	Avoid alcohol while taking medication and for 3 days after finishing course of medication
	Cross allergy with penicillins (cephalosporins should not be given to clients with a severe penicillin allergy)
	Monitor renal and hepatic function
	Monitor for Thrombophlebitis

ANTI-INFECTIVE: FLUOROQUINOLONES MEDICATION	
Examples	Ciprofloxacin
	Levofloxacin
Actions	Bactericidal; interferes with DNA replication in Gram-negative bacteria
Indications	Treatment of infection caused *by E. coli* and other bacteria, chronic bacterial prostatitis, acute sinusitis, postexposure inhalation anthrax
Adverse effects	Headache
	Nausea
	Diarrhea
	Elevated BUN, AST, ALT, serum creatinine, alkaline phosphatase
	Decreased WBC and hematocrit
	Rash
	Photosensitivity
	Achilles tendon rupture
Nursing considerations	Culture and sensitivity before starting therapy
	Take 1 h before or 2 h after meals with glass of water
	Encourage fluids
	If needed administer antacids 2 h after medication
	Take full course of therapy

ANTI-INFECTIVE: GLYCOPEPTIDE MEDICATIONS

Example	Vancomycin
Action	Bacteriocidal Binds to bacterial cell wall, stopping its synthesis
Indications	Treatment of resistant staph infections, pseudomembranous entero-colitis due to c. *difficile* infection
Adverse effects	Thrombophlebitis Abscess formation Nephrotoxicity Ototoxicity
Nursing considerations	Monitor renal function and hearing Poor absorption orally; administer IV: peak 5 minutes, duration 12–24 hours Avoid extravasation during therapy; it may cause necrosis Give antihistamine if "red man syndrome": decreased blood pressure, flushing of face and neck Contact health care provider if signs of superinfection: sore throat, fever, fatigue

ANTI-INFECTIVE: LINCOSAMIDE MEDICATIONS

Example	Clindamycin HCl Phosphate
Action	Both bacteriostatic and bactericidal, it suppresses protein synthesis by preventing peptide bond formation
Indications	Staph, strep, and other infections
Adverse effects	Diarrhea Rash Liver toxicity
Nursing considerations	Administer oral med with a full glass of water to prevent esophageal ulcers Monitor for persistent vomiting, diarrhea, fever, or abdominal pain and cramping, superinfectious

ANTIBIOTICS/ANTI-INFECTIVE: MACROLIDE MEDICATIONS

Examples	Erythromycin AzIthromycin
Actions	Bacteriostatic; bactericidal; binds to cell membrane and causes changes in protein function
Indications	Acute infections Acne and skin infections Upper respiratory tract infections Prophylaxis before dental procedures for clients allergic to PCN with valvular heart disease

ANTIBIOTICS/ANTI-INFECTIVE: MACROLIDE MEDICATIONS *(CONTINUED)*	
Adverse effects	Abdominal cramps, diarrhea
	Confusion, uncontrollable emotions
	Hepatotoxicity
	Superinfections
Nursing considerations	Take oral med 1 h before or 2-3 h after meals with full glass of water
	Take around the clock to maximize effectiveness
	Monitor liver function
	Take full course of therapy

ANTI-INFECTIVE: PENICILLIN MEDICATIONS	
Examples	Amoxicillin
	Ampicillin
	Methicillin
	Nafcillin
	Penicillin G
	Penicillin V
Actions	Bactericidal; inhibit synthesis of cell wall of sensitive organisms
Indications	Effective against gram positive organisms
	Moderate to severe infections
	Syphilis
	Gonococcal infections
	Lyme disease
Adverse effects	Glossitis, stomatitis
	Gastritis
	Diarrhea
	Superinfections
	Hypersensitivity reactions
Nursing considerations	Culture and sensitivity before treatment
	Monitor serum electrolytes and cardiac status if given IV
	Monitor and rotate injection sites
	Good mouth care
	Yogurt or buttermilk if diarrhea develops
	Instruct client to take missed drugs as soon as possible; do not double dose

ANTI–INFECTIVE: SULFONAMIDE MEDICATIONS	
Example	Sulfasalazine
	Trimethoprim/Sulfamethoxazole
Actions	Bacteriostatic; competitively antagonize paraminobenzoic acid, essential component of folic acid synthesis, causing cell death
Indications	Ulcerative colitis, Crohn's disease
	Otitis media
	Conjunctivitis
	Meningitis
	Toxoplasmosis
	UTIs
	Rheumatoid arthritis
Adverse effects	Peripheral neuropathy
	Crystalluria, proteinuria
	Photosensitivity
	GI upset
	Stomatitis
	Hypersensitvity reaction
Nursing considerations	Culture and sensitivity before therapy
	Take with a full glass of water
	Take around the clock
	Encourage fluid intake (8 glasses of water/day)
	Protect from exposure to light (sunscreen, protective clothing)
	Good mouth care

ANTI-INFECTIVE: TETRACYCLINE MEDICATIONS	
Examples	Doxycycline Minocycline HCL Tetracycline HCl
Actions	Bacteriostatic; inhibits protein synthesis of susceptible bacteria
Indications	Treatment of syphilis, chlamydia, gonorrhea, malaria prophylaxis, chronic periodontitis, acne; treatment of anthrax (doxycycline); as part of combination therapy to eliminate *H. pylori* infections; drug of choice for stage 1 Lyme disease (tetracycline HCl)
Adverse effects	Discoloration and inadequate calcification of primary teeth of fetus if taken during pregnancy Glossitis Dysphagia Diarrhea Phototoxic reactions Rash Superinfections
Nursing considerations	Take 1 h before or 2-3 h after meals Do not take with antacids, milk, iron preparations (give 3 h after medication) Note expiration date (becomes highly nephrotoxic) Protect from sunlight Monitor renal function Topical applications may stain clothing Use contraceptive method in addition to oral contraceptives

ANTI-INFECTIVE MEDICATIONS: VANCOMYCIN	
Examples	Vancomycin
Action	Bacteriocidal Binds to bacterial cell wall, stopping its synthesis
Indications	Treatment of resistant staph infections, pseudomembranous enterocolitis due to c. difficile infection
Adverse effects	Thrombophlebitis Abscess formation Nephrotoxicity Ototoxicity
Nursing considerations	Monitor renal function and hearing Poor absorption orally; administer IV: peak 5 minutes, duration 12–24 hours Avoid extravasation during therapy; it may cause necrosis Give antihistamine if "red man syndrome": decreased blood pressure, flushing of face and neck Contact health care provider if signs of superinfection: sore throat, fever, fatigue

ANTI-INFECTIVE MEDICATION OVERVIEW		
MEDICATION	**ADVERSE EFFECTS**	**NURSING CONSIDERATIONS**
Penicillins Amoxicillin Ampicillin Methicillin Penicillin G Penicillin V	Skin rashes, diarrhea Allergic reactions Renal, hepatic, hematological abnormalities Nausea, vomiting	Obtain C and S before first dose Take careful history of penicillin reaction Observe for 20 minutes post IM injection Give 1-2 h ac or 2-3 h pc to reduce gastric acid destruction of drug Monitor for loose, foul-smelling stool and change in tongue Teach to continue medication for entire time prescribed, even if symptoms resolve Check for hypersensitivity to other drugs, especially cephalosporins
Sulfonamides Sulfisoxazole	Headache, GI disturbances Allergic rash Urinary crystallization	Monitor I and 0, force fluids Maintain alkaline urine Bicarbonate may be indicated to elevate pH Avoid vitamin C, which acidifies urine
Sulfasalazine	Nausea, vomiting Skin eruption Agranulocytosis	Advise client to avoid exposure to sunlight Maintain fluid intake at 3,000 mL/day to avoid crystal formation
Trimethoprim/ Sulfamethoxazole	Hypersensitivity reaction Blood dyscrasias Rash	Obtain C and S before first dose IV solution must be given slowly over 60-90 minutes Never administer IM Encourage fluids to 3,000/day
Tetracylines Tetracycline	Photosensitivity GI upset, renal, hepatic, hematological abnormalities Dental discoloration of deciduous ("baby") teeth, enamel hypoplasia	Give between meals If GI symptoms occur, administer with food EXCEPT milk products or other foods high in calcium (interferes with absorption) Assess for change in bowel habits, perineal rash, black "hairy" tongue Good oral hygiene Avoid during tooth and early development periods (fourth month prenatal to 8 years of age) Monitor I and 0 Caution client to avoid sun exposure Decomposes to toxic substance with age and exposure to light
Doxycycline	Photosensitivity	Check client's tongue for *Monilia* infection
Aminogylcosides Gentamicin	Ototoxicity cranial nerve VIII Nephrotoxicity	Check creatinine and BUN Check peak—2 h after med given Check trough—at time of dose/prior to med Monitor for symptoms of bacterial overgrowth, photosensitivity Teach to immediately report tinnitus, vertigo, nystagmus, ataxia Monitor I and 0 Audiograms if given long-term

ANTI-INFECTIVE MEDICATION OVERVIEW (CONTINUED)		
MEDICATION	**ADVERSE EFFECTS**	**NURSING CONSIDERATIONS**
Neomycin sulfate	Hypersensitivity reactions	Ophthalmic—remove infective exudate around eyes before administration of ointment
Fluoroquinolones Ciprofloxacin	Seizures GI upset Rash	Contraindicated in children less than 18 years of age Give 2 hours pc or 2 hours before an antacid or iron preparation Avoid caffeine Encourage fluids
Macrolides Azithromycin Erythromycin	Pain at injection site Nausea, diarrhea	Can be used in clients with compromised renal function because excretion is primarily through the bile
Cephalosporins	Diarrhea, nausea Dizziness, abdominal pain Eosinophilia, superinfections Allergic reactions	Can cause false-positive Coombs' test (which will complicate transfusion cross-matching procedure) Cross-sensitivity with penicillins Take careful history of penicillin reactions
Glycopeptides Vancomycin	Liver damage	Poor absorption orally, but IV peak 5 minutes, duration 12–24 hours Avoid extravasation during therapy—may cause necrosis Give antihistamine if "red man syndrome": decreased blood pressure, flushing of face and neck Contact health care provider if signs of superinfection: sore throat, fever, fatigue
Lincosamides Clindamycin HCl phosphate	Nausea Vaginitis Colitis may occur 2–9 days or several weeks after starting meds	Administer oral med with a full glass of water to prevent esophageal ulcers Monitor for persistent vomiting, diarrhea, fever, or abdominal pain and cramping

ANTI-INFECTIVE MEDICATIONS: TOPICAL		
MEDICATION	**ADVERSE EFFECTS**	**NURSING CONSIDERATIONS**
Bacitracin ointment	Nephrotoxicity Ototoxicity	Overgrowth of nonsusceptible organisms can occur
Neosporin cream	Nephrotoxicity Ototoxicity	Allergic dermatitis may occur
Povidone-iodine solution	Irritation	Don't use around eyes May stain skin Don't use full-strength on mucous membranes
Silver sulfadiazine cream	Neutropenia Burning	Use cautiously if sensitive to sulfonamides

ANTI-INFECTIVE MEDICATIONS: TOPICAL *(CONTINUED)*		
MEDICATION	ADVERSE EFFECTS	NURSING CONSIDERATIONS
Tolna flake cream	Irritation	Use small amount of medication Use medication for duration prescribed
Nystatin cream	Contact dermatitis	Do not use occlusive dressings

ANTIHYPERTENSIVE MEDICATIONS: ANGIOTENSIN II RECEPTOR ANTAGONISTS (ACE RECEPTOR BLOCKERS/ARBS)	
Examples	Candesartan Eprosartan Irbesartan Losartan Valsartan
Indications	Hypertension Heart failure Diabetic neuropathy Myocardial infarction Stroke prevention
Adverse effects	Angioedema Renal failure Orthostatic hypotension
Nursing considerations	Instruct client about position changes Monitor for edema Instruct client to notify health care provider if edema occurs

ANTIHYPERTENSIVE MEDICATIONS: ACE INHIBITORS (ANGIOTENSIN-CONVERTING ENZYME)	
Example	Captopril Enalapril Lisinopril Benazepril Fosinopril Quinapril Ramipril
Actions	Blocks ACE in lungs from converting angiotensin I to angiotensin II (powerful vasoconstrictor); causes decreased BP, decreased aldosterone secretion, sodium and fluid loss
Indications	Hypertension CHF

ANTIHYPERTENSIVE MEDICATIONS: ACE INHIBITORS (ANGIOTENSIN-CONVERTING ENZYME) *(CONTINUED)*	
Adverse effects	Gastric irritation, peptic ulcer, orthostatic hypotension
	Tachycardia
	Myocardial infarction
	Proteinuria
	Rash, pruritis
	Persistent dry nonproductive cough
	Peripheral edema
Nursing considerations	Decreased absorption if taken with food—give 1 h ac or 2 h pc
	Small, frequent meals
	Frequent mouth care
	Change position slowly
	Can be used with thiazide diuretics

ANTIHYPERTENSIVE MEDICATIONS: ALPHA-1 ADRENERGIC BLOCKERS	
Examples	Doxazosin
	Prazosin
	Terazosin
Actions	Selective blockade of alpha-1 adrenergic receptors in peripheral blood vessels
Indications	Hypertension
	Benign prostatic hypertrophy
	Pheochromocytoma
	Raynaud's disease
Adverse effects	Orthostatic hypotension
	Reflex tachycardia
	Nasal congestion
	Impotence
Nursing considerations	Administer first dose at bedtime to avoid fainting
	Change positions slowly to prevent orthostatic hypotension
	Monitor BP, weight, BUN/creatinine, edema

ANTIHYPERTENSIVE MEDICATIONS: BETA-ADRENERGIC BLOCKERS	
Examples	Atenolol
	Nadolol
	Propranolol
	Metoprolol
	Acebutolol
	Carvedilol
	Pindolol
Actions	Blocks beta-adrenergic receptors in heart; decreases excitability of heart; reduces cardiac workload and oxygen consumption; decreases release of renin; lowers blood pressure by reducing CNS stimuli
Indications	Hypertension (used with diuretics)
	Angina
	Supraventricular tachycardia
	Prevent recurrent MI
	Migraine headache (propranolol)
	Stage fright (propranolol)
	Heart failure
Adverse effects	Gastric pain
	Bradycardia/tachycardia
	Acute severe heart failure
	Cardiac dysrhythmias
	Impotence
	Decreased exercise tolerance
	Nightmares, depression
	Dizziness
	Bronchospasm (nonselective beta blockers)
Nursing considerations	Do not discontinue abruptly, taper gradually over 2 weeks
	Take with meals
	Provide rest periods
	For diabetic clients, blocks normal signs of hypoglycemia (sweating, tachycardia); monitor blood glucose
	Medications have antianginal and antiarrhythmic actions

ANTIHYPERTENSIVE MEDICATIONS: CALCIUM-CHANNEL BLOCKERS	
Examples	Nifedipine
	Verapamil
	Diltiazem
	Amlodipine
	Felodipine
Actions	Inhibits movement of calcium ions across membrane of cardiac and arterial muscle cells; results in slowed impulse conduction, depression of myocardial contractility, dilation of coronary arteries; decreases cardiac workload and energy consumption, increases oxygenation of myocardial cells

ANTIHYPERTENSIVE MEDICATIONS: CALCIUM–CHANNEL BLOCKERS *(CONTINUED)*	
Indications	Angina Hypertension Dysrhythmias Interstitial cystitis Migraines
Adverse effects	Dizziness Headache Nervousness Peripheral edema Angina Bradycardia AV block Flushing, rash Impotence
Nursing considerations	Monitor vital signs Do not chew or divide sustained-release tablets Medications also have antianginal actions Contraindicated in heart block Contact health care provider if blood pressure less than 90/60 Instruct client to avoid grapefruit juice (verapamil) Monitor for signs of heart failure

ANTIHYPERTENSIVE MEDICATIONS: CENTRALLY ACTING ALPHA-ADRENERGICS	
Examples	Clonidine Methyldopa
Actions	Stimulates alpha receptors in medulla, causing reduction in sympathetic action in heart; decreases rate and force of contraction, decreasing cardiac output
Indications	Hypertension
Adverse effects	Drowsiness, sedation Orthostatic hypotension CHF
Nursing considerations	Don't discontinue abruptly Monitor for fluid retention Older adults: potential for orthostatic hypotension and CNS adverse effects

ANTIHYPERTENSIVE MEDICATIONS: DIRECT-ACTING VASODILATORS	
Examples	Hydralazine Minoxidil
Actions	Relaxes smooth muscle of blood vessels, lowering peripheral resistance
Indications	Hypertension
Adverse effects	Same as centrally acting alpha adrenergics
Nursing considerations	Same as centrally acting alpha adrenergics

ANTIHYPERTENSIVE MEDICATIONS OVERVIEW		
MEDICATION	**ADVERSE EFFECTS**	**NURSING CONSIDERATIONS**
Methyldopa	Drowsiness, dizziness, bradycardia, hemolytic anemia, fever, orthostatic hypotension	Monitor CBC Monitor liver function Take at hs to minimize daytime drowsiness Change position slowly
Clonidine	Drowsiness, dizziness Dry mouth, headache Dermatitis Severe rebound hypertension	Don't discontinue abruptly Apply patch to nonhairy area (upper outer arm, anterior chest)
Atenolol	Bradycardia Hypotension Bronchospasm	Once-a-day dose increases compliance Check apical pulse; if less than 60 bpm hold drug and call health care provider Don't discontinue abruptly Masks signs of shock and hypoglycemia
Metoprolol	Bradycardia, hypotension, heart failure, depression	Give with meals Teach client to check pulse before each dose; take apical pulse before administration Withhold if pulse less than 60 bpm
Nadolol	Bradycardia, hypotension, heart failure	Teach client to check pulse before each dose; check apical pulse before administering Withhold if pulse less than 60 bpm Don't discontinue abruptly
Hydralazine	Headache, palpitations, edema, tachycardia, lupus erythematosus-like syndrome	Give with meals Observe mental status Check for weight gain, edema
Minoxidil	Tachycardia, angina pectoris, edema, increase in body hair	Teach client to check pulse; check apical pulse before administration Monitor I and 0, weight

ANTIHYPERTENSIVE MEDICATIONS OVERVIEW *(CONTINUED)*		
MEDICATION	ADVERSE EFFECTS	NURSING CONSIDERATIONS
Captopril Enalapril Lisinopril	Dizziness Orthostatic hypotension	Report swelling of face, lightheadedness ACE-inhibitor medication
Propranolol	Weakness Hypotension Bronchospasm Bradycardia Depression	Beta blocker: blocks sympathetic impulses to heart Client takes pulse at home before each dose Dosage should be reduced gradually before discontinued
Nifedipine Verapamil Diltiazem	Hypotension Dizziness GI distress Liver dysfunction Jitteriness	Calcium-channel blocker: reduces workload of left ventricle Coronary vasodilator; monitor blood pressure during dosage adjustments Assist with ambulation at start of therapy
Herbal interaction	Ma-huang (ephedra) decreases effect of antihypertensive drugs Ephedra increases hypertension when taken with beta blockers Black cohosh increases hypotensive effects of antihypertensives Goldenseal counteracts effects of antihypertensives	

ANTILIPEMIC MEDICATIONS		
MEDICATION	ADVERSE EFFECTS	NURSING CONSIDERATIONS
Bile acid sequestrants Cholestyramine Colestipol HMG-COA reductase inhibitors Folic acid derivatives Nicotinic acid	Constipation Rash Fat-soluble vitamin deficiency Abdominal pain and bloating	Increases loss of bile acid in feces; decreases cholesterol Sprinkle powder on noncarbonated beverage or wet food, let stand 2 min, then stir slowly Administer 1 h before or 4–6 h after other medication to avoid blocking absorption Instruct client to report constipation immediately
HMG-CoA reductase inhibitors (statins) Lovostatin Pravastatin Simvastatin Atorvastatin Fluvastatin Rosuvastatin	Myopathy Increased liver enzyme levels	Decreases LDL cholesterol levels; causes peripheral vasodilation Take with food; absorption is reduced by 30% on an empty stomach; avoid alcohol Contact health care provider if unexplained muscle pain, especially with fever or malaise Take at night Give with caution with ↓ liver function

ANTILIPEMIC MEDICATIONS *(CONTINUED)*

MEDICATION	ADVERSE EFFECTS	NURSING CONSIDERATIONS
Nicotinic acid Niacin	Flushing Hyperglycemia Gout Upper GI distress Liver damage	Decreases total cholesterol, LDL, triglycerides, increases HDL Flushing will occur several hours after med is taken, will decrease over 2 wk Also used for pellagra and peripheral vascular disease Avoid alcohol
Folic acid derivatives Fenofibrate Gemfibrozil	Abdominal pain Increased risk gallbladder disease Myalgia and swollen joints	Decreases total cholesterol, VLDL, and triglycerides Administer before meals Instruct clients to notify health care provider if muscle pain occurs
Action	Inhibits cholesterol and triglyceride synthesis; decreases serum cholesterol and LDLs	
Indications	Elevated total and LDL cholesterol Primary hypercholesterolemia Reduce incidence of cardiovascular disease	
Adverse effects	Varies with medication	
Nursing considerations	Medication should be used with dietary measures, physical activity, and cessation of tobacco use Lipids should be monitored every 6 wk until normal, then every 4–6 mo	
Herbals used to lower cholesterol	Flax or flax seed—decreases the absorption of other medications Garlic—increases the effects of anticoagulants; increases the hypoglycemic effects of insulin Green tea—produces a stimulant effect with the tea contains caffeine Soy	

ANTINEOPLASTIC MEDICATIONS: ANTIMETABOLITES

Examples	Cytarabine Fluorouracil Pemetrexed Mercaptopurine Methotrexate
Actions	Closely resembles normal metabolites, "counterfeits" fool cells; cell division halted
Indications	Acute lymphatic leukemia Rheumatoid arthritis Psoriasis Cancer of colon, breast, stomach, pancreas Sickle cell anemia

ANTINEOPLASTIC MEDICATIONS: ANTIMETABOLITES *(CONTINUED)*	
Adverse effects	Nausea, vomiting
	Diarrhea
	Stomatitis and oral ulceration
	Hepatic dysfunction
	Bone marrow suppression
	Renal dysfunction
	Alopecia
Nursing considerations	Monitor hematopoietic function
	Good mouth care
	Small frequent feedings
	Counsel about body image changes (alopecia); provide wig
	Good skin care
	Photosensitivity precautions
	Infection control precautions

ANTINEOPLASTIC MEDICATIONS: ANTIBIOTICS	
Examples	Bleomycin
	Dactinomycin
	Doxorubicin
Actions	Interferes with DNA and RNA synthesis
Indications	Hodgkin's disease
	Non-Hodgkin's lymphoma
	Leukemia
	Many cancers
Adverse effects	Bone marrow depression
	Nausea, vomiting
	Alopecia
	Stomatitis
	Heart failure
	Septic shock
Nursing considerations	Monitor closely for septicemic reactions
	Monitor for manifestations of extravasation at injection site (severe pain or burning that lasts minutes to hours, redness after injection is completed, ulceration after 48 hours)

ANTINEOPLASTIC MEDICATIONS: CYTOXIC MEDICATIONS	

Examples	Busulfan
	  Chlorambucil
	  Cisplatin platinol-AQ
	  Cyclophosphamide

Actions	Interferes with rapidly reproducing cell DNA
Indications	Leukemia Multiple myeloma
Adverse effects	Bone marrow suppression Nausea, vomiting Stomatitis Alopecia Gonadal suppression Renal toxicity (cisplatin) Ototoxicity
Nursing considerations	Used with other chemotherapeutic medications Check hematopoietic function weekly Encourage fluids (10-12 glasses/day)

ANTINEOPLASTIC MEDICATIONS: HORMONAL MEDICATIONS	
Examples	Tamoxifen Anastrozole Letrozole Leuprolide Degarelix Testolactone Testosterone
Actions	Tamoxifen–antiestrogen (competes with estrogen to bind at estrogen receptor sites on malignant cells) Leuprolide–progestin (causes tumor cell regression by unknown mechanism) Testolactone–androgen (used for palliation in advanced breast cancer)
Indications	Breast cancer
Adverse effects	Hypercalcemia Jaundice Increased appetite Masculinization or feminization Sodium and fluid retention Nausea, vomiting Hot flashes Vaginal dryness

Nursing considerations	Baseline and periodic gyn exams recommended
	  Not given IVLK
	  Discuss pregnancy prevention

ANTINEOPLASTIC MEDICATIONS: TOPOISOMERASE

Examples	Irinotecan Topotecan
Actions	Binds to enzyme that breaks the DNA strands
Indications	Ovary, lung, colon, and rectal cancers
Adverse effects	Bone marrow suppression Diarrhea Nausea, vomiting Hepatotoxicity

ANTINEOPLASTIC MEDICATIONS: VINCA ALKALOIDS

Examples	Vinblastine Vincristine
Actions	Interferes with cell division
Indications	Hodgkin's disease Lymphoma Cancers
Adverse effects	Bone marrow suppression (mild with VCR) Neuropathies (VCR) Stomatitis
Nursing considerations	Same as antitumor antibiotics

ANTINEOPLASTIC MEDICATION: NURSING IMPLICATIONS FOR ADVERSE EFFECTS

Bone marrow suppression	Monitor bleeding: bleeding gums, bruising, petechiae, guaiac stools, urine and emesis Avoid IM injections and rectal temperatures Apply pressure to venipuncture sites
Nausea, vomiting	Monitor intake and output ratios, appetite and nutritional intake Prophylactic antiemetics may be used Smaller, more frequent meals
Altered immunologic response	Prevent infection by handwashing Timely reporting of alterations in vital signs or symptoms indicating possible infection
Impaired oral mucous membrane; stomatis	Oral hygiene measures
Fatigue	Encourage rest and discuss measures to conserve energy Use relaxation techniques, mental imagery

ANTIPARKINSON MEDICATIONS		
MEDICATION	**ADVERSE EFFECTS**	**NURSING CONSIDERATIONS**
Trihexyphenidyl	Dry mouth Blurred vision Constipation, urinary hesitancy Decreased mental acuity, difficulty concentrating, confusion, hallucination	Acts by blocking acetylcholine at cerebral synaptic sites Intraocular pressure should be monitored Supervise ambulation Causes nausea if given before meals Suck on hard candy for dry mouth
Levodopa	Nausea and vomiting, anorexia Postural hypotension Mental changes: confusion, agitation, mood alterations Cardiac arrhythmias Twitching	Precursor of dopamine Thought to restore dopamine levels in extrapyramidal centers Administered in large prolonged doses Contraindicated in glaucoma, hemolytic anemia Give with food Monitor for postural hypotension Avoid OTC meds and foods that contain vitamin B_6 (pyridoxine); reverses effects
Bromocriptine mesylate Pergolide	Dizziness, headache, hypotension Tinnitus Nausea, abdominal cramps Pleural effusion Orthostatic hypotension	Give with meals May lead to early postpartum conception Monitor cardiac, hepatic, renal, hematopoietic function
Carbidopa–Levodopa	Hemolytic anemia Dystonic movements, ataxia Orthostatic hypotension Dysrhythmias GI upset, dry mouth	Stimulates dopamine receptors Don't use with MAO inhibitors Advise to change positions slowly Take with food
Amantadine	CNS disturbances, hyperexcitability Insomnia, vertigo, ataxia Slurred speech, convulsions	Enhances effect of L-Dopa Contraindicated in epilepsy, arteriosclerosis Antiviral
Action	Levodopa—precursor to dopamine that is converted to dopamine in the brain Bromocriptine—stimulates postsynaptic dopamine receptors	
Indications	Parkinson's disease	

ANTIPARKINSON MEDICATIONS (CONTINUED)

MEDICATION	ADVERSE EFFECTS	NURSING CONSIDERATIONS
Adverse effects	Dizziness Ataxia Confusion Psychosis Hemolytic anemia	
Nursing considerations	Monitor for urinary retention Large doses of pyridoxine (vitamin B_6) decrease or reverse effects of medication Avoid use of other CNS depressants (alcohol, narcotics, sedatives) Anticholinergics, dopamine agonists, MAO inhibitors, catechol-O-methyltransferase (COMT) inhibitors, and antidepressants may also be used	

ANTIPLATELET MEDICATIONS

MEDICATION	ADVERSE EFFECTS	NURSING CONSIDERATIONS
Adenosine diphosphate receptor antagonists Ticlodipine Clopidrogrel	Thrombocytopenic purpura GI upset	Prevents platelet aggregation Higher risk of hemorrhage with ticlopidine
Dipyridamole Dipyridamole plus aspirin	Headache Dizziness EKG changes Hypertension, hypotension	Administer 1 h ac or with meals Monitor BP Check for signs of bleeding
Glycoprotein IIb and IIIa receptor antagonists Eptifibatide Abciximab	GI, retroperitoneal, and urogenital bleeding	Does not increase risk of fatal hemorrhage or hemorrhagic stroke
Asprin	Short-term use—GI bleeding, heartburn, occasional nausea Prolonged high dosage—salicylism: metabolic acidosis, respiratory alkalosis, dehydration, fluid and electrolyte imbalance, tinnitus	Observe for bleeding gums, bloody or black stools, bruises Give with milk, water, or food, or use enteric-coated tablets to minimize gastric distress Contraindications—GI disorders, severe anemia, vitamin K deficiency Anti-inflammatory, analgesic, antipyretic
Action	Interferes with platelet aggregation	
Indications	Venous thrombosis Pulmonary embolism CVA and acute coronary prevention Post-cardiac surgery; post-percutaneous coronary interventions Acute coronary syndrome	

ANTIPLATELET MEDICATIONS *(CONTINUED)*		
MEDICATION	**ADVERSE EFFECTS**	**NURSING CONSIDERATIONS**
Adverse effects	Hemorrhage, bleeding Thrombocytopenia Hematuria Hemoptysis	
Nursing considerations	Teach client to check for signs of bleeding Inform health care provider or dentist before procedures Older adults at higher risk for ototoxicity Instruct client to contact health care provider before taking any over-the-counter medications Instruct client to avoid gingko, garlic and ginger herbal preparations	
Gerontologic considerations	Dipyridamole causes orthostatic hypotention in older adults Ticlopidine–greater risk of toxicity with older adults	

ANTIPSYCHOTIC MEDICATIONS		
MEDICATION	**ADVERSE EFFECTS**	**NURSING CONSIDERATIONS**
High potency (traditional) Haloperidol Haloperidol decanoate Fluphenazine Fluphenazine decanoate	Low sedative effect Low incidence of hypotension High incidence of extrapyramidal adverse effects	Used in large doses for assaultive clients Used with elderly (risk of falling reduced) Decanoate: long-acting form given every 2–4 wk; IM into deep muscle Z-track
Medium potency (traditional) Perphenazine	Orthostatic hypotension Dry mouth Constipation	Can help control severe vomiting Medication is available PO, IM, and IV
Low potency (traditional) Chlorpromazine	High sedative effect High incidence of hypotension Irreversible retinitis pigmentosus at 800 mg/day	Educate client about increased sensitivity to sun (as with other phenothiazines) No tolerance or potential for abuse
Atypical		
Risperidone	Moderate orthostatic hypotension Moderate sedation Significant weight gain Doses over 6 mg can cause tardive dyskinesia	Chosen as first-line antipsychotic due to mild EPS and very low anticholinergic adverse effects
Quetiapine	Moderate orthostatic hypotension Moderate sedation Very low risk of tardive dyskinesia and neuroleptic malignant syndrome	Chosen as first-line antipsychotic due to mild EPS and very low anticholinergic adverse effects

ANTIPSYCHOTIC MEDICATIONS *(CONTINUED)*		
MEDICATION	ADVERSE EFFECTS	NURSING CONSIDERATIONS
Ziprasidone Aripiprazole Clozapine Olanzapine	ECG changes—QT prolongation	Effective with depressive symptoms of schizophrenia Low propensity for weight gain
Indications	Acute and chronic psychosis	
Adverse effects	Akathisia (motor restlessness) Dyskinesia (abnormal voluntary movements) Dystonias (abnormal muscle tone producing spasms of tongue, face, neck) Parkinson syndrome (shuffling gait, rigid muscles, excessive salivation, tremors, mask-like face, motor retardation) Tardive dyskinesia (involuntary movements of mouth, tongue, trunk, extremities; chewing motions, sucking, tongue thrusting) Photosensitivity Orthostatic hypotension Neuroleptic malignant syndrome	
Nursing considerations	Lowers seizure threshold May slow growth rate in children Monitor for urinary retention and decreased GI motility Avoid alcohol May cause hypotension if taken with antihypertensives, nitrates Phenothiazines also used	

ANTIPSYCHOTIC MEDICATION ADVERSE EFFECTS		
MEDICATION	**ADVERSE EFFECTS**	**NURSING CONSIDERATIONS**
Extrapyramidal	Pseudoparkinsonism Dystonia (muscle spasm) Acute dystonic reaction Early signs: tightening of jaw, stiff neck, swollen tongue Late signs: swollen airway, oculogyric crisis Akathisia (inability to sit or stand still, foot tap, pace) Tardive dyskinesia (abnormal, involuntary movements); may be irreversible	Pharmacologic management of Parkinsonian adverse effects: benztropine or trihexyphenidyl Recognize early symptoms of acute dystonic reaction Notify health care provider for IM diphenhydramine protocol
Anticholinergic	Blurred vision Dry mouth Nasal congestion Constipation Acute urinary retention	Educate client that some anticholinergic adverse effects often diminish over time Maintain adequate fluid intake and monitor I and O
Sedative	Sleepiness Possible danger if driving or operating machinery	Monitor sedative effects and maintain client safety
Hypotensive	Orthostatic hypotension is common	Frequent monitoring of BP and advise client to rise slowly
Other	Phototoxicity	Educate client regarding need for sunscreen
Neuroleptic malignant syndrome	Rigidity Fever Sweating Autonomic dysfunction (dysrhythmias, fluctuations in BP) Confusion Seizures, coma	Immediately withdraw antipsychotics Control hyperthermia Hydration Dantrolene (muscle relaxant) used for rigidity and severe reactions Bromocriptine (dopamine receptor antogonist) used for CNS toxicity and mild reactions
Atropine psychosis	Skin hot to touch without fever–"red as a beet" (flushed face) Dehydration–"dry as a bone" Altered mental status–"mad as a hatter"	Reduce or discontinue medication Hydration Stay with client while confused for safety

ANTIPSYCHOTIC: DEGREE OF ADVERSE EFFECTS	
Action	Blocks postsynaptic dopamine receptors in brain
Indications	Psychotic disorders
	Severe nausea and vomiting
Adverse effects	Drowsiness
	Pseudoparkinsonism
	Dystonia
	Akathisia
	Tardive dyskinesia
	Neuroleptic malignant syndrome
	Dysrhythmias
	Photophobia
	Blurred vision
	Photosensitivity
	Lactation
	Discolors urine pink to red-brown
Nursing considerations	May cause false-positive pregnancy tests
	Dilute oral concentrate with water, saline, 7-Up, homogenized milk, carbonated orange drink, fruit juices (pineapple, orange, apricot, prune, V-8, tomato, grapefruit); use 60 mL for each 5 mL of medication
	Do not mix with beverages that contain caffeine (coffee, tea, cola) or apple juice; incompatible
	Monitor vital signs
	Takes 4-6 weeks to achieve steady plasma levels
	Monitor bowel function
	Monitor elderly for dehydration (sedation and decreased thirst sensation)
	Avoid activities requiring mental alertness
	Avoid exposure to sun
	Maintain fluid intake
	May have anticholinergic and antihistamine actions

ANTIPSYCHOTIC: DEGREE OF ADVERSE EFFECTS				
MEDICATION	**EXTRAPYRAMIDAL**	**ANTICHOLINERGIC**	**SEDATIVE**	**HYPOTENSIVE**
Chlorpromazine	↑	↑↑	↑↑↑	↑↑↑
Thioridazine	↑	↑↑↑	↑↑↑	↑↑
Trifluoperazine	↑↑↑	↑	↑	↑
Fluphenazine	↑↑↑	↑	↑	↑
Perphenazine	↑↑↑	↑	↑↑	↑
Haloperidol	↑↑↑	↑	↑	↑
Thiothixene	↑↑	↑	↑	↑↑
KEY: ↑ mild; ↑↑ moderate; ↑↑↑ severe				

ANTIPYRETIC MEDICATIONS		
MEDICATION	ADVERSE EFFECTS	NURSING CONSIDERATIONS
Acetaminophen	Overdosage may be fatal GI adverse effects are not common	Do not exceed recommended dose
Asprin	Short-term use—GI bleeding, heartburn, occasional nausea Prolonged high dosage—salicylism: metabolic acidosis, respiratory alkalosis, dehydration, fluid and electrolyte imbalance, tinnitus	Observe for bleeding gums, bloody or black stools, bruises Give with milk, water, or food, or use enteric-coated tablets to minimize gastric distress Contraindications—GI disorders, severe anemia, vitamin K deficiency Anti-inflammatory, analgesic, antipyretic
Action	Antiprostaglandin activity in hypothalamus reduces fever; causes peripheral vasodilation; anti-inflammatory actions	
Indications	Fever	
Adverse effects	GI irritation Occult bleeding Tinnitus Dizziness Confusion Liver dysfunction (acetaminophen)	
Nursing considerations	Aspirin contraindicated for client less than 21 years old due to risk of Reye's syndrome Aspirin contraindicated for clients with bleeding disorders due to anticlotting activity NSAIDS are also used for fever	

ANTIPYRETIC MEDICATIONS		
MEDICATION	ADVERSE EFFECTS	NURSING CONSIDER-ATIONS
Acetaminophen	Overdosage may be fatal GI adverse effects are not common	Do not exceed recommended dose
Salicylates	Short-term use—GI bleeding, heartburn, occasional nausea Prolonged high dosage—salicylism: metabolic acidosis, respiratory alkalosis, dehydration, fluid and electrolyte imbalance, tinnitus	Observe for bleeding gums, bloody or black stools, bruises Give with milk, water, or food, or use enteric-coated tablets to minimize gastric distress Contraindications—GI disorders, severe anemia, vitamin K deficiency Anti-inflammatory, analgesic, antipyretic

ANTIPYRETIC MEDICATIONS *(CONTINUED)*		
MEDICATION	**ADVERSE EFFECTS**	**NURSING CONSIDER-ATIONS**
Action	Antiprostaglandin activity in hypothalamus reduces fever; causes peripheral vasodilation; anti-inflammatory actions	
Indications	Fever	
Adverse effects	GI irritation Occult bleeding Tinnitus Dizziness Confusion Liver dysfunction (acetaminophen)	
Nursing considerations	Aspirin contraindicated for client less than 21 years old due to risk of Reye's syndrome Aspirin contraindicated for clients with bleeding disorders due to anticlotting activity NSAIDS are also used for fever	

ANTITHYROID MEDICATIONS		
MEDICATION	**ADVERSE EFFECTS**	**NURSING CONSIDERATIONS**

Methimazole
Propylthiouracil
	Leukopenia,
	  fever,
	  rash,
	  sore throat, jaundice
		Inhibits synthesis of thyroid hormone by thyroid gland
		
		Check CBC and hepatic function
		
		Give with meals
		
		Report fever, sore throat to health care provider

Lugol's iodine solution Potassium iodide	Nausea, vomiting, metallic taste Rash	Iodine preparation Used 2 weeks prior to surgery; decreases vascularity, decreases hormone release Only effective for a short period Give after meals Dilute in water, milk, or fruit juice Stains teeth Give through straw
Radioactive iodine (^{131}I)	Feeling of fullness in neck Metallic taste Leukemia	Destroys thyroid tissue Contraindicated for women of childbearing age Fast overnight before administration Urine, saliva, vomit radioactive 3 days Use full radiation precautions Encourage fluids

ANTITHYROID MEDICATIONS *(CONTINUED)*		
MEDICATION	**ADVERSE EFFECTS**	**NURSING CONSIDERATIONS**
Action	Antithyroid agents—inhibits oxidation of iodine Iodines—reduces vascularity of thyroid gland; increases amount of inactive (bound) hormone; inhibits release of thyroid hormones into circulation	
Indications	Hyperthyroidism Thyrotoxic crisis	
Adverse effects	Nausea, vomiting Diarrhea Rashes Thrombocytopenia Leukopenia	
Nursing considerations	Changes in vital signs or weight and appearance may indicate adverse reactions, which should lead to evaluation of continued medication use	

THYROID REPLACEMENT MEDICATIONS		
MEDICATION	**ADVERSE EFFECTS**	**NURSING CONSIDERATIONS**
Levothyroxine	Nervousness, tremors Insomnia Tachycardia, palpitations Dysrhythmias, angina	Tell client to report chest pain, palpitations, sweating, nervousness, shortness of breath to health care provider
Liothyronine sodium	Excessive dosages produce symptoms of hyperthyroidism	Take at same time each day Take in AM Monitor pulse and BP
Action	Increases metabolic rate of body	
Indications	Hypothyroidism	
Adverse effects	Nervousness Tachycardia Weight loss	
Nursing considerations	Obtain history of client's medications Enhances action of oral anticoagulants, antidepressants Decreases action of insulin, digitalis Obtain baseline vital signs Monitor weight Avoid OTC drugs	

ANTITUBERCULOTIC MEDICATION		
MEDICATION	ADVERSE EFFECTS	NURSING CONSIDERATIONS
First-line medications		
Isoniazid	Hepatitis Peripheral neuritis Rash Fever	Pyridoxine (B6): 10–50 mg as prophylaxis for neuritis; 50-100 mg as treatment Teach signs of hepatitis Check liver function tests Alcohol increases risk of hepatic complications Therapeutic effects can be expected after 2–3 weeks of therapy Monitor for resolution of symptoms (fever, night sweats, weight loss); hypotension (orthostatic) may occur initially, then resolve; caution client to change position slowly Give before meals Do not combine with phenytoin, causes phenytoin toxicity
Ethambutol	Optic neuritis	Use cautiously with renal disease Check visual acuity
Rifampin	Hepatitis Fever	Orange urine, tears, saliva Check liver function tests Can take with food
Streptomycin	Nephrotoxicity VIII nerve damage	Check creatinine and BUN Audiograms if given long-term
Second-line medications		
Para-amino- salicyclic acid	GI disturbances Hepatotoxicity	Check for ongoing GI adverse effects
Pyrazinamide	Hyperuricemia Anemia Anorexia	Check liver function tests, uric acid, and hematopoietic studies
Action	Inhibits cell wall and protein synthesis of *Mycobacterium tuberculosis*	
Indications	Tuberculosis INH–used to prevent disease in person exposed to organism	

ANTITUBERCULOTIC MEDICATION *(CONTINUED)*		
MEDICATION	ADVERSE EFFECTS	NURSING CONSIDERATIONS
Adverse effects	Hepatitis Optic neuritis Seizures Peripheral neuritis	
Nursing considerations	Used in combination (2 medications or more) Monitor for liver damage and hepatitis With active TB, the client should cover mouth and nose when coughing, confine used tissues to plastic bags, and wear a mask with crowds until three sputum cultures are negative (no longer infectious) In inpatient settings, client is placed under airborne precautions and workers wear a N95 or high-efficiency particulate air (HEPA) respirator until the client is no longer infectious	

ANTITUSSIVE/EXPECTORANT MEDICATIONS		
MEDICATION	ADVERSE EFFECTS	NURSING CONSIDERATIONS
Dextromethorphan hydrobromide	Drowsiness Dizziness	Antitussive Onset occurs within 30 min, lasts 3-6 h Monitor cough type and frequency
Guaifenesin	Dizziness Headache Nausea, vomiting	Expectorant Monitor cough type and frequency Take with glass of water
Action	Antitussives—suppresses cough reflex by inhibiting cough center in medulla Expectorants—decreases viscosity of bronchial secretions	
Indications	Coughs due to URI and/or COPD	
Adverse effects	Respiratory depression Hypotension Bradycardia Anticholinergic effects Photosensitivity	
Nursing considerations	Elderly clients may need reduced dosages Avoid alcohol	

ANTIVIRAL MEDICATIONS		
MEDICATION	ADVERSE EFFECTS	NURSING CONSIDERATIONS
Acyclovir	Headaches, dizziness Seizures Diarrhea	Used for herpes simplex and herpes zoster Given PO, IV, topically Does not prevent transmission of disease Slows progression of symptoms Encourage fluids Check liver and renal function tests
Ribavarin	Worsening of pulmonary status, bacterial pneumonia Hypotension, cardiac arrest	Used for severe lower respiratory tract infections in infants and children Must use special aerosol-generating device for administration Can precipitate Contraindicated in females who may become pregnant during treatment
Zidovudine	Anemia Headache Anorexia, diarrhea, nausea, GI pain Paresthesias, dizziness Insomnia Agranulocytosis	Used for HIV infection Teach clients to strictly comply with dosage schedule
Zalcitabine	Oral ulcers Peripheral neuropathy, headache Vomiting, diarrhea CHF, cardiomyopathy	Used in combination with zidovudine for advanced HIV
Didanosine	Headache Rhinitis, cough Diarrhea, nausea, vomiting Pancreatitis, granulocytopenia Peripheral neuropathy Seizures Hemorrhage	Used for HIV infection Monitor liver and renal function studies Note baseline vital signs and weight Take on empty stomach Chew or crush tablets
Famciclovir	Fatigue, fever Nausea, vomiting, diarrhea, constipation Headache, sinusitis	Used for acute herpes zoster (shingles) Obtain baseline CBC and renal function studies Remind clients they are contagious when lesions are open and draining

ANTIVIRAL MEDICATIONS *(CONTINUED)*		
MEDICATION	**ADVERSE EFFECTS**	**NURSING CONSIDERATIONS**
Ganciclovir	Fever Rash Leukemia Seizures GI hemorrhage MI, stroke	Used for retinitis caused by cytomegalovirus Check level of consciousness Monitor CBC, I and O Report any dizziness, confusions, seizures immediately Need regular eye exams
Amantadine	Dizziness Nervousness Insomnia Orthostatic hypotension	Used for prophylaxis and treatment of influenza A Orthostatic hypotension precautions Instruct clients to avoid hazardous activities
Oseltamivir Zanamivir	Nausea, vomiting Cough and throat irritation	Used for the treatment of Types A and B influenza Best effect if given within 2 days of infection Instruct clients that medication will reduce flu-symptom duration
Action	Inhibits DNA or RNA replication in virus	
Indications	Recurrent HSV 1 and 2 in immunocompromised clients Encephalitis Herpes zoster HIV infections	
Adverse effects	Vertigo Depression Headache Hematuria	
Nursing considerations	Encourage fluids Small, frequent feedings Good skin care Wear glove when applying topically Not a cure, but relieves symptoms	

ATTENTION–DEFICIT HYPERACTIVITY DISORDER MEDICATIONS		
MEDICATION	ADVERSE EFFECTS	NURSING CONSIDERATIONS
Methylphenidate	Nervousness, palpitations Insomnia Tachycardia Weight loss, growth suppression	May precipitate Tourette's syndrome Monitor CBC, platelet count Has paradoxical calming effect in ADD Monitor height/weight in children Monitor BP Avoid drinks with caffeine Give at least 6 h before bedtime Give pc
Dextroamphetamine sulfate	Insomnia Tachycardia, palpitations	Controlled substance May alter insulin needs Give in AM to prevent insomnia Don't use with MAO inhibitor (possible hypertensive crisis)
Action	Increases level of catecholamines in cerebral cortex and reticular activating system	
Indications	Attention-deficit hyperactivity disorder (ADHD) Narcolepsy	
Adverse effects	Restlessness Insomnia Tremors Tachycardia Seizures	
Nursing considerations	Monitor growth rate in children	

BIPOLAR DISORDER MEDICATIONS		
MEDICATION	ADVERSE EFFECTS	NURSING CONSIDERATIONS
Lithium	Dizziness Headache Impaired vision Fine hand tremors Reversible leukocytosis	Use for control of manic episodes in the syndrome of manic-depressive psychosis; mood stabilizer Blood levels must be monitored frequently GI symptoms can be reduced if taken with meals Therapeutic effects preceded by lag of 1-2 weeks Signs of intoxication—vomiting, diarrhea, drowsiness, muscular weakness, ataxia Dosage is usually halved during depressive stages of illness Normal blood target level = 1-1.5 mEq/L Check serum levels 2-3 times weekly when started and monthly while on maintenance; serum levels should be drawn in AM prior to dose Should have fluid intake of 2,500-3,000 mL/day and adequate salt intake
Carbamazepine	Dizziness, vertigo Drowsiness Ataxia CHF Aplastic anemia, thrombocytopenia	Mood stablizer used with bipolar disorder Traditionally used for seizures and trigeminal neuralgia Obtain baseline urinalysis, BUN, liver function tests, CBC Shake oral suspension well before measuring dose When giving by NG tube, mix with equal volume of water, 0.9% NaCl or D_5 W, then flush with 100 mL after dose Take with food Drowsiness usually disappears in 3-4 days

BIPOLAR DISORDER MEDICATIONS *(CONTINUED)*		
MEDICATION	ADVERSE EFFECTS	NURSING CONSIDERATIONS
Divalproex sodium	Sedation Pancreatitis Indigestion Thrombocytopenia Toxic hepatitis	Mood stablizers used with bipolar disorder Traditionally used for seizures Monitor liver function tests, platelet count before starting med and periodically after med Teach client symptoms of liver dysfunction (e.g., malaise, fever, lethargy) Monitor blood levels Take with food or milk Avoid hazardous activities
Action	Reduces amount of catecholamines released into synapse and increases reuptake of norepinephrine and serotonin from synaptic space; competes with Na^+ and K^+ transport in nerve and muscle cells	
Indications	Manic episodes	
Adverse effects	GI upset Tremors Polydipsia, polyuria	
Nursing considerations	Monitor serum levels carefully Severe toxicity: exaggerated reflexes, seizures, coma, death	

BONE-RESORPTION INHIBITOR (BISPHOSPHONATE) MEDICATIONS		
MEDICATION	ADVERSE EFFECTS	NURSING CONSIDERATIONS
Alendronate Risedronate Ibandronate	Esophagitis Arthralgia Nausea, diarrhea	Prevention and treatment of postmenopausal osteoporosis, Paget's disease, glucocorticoid-induced osteoporosis Instruct clients to take medication in the morning with 6–8 ounces of water before eating and to remain in upright position for 30 minutes Bone density tests may be monitored

BRONCHODILATORS/LEUKOTRIENE-RECEPTOR BLOCKER MEDICATIONS		
MEDICATION	**ADVERSE EFFECTS**	**NURSING CONSIDERATIONS**
Aminophylline	Nervousness Nausea Dizziness Tachycardia Seizures	IM injection causes intense pain Coffee, tea, cola increase risk of adverse reactions Monitor blood levels IV–incompatible with multiple medications
Terbutaline sulfate	Nervousness, tremor Headache Tachycardia Palpitations Fatigue	Short-acting beta agonist most useful when about to enter environment or begin activity likely to induce asthma attack Pulse and blood pressure should be checked before each dose
Ipratropium bromide Tiotropium	Nervousness Tremor Dry mouth Palpitations	Cholinergic antagonist Don't mix in nebulizer with cromolyn sodium Not for acute treatment Teach use of metered dose inhaler: inhale, hold breath, exhale slowly
Albuterol	Tremors Headache Hyperactivity Tachycardia	Short-acting beta agonist most useful when about to enter environment or begin activity likely to induce asthma attack Monitor for toxicity if using tablets and aerosol Teach how to correctly use inhaler
Epinephrine	Cerebral hemorrhage Hypertension Tachycardia	When administered IV monitor BP, heart rate, EKG If used with steroid inhaler, use bronchodilator first, then wait 5 minutes before using steroid inhaler (opens airway for maximum effectiveness)
Salmeterol	Headache Pharyngitis Nervousness Tremors	Dry powder preparation Not for acute bronchospasm or exacerbations
Montelukast sodium Zafirlukast Zileuton	Headache GI distress	Used for prophylactic and maintenance therapy of asthma Liver tests may be monitored Interacts with theophylline

CARBONIC ANHYDRASE INHIBITOR MEDICATIONS		
MEDICATION	ADVERSE EFFECTS	NURSING CONSIDERATIONS
Acetazolamide	Lethargy, depression Anorexia, weakness Decreased K$^+$ level, confusion	Used for glaucoma Assess client's mental status before repeating dose
Action	Decreases production of aqueous humor in ciliary body	
Indications	Open-angle glaucoma	
Adverse effects	Blurred vision Lacrimation Pulmonary edema	
Nursing considerations	Monitor client for systemic effects	

CARDIAC GLYCOSIDE MEDICATION		
MEDICATION	ADVERSE EFFECTS	NURSING CONSIDERATIONS
Digoxin	Anorexia Nausea Bradycardia Visual disturbances Confusion Abdominal pain	Administer with caution to elderly or clients with renal insufficiency Monitor renal function and electrolytes Instruct clients to eat high-potassium foods Take apical pulse for 1 full minute before administering Notify health care provider if AP less than 60 (adult), less than 90-110 (infants and young children), less than 70 (older children) Rapid digitalization–0.5 to 0.75 mg po, then 0.125 mg - 0.375mg cautiously until adequate effect is noted Gradual digitalization–0.25 to 0.5 mg may increase dosage every 2 weeks until desired clinical effect achieved Digoxin immune fab (Digibind)–used for treatment of life-threatening toxicity Maintenance dose 0.125-0.5 mg IV or PO (average is 0.25 mg) Teach client to check pulse rate and discuss adverse effects Low K$^+$ increases risk of digitalis toxicity Serum therapeutic blood levels 0.5–2 nanograms/mL Toxic blood levels 9 2 nanograms/mL
Action	Increases force of myocardial contraction and slows heart rate by stimulating the vagus nerve and blocking the AV node	
Indications	Heart failure, Dysrhythmias	
Adverse effects	Tachycardia, bradycardia, heart block Anorexia, nausea, vomiting Halos around dark objects, blurred vision, halo vision Dysrhythmias, heart block	

CARDIAC GLYCOSIDE MEDICATION *(CONTINUED)*		
MEDICATION	ADVERSE EFFECTS	NURSING CONSIDERATIONS
Nursing considerations	Instruct client to eat high potassium foods	
	Monitor for digitalis toxicity	
	Risk of digitalis toxicity increases if client is hypokalemic	
Herbal interactions	Licorice can potentiate action of digoxin by promoting potassium loss	
	Hawthorn may increase effects of digoxin	
	Ginseng may falsely elevate digoxin levels	
	Ma-huang (ephedra) increases risk of digitalis toxicity	

CYTOPROTECTIVE MEDICATIONS		
MEDICATION	ADVERSE EFFECTS	NURSING CONSIDERATIONS
Sucralfate	Constipation	Take medication 1 hour ac
	Dizziness	Should not be taken with antacids or H_2 blockers
Action	Adheres to and protects ulcer's surface by forming a barrier	
Indications	Duodenal ulcer	
Adverse effects	Constipation	
	Vertigo	
	Flatulence	
Nursing considerations	Action lasts up to 6 h	
	Give 2 hours before or after most medications to prevent decreased absorption	

DISEASE-MODIFYING ANTIRHEUMATIC MEDICATIONS(DMARDS)		
MEDICATION	ADVERSE EFFECTS	NURSING CONSIDERATIONS
Nonbiologic DMARDs Methotrexate Hydroxychloroquine sulfate Sulfasalazine Cyclosporine	GI track irritation Hematuria Leukopenia Thrombocytopenia Respiratory involvement	Assess hepatic Notify HCP if dry non-productive cough noted or renal function Assess severe skin reactions Assess for opportunistic infections
Biologic DMARDs Entanercept Infliximab Adalimumab Anakinra Rituximab Abatacept	Leukopenia Neutropenia Thrombocytopenia Intestinal obstruction Fatigue	Assess for infusion related reactions (fever chills, dyspnea, chest discomfort) Assess for CNS adverse reactions Assessfor lymphoma and infection Assess for opportunistic infections
Action	Non-biologic DMARDs: Interfere with immune system Indirect and nonspecific effect Biologic DMARDs: Interfere with immune system (tumor necrosis factor, interleukins, T- or B-cell lymphocytes)	
Indications	Rheumatoid arthritis Psoriasis Inflammatory bowel disease	
Adverse effects	Stomatitis Liver toxicity Bleeding Anemia Infections Hypersensitivity Kidney failure	
Nursing considerations	Precautions: infections, bleeding disorders Monitor liver function tests Monitor BUN and creatinine Monitor for signs of infection Monitor response to medication Teach client about risk of live vaccines Teach client to avoid alcohol Teach client about risk of infection	

DIURETIC MEDICATIONS		
MEDICATION	**ADVERSE EFFECTS**	**NURSING CONSIDERATIONS**
Thiazide diuretics Hydrochlorothiazide Chlorothiazide	Hypokalemia Hyperglycemia Blurred vision Loss of Na^+ Dry mouth Hypotension	Monitor electrolytes, especially potassium I and O Monitor BUN and creatinine Don't give at hs Weigh client daily Encourage potassium-containing foods
Potassium sparing Spironlactone	Hyperkalemia Hyponatremia Hepatic and renal damage Tinnitus Rash	Used with other diuretics Give with meals Avoid salt substitutes containing potassium Monitor I and O
Loop diuretics Furosemide Ethacrynic acid	Hypotension Hypokalemia Hyperglycemia GI upset Weakness	Monitor BP, pulse rate, I and O Monitor potassium Give IV dose over 1-2 minutes, causes diuresis in 5-10 min After PO dose diuresis in about 30 min Weigh client daily Don't give at hs Encourage potassium-containing foods
Ethacrynic acid bumetanide	Potassium depletion Electrolyte imbalance Hypovolemia Ototoxicity	Supervise ambulation Monitor blood pressure and pulse Observe for signs of electrolyte imbalance
Osmotic diuretic Mannitol	Dry mouth Thirst	I and O must be measured Monitor vital signs Monitor for electrolyte imbalance
Other Chlorthalidone	Dizziness Aplastic anemia Orthostatic hypotension	Acts like a thiazide diuretic Acts in 2-3 h, peak 2-6 h, lasts 2-3 days Administer in AM Monitor output, weight, BP, electrolytes Increase K^+ in diet Monitor glucose levels in diabetic clients Change position slowly

DIURETIC MEDICATIONS *(CONTINUED)*		
MEDICATION	ADVERSE EFFECTS	NURSING CONSIDERATIONS
Action	Thiazides—inhibits reabsorption of sodium and chloride in distal renal tubule	
	Loop—inhibits reabsorption of sodium and chloride in loop of Henle and distal renal tubules	
	Potassium-sparing—blocks effect of aldosterone on renal tubules, causing loss of sodium and water and retention of potassium	
	Osmotic—pulls fluid from tissues due to hypertonic effect	
Indications	Heart failure	
	Hypertension	
	Renal diseases	
	Diabetes insipidus	
	Reduction of osteoporosis in postmenopausal women	
Adverse effects	Dizziness, vertigo	
	Dry mouth	
	Orthostatic hypotension	
	Leukopenia	
	Polyuria, nocturia	
	Photosensitivity	
	Impotence	
	Hypokalemia (except for potassium-sparing)	
	Hyponatremia	
Nursing considerations	Take with food or milk	
	Take in A.M.	
	Monitor weight and electrolytes	
	Protect skin from the sun	
	Diet high in potassium for loop and thiazide diuretics	
	Limit potassium intake for potassium-sparing diuretics	
	Used as first-line drugs for hypertension	
Herbal interactions	Licorice can promote potassium loss, causing hypokalemia	
	Aloe can decrease serum potassium level, causing hypokalemia	
	Gingko may increase blood pressure when taken with thiazide diuretics	

ELECTROLYTES AND REPLACEMENT SOLUTIONS		
MEDICATION	ADVERSE EFFECTS	NURSING CONSIDERATIONS
Calcium carbonate Calcium chloride	Dysrhythmias Constipation	Foods containing oxalic acid (rhubarb, spinach), phytic acid (bran, whole cereals), and phosphorus (milk, dairy products) interfere with absorption Monitor EKG Take 1–1.5 h pc if GI upset occurs
Magnesium chloride	Weak or absent deep tendon reflexes Hypotension Respiratory paralysis	Respirations should be greater than 16/min before medication given IV Test knee-jerk and patellar reflexes before each dose Monitor I and 0
Potassium chloride Potassium gluconate	Dysrhythmias, cardiac arrest Adominal pain Respiratory paralysis	Monitor EKG and serum electrolytes Take with or after meals with full glass of water or fruit juice
Sodium chloride	Pulmonary edema	Monitor serum electrolytes

ELECTROLYTES/ELECTROLYTE MODIFIER MEDICATIONS	
Action	Alkalinizing agents—release bicarbonate ions in stomach and secrete bicarbonate ions in kidneys
	Calcium salts—provide calcium for bones, teeth, nerve transmission, muscle contraction, normal blood coagulation, cell membrane strength
	Hypocalcemic medications—decrease blood levels of calcium
	Hypophosphatemic agents—bind phosphates in GI tract lowering blood levels; neutralize gastric acid, inactivate pepsin
	Magnesium salts—provide magnesium for nerve conduction and muscle activity and activate enzyme reactions in carbohydrate metabolism
	Phosphates—provide body with phosphorus needed for bone, muscle tissue, metabolism of carbohydrates, fats, proteins, and normal CNS function
	Potassium exchange resins—exchange Na^+ for K^+ in intestines, lowering K^+ levels
	Potassium salts—provide potassium needed for cell growth and normal functioning of cardiac, skeletal, and smooth muscle
	Replacement solution—provide water and Na^+ to maintain acid-base and water balance, maintain osmotic pressure
	Urinary acidifiers—secrete H^+ ions in kidneys, making urine acidic
	Urinary alkalinizers—convert to sodium bicarbonate, making the urine alkaline
Indications	Fluid and electrolyte imbalances
	Renal calculi
	Peptic ulcers
	Osteoporosis
	Metabolic acidosis or alkalosis
Adverse effects	See individual medications
Nursing considerations	Monitor clients with CHF, hypertension, renal disease

GENITOURINARY MEDICATIONS		
MEDICATION	ADVERSE EFFECTS	NURSING CONSIDERATIONS
Nitrofurantoin	Diarrhea Nausea, vomiting Asthma attacks	Anti-infective Check CBC Give with food or milk Avoid acidic foods (cranberry juice, prunes, plums) which increase drug action Check I and O Monitor pulmonary status
Phenazopyridine	Headache Vertigo	Urinary tract analgesic, spasmolytic Inform client that urine will be bright orange Take with meals

GENITOURINARY MEDICATIONS *(CONTINUED)*		
MEDICATION	ADVERSE EFFECTS	NURSING CONSIDERATIONS
Anticholinergics Oxybutynin Hyoscyamine Propantheline Darifenacin Solifenacin Tolterodine	Drowsiness Blurred vision Dry mouth Constipation Urinary retention	Used to reduce bladder spasms and treat urinary incontinence Increase fluids and fiber in diet Oxybutynin–older adults require higher dose and have greater incidence of adverse effects
Anti-impotence Sildenafil Vardenafil Tadalafil	Headache Flushing Hypotension Priapism	Treatment of erectile dysfunction Take 1 hour before sexual activity Never use with nitrates—could have fatal hypotension Do not take with alpha blockers, e.g., doxazosin –risk of hypotension Do not drink grapefruit juice
Testosterone inhibitors Finasteride	Decreased libido Impotence Breast tenderness	Treatment of benign prostatic hyperplasia (BPH), male hair loss Pregnant women should avoid contact with crushed drug or client's semen—may adversely affect male fetus

GI ULCER MEDICATIONS		
MEDICATION	ADVERSE EFFECTS	NURSING CONSIDERATIONS
H2-antagonists Cimetidine Ranitidine Famotidine Nizatidine	Diarrhea Confusion and dizziness (esp. in elderly with large doses) Headache	Bedtime dose suppresses nocturnal acid production Compliance may increase with single-dose regimen Avoid antacids within 1 hour of dose Dysrhythmias Cimetidine–greater incidence of confusion and agitation with older adults
Antisecretory Omeprazole Lansoprazole Rabeprazole Esomeprazole Pantoprazole	Dizziness Diarrhea	Bedtime dose suppresses nocturnal acid production Do not crush sustained-release capsule; contents may be sprinkled on food or instilled with fluid in NG tube

GI ULCER MEDICATIONS *(CONTINUED)*		
MEDICATION	ADVERSE EFFECTS	NURSING CONSIDERATIONS
Prostaglandin analogs Misoprostol	Abdominal pain Diarrhea (13%) Miscarriage	Notify health care provider if diarrhea more than 1 week or severe abdominal pain or black, tarry stools
Nursing considerations	Other medications may be prescribed, included antacids (time administration to avoid canceling med effect) and antimicrobials to eradicate *H. pylori* infections Client should avoid smoking, alcohol, ASA, and caffeine, all of which increase stomach acid	

EYE MEDICATIONS: MIOTIC		
MEDICATION	ADVERSE EFFECTS	NURSING CONSIDERATIONS
Pilocarpine	Painful eye muscle spasm, blurred or poor vision in dim lights Photophobia, cataracts, or floaters	Teach to apply pressure on lacrimal sac for 1 min following instillation Used for glaucoma Caution client to avoid sunlight and night driving
Carachol	Headache If absorbed systemically, can cause sweating, abdominal cramps, and decreased blood pressure	Cholinergic (ophthalmic) Similar to acetylcholine in action Produces pupillary miosis during ocular surgery
Action	Causes contraction of sphincter muscles of iris, resulting in miosis	
Indications	Pupillary miosis in ocular surgery Primary open-angle glaucoma	
Adverse effects	Headache Hypotension Bronchoconstriction	
Nursing considerations	Teach how to instill eye drops correctly Apply light pressure on lacrimal sac for 1 minute after medication instilled Avoid hazardous activities until temporary blurring disappears Transient brow pain and myopia are common initially, disappear within 10-14 days	

EYE MEDICATIONS: MYDRIATIC AND CYCLOPLEGIC		
MEDICATION	ADVERSE EFFECTS	NURSING CONSIDERATIONS
Atropine sulfate	Blurred vision, photophobia Flushing, tachycardia Dry mouth	Contraindicated with narrow-angle glaucoma Suck on hard candy for dry mouth
Cyclopentolate	Photophobia, blurred vision Seizures Tachycardia	Contraindicated in narrow-angle glaucoma Burns when instilled
Action	Anticholinergic action leaves the pupil under unopposed adrenergic influence, causing it to dilate	
Indications	Diagnostic procedures Acute iritis, uveitis	
Adverse effects	Headache Tachycardia Blurred vision Photophobia Dry mouth	
Nursing considerations	Mydriatics cause pupil dilation; cycloplegics paralyze the iris sphincter Watch for signs of glaucoma (increased intraocular pressure, headache, progressive blurring of vision) Apply light pressure on lacrimal sac for 1 minute after instilling medication Avoid hazardous activities until blurring of vision subsides Wear dark glasses	

EYE MEDICATIONS: OVERVIEW		
MEDICATION	ADVERSE EFFECTS	NURSING CONSIDERATIONS
Methylcellulose	Eye irritation if excess is allowed to dry on eyelids	Lubricant Use eyewash to rinse eyelids of "sandy" sensation felt after administration
Polyvinyl alcohol	Blurred vision Burning	Artificial tears Applied to contact lenses before insertion
Tetrahydrozoline	Cardiac irregularities Pupillary dilation, increased intraocular pressure Transient stinging	Used for ocular congestion, irritation, allergic conditions Rebound congestion may occur with frequent or prolonged use Apply light pressure on lacrimal sac for 1 min instillation
Timolol maleate Levobunolol	Eye irritation Hypotension	Beta-blocking agent Reduces intraocular pressure in management of glaucoma Apply light pressure on lacrimal sac for 1 min following instillation Monitor BP and pulse
Proparacaine HCl Tetracaine HCl, cocaine	Corneal abrasion	Topical anesthetic Remind client not to touch or rub eyes while anesthetized Patch the eye to prevent corneal abrasion
Prednisolone acetate	Corneal abrasion	Topical steroid Steroid use predisposes client to local infection
Gentamicin Tobramycin	Eye irritation; itching, redness	Anti-infective agent Clean exudate from eyes before use
Idoxuridine	Eye irritation Itching lids	Topical antiviral agent Educate client about possible adverse effects
Dipivefrin HCl	Increase in heart rate and blood pressure	Adrenergic Monitor vital signs because of systemic absorption
Flurbiprofen	Platelet aggregation disorder	Nonsteroidal anti-inflammatory medications Monitor client for eye hemorrhage Client should not continue wearing contact lens
Nursing considerations	Place pressure on tear ducts for one minute Wash hands before and after installation Do not touch tip of dropper to eye or body	

HEAVY METAL ANTAGONIST MEDICATIONS		
MEDICATION	ADVERSE EFFECTS	NURSING CONSIDERATIONS
Deferoxamine mesylate	Pain and induration at injection site Urticaria Hypotension Generalized erythema	Used for acute iron intoxication, chronic iron overload
Dimercaprol	Hypertension Tachycardia Nausea, vomiting Headache	Used for treatment of arsenic, gold, and mercury poisoning; acute lead poisoning when used with edetate calcium disodium Administered as initial dose because of its improved efficiency in removing lead from brain tissue
Edetate calcium disodium (EDTA)		Used for acute and chronic lead poisoning, lead encephalopathy Renal tubular necrosis Multiple deep IM doses or IV Very painful—local anesthetic procaine is injected with the drug (drawn into syringe last, after which the syringe is maintained with needle held slightly down so that it is administered first); rotate sites; provide emotional support and play therapy as outlet for frustration Ensure adequate hydration and monitor I and O and kidney function—$CaNa_2$ EDTA and lead are toxic to kidneys Seizure precautions—initial rapid mobilization of lead may cause an increase in brain lead levels, exacerbating symptoms
Action	Forms stable complexes with metals	
Indications	Poisoning (gold, arsenic) Acute lead encephalopathy	
Adverse effects	Tachycardia Burning sensation in lips, mouth, throat Abdominal pain	
Nursing considerations	Monitor I and O, BUN, EKG Encourage fluids	

IMMUNOSUPPRESSANT MEDICATIONS		
MEDICATION	ADVERSE EFFECTS	NURSING CONSIDERATIONS
Cyclosporine	Nephrotoxicity Headache Seizures Hypertension Gingival hyperplasia Leukopenia Thrombocytopenia Infections Tremor	Take once daily in AM Measure dosage carefully in oral syringe Mix with whole milk, chocolate milk, fruit juice Always used with adrenal corticosteroids Monitor BUN, serum creatinine, liver function tests To prevent thrush, swish and swallow nystatin QID Use mechanical contraceptives, not oral contraceptives
Action	Prevents production of T cells and their response to interleukin-2; recognizes antigens foreign to body	
Indications	Prevent rejection for transplanted organs	
Adverse effects	Nausea, vomiting Diarrhea Hepatotoxicity Nephrotoxicity Infection Myocardial fibrosis	
Nursing considerations	Monitor carefully for infections	

IMMUNOMODULATOR MEDICATIONS	
MEDICATION	ADVERSE EFFECTS
Beta interferons	"Flu-like" symptoms Liver dysfunction Bone marrow depression Injection site reactions Photosensitivity Central nervous system infection (natalizumab)
Interferon beta-1a Interferon beta-1b	
Glatiramer acetate Natalizumab	
Action	Modify the immune response Decrease the movement of leukocytes into the central nervous system neurons
Indications	Multiple sclerosis

IMMUNOMODULATOR MEDICATIONS *(CONTINUED)*	
MEDICATION	**ADVERSE EFFECTS**
Adverse effects	"Flu-like" symptoms
	Liver dysfunction
	Bone marrow depression
	Injection site reactions
	Photosensitivity
	Central nervous system infection (natalizumab)
Nursing considerations	Monitor liver function tests
	Monitor complete blood count
	Subcutaneous injection: rotate injection sites, apply ice, and then use warm compresses, analgesics for discomfort
	Photosensitivity precautions

IRON PREPARATION MEDICATION		
MEDICATION	**ADVERSE EFFECTS**	**NURSING CONSIDERATIONS**
Ferrous sulfate	Nausea Constipation Black stools	Food decreases absorption but may be necessary to reduce GI effects Monitor Hgb, Hct Dilute liquid preparations in juice, but not milk or antacids Use straw for liquid to avoid staining teeth
Iron dextran	Nausea Constipation Black stools	IM injections cause pain and skin staining; use the Z-track technique to put med deep into buttock; IV administration is preferred
Action	Iron salts increase availability of iron for hemoglobin	
Indications	Iron-deficiency anemia	
Adverse effects	Constipation, diarrhea Dark stools Tooth enamel stains Seizures Flushing, hypotension Tachycardia	
Nursing considerations	Take iron salts on empty stomach (absorption is reduced by one-third when taken with food) Absorption of iron decreased when administered with tetracyclines, antacids, coffee, tea, milk, eggs (bind to iron) Concurrent use of iron decreases effectiveness of tetracyclines and quinolone antibiotics Vitamin C increases absorption of iron salts Vitamin E delays therapeutic responses to iron salts	

LAXATIVES AND STOOL SOFTENER MEDICATIONS		
MEDICATION	ADVERSE EFFECTS	NURSING CONSIDERATIONS
Cascara	Anorexia, nausea, abdominal cramps, hypokalemia, calcium deficiency	Avoid exposure to sunlight Should be taken with full glass of water Relieves constipation and softens stool in about 8 hours
Bisacodyl	Mild cramps, rash, nausea, diarrhea	Stimulant Tablets should not be taken with milk or antacids (causes dissolution of enteric coating and loss of cathartic action) Can cause gastric irritation Effects in 6-12 hours
Phenolphthalein	Urticaria, rash, electrolyte imbalance Allergic reactions, skin eruption	Caution clients against prolonged use Will turn alkaline urine a pink-red color
Mineral oil	Pruritus ani, anorexia, nausea	Lubricant Administer in upright position Prolonged use can cause fat-soluble vitamin malabsorption
Docusate	Few adverse effects Abdominal cramps	Stool softener Contraindicated in atonic bowel, nausea, vomiting, GI pain Effects in 1-3 days
Milk of Magnesia (Magnesium hydroxide)	Hypermagnesemia, dehydration	Saline agent Na^+ salts can exacerbate heart failure
Psyllium hydrophilic mucilloid	Obstruction of GI tract	Take with a full glass of water; do not take dry Report abdominal distention or unusual amount of flatulence
Polyethylene glycol and electrolytes	Nausea and bloating	Large-volume product—allow time to consume it safely
Action	Bulk-forming—absorbs water into stool mass, making stool bulky, thus stimulating peristalsis Lubricants—coat surface of stool and soften fecal mass, allowing for easier passage Osmotic agents and saline laxatives—draw water from plasma by osmosis, increasing bulk of fecal mass, thus promoting peristalsis Stimulants—stimulate peristalsis when they come in contact with intestinal mucosa Stool softeners—soften fecal mass	
Indications	Constipation Preparation for procedures or surgery	

LAXATIVES AND STOOL SOFTENER MEDICATIONS *(CONTINUED)*		
MEDICATION	ADVERSE EFFECTS	NURSING CONSIDERATIONS
Adverse effects	Diarrhea Dependence	
Nursing considerations	Contraindicated for clients with abdominal pain, nausea and vomiting, fever (acute abdomen) Chronic use may cause hypokalemia	

MINERALS		
MEDICATION	ADVERSE EFFECTS	NURSING CONSIDERATIONS
Calcium	Cardiac dysrhythmias Constipation Hypercalcemia Renal calculi	Give 1 h before meals Give 1/3 dose at bedtime Monitor for urinary stones
Vitamin D (Ergocalciferol)	Seizures Impaired renal function Hypercalcemia Renal calculi	Treatment of vitamin D deficiency, rickets, psoriasis, rheumatoid arthritis Check electrolytes Restrict use of antacids containing Mg
Sodium fluoride	Bad taste Staining of teeth Nausea, vomiting	Observe for synovitis
Potassium	Nausea, vomiting Cramps, diarrhea	Prevention and treatment of hypokalemia Report hyperkalemia: lethargy, confusion, fainting, decreased urine output Report continued hypocalcemia: fatigue, weakness, polyuria, polydipsia, cardiac changes

MUSCULOSKELETAL MEDICATIONS		
MEDICATION	**ADVERSE EFFECTS**	**NURSING CONSIDERATIONS**
Edrophonium	Seizures Hypotension Diarrhea Bronchospasm Respiratory paralysis	Diagnostic test for myasthenia gravis Increased muscular strength within 30-60 seconds confirms diagnosis, lasts 4-5 minutes Monitor respirations closely Have atropine 0.5 mg injection available
Neostigmine	Nausea, vomiting Abdominal cramps Respiratory depression Bronchoconstriction Hypotension Bradycardia	Monitor vital signs frequently Have atropine injection available Observe for improvement in strength, vision, ptosis 45 min after each dose Schedule dose before periods of fatigue (e.g., ac) Take with milk or food Potentiates action of morphine Diagnostic test for myasthenia gravis
Pyridostigmine bromide	Seizures Bradycardia Hypotension Bronchoconstriction	Monitor vital signs frequently Have atropine injection available Take extended-release tablets same time each day at least 6 h apart Drug of choice for myasthenia gravis to improve muscle strength
Alendronate sodium	Vitamin D deficiency Osteomalacia	Prevents and treats osteoporosis Longer-lasting treatment for Paget's disease Take in A.M. at least 30 min before other medication, food, water, or other liquids Should sit up for 30 min after taking medication Use sunscreen and wear protective clothing
Glucosamine	Nausea, heartburn, diarrhea	Antirheumatic Contraindicated with shellfish allergy, pregnancy, and lactation May worsen glycemic control Must be taken on regular basis to be effective

MUSCULOSKELETAL MEDICATIONS *(CONTINUED)*		
MEDICATION	**ADVERSE EFFECTS**	**NURSING CONSIDERATIONS**
Action	Inhibits destruction of acetylcholine released from parasympathetic and somatic efferent nerves	
Indications	Myasthenia gravis Postoperative and postpartum functional urinary retention	
Adverse effects	Bronchoconstriction Diarrhea Respiratory paralysis Muscle cramps	
Nursing considerations	Give with milk or food Administer exactly as ordered and on time Doses vary with client's activity level Monitor vital signs, especially respirations	

NITRATES/ANTIANGINAL MEDICATIONS		
MEDICATION	**ADVERSE EFFECTS**	**NURSING CONSIDERATIONS**
Nitroglycerin	Flushing Hypotension Headache Tachycardia Dizziness Blurred vision	Renew supply every 3 months Avoid alcoholic beverages Sublingual dose may be repeated every 5 minutes for 3 doses Protect drug from light Should wet tablet with saliva and place under tongue
Isosorbide	Headache Orthostatic hypotension	Change position slowly Take between meals Don't discontinue abruptly
Action	Relaxes vascular smooth muscle; decreases venous return; decreases arterial blood pressure; reduces myocardial oxygen consumption	
Indications	Angina Perioperative hypertension CHF associated with MI Raynaud's disease (topical)	

NITRATES/ANTIANGINAL MEDICATIONS *(CONTINUED)*		
MEDICATION	ADVERSE EFFECTS	NURSING CONSIDERATIONS
Adverse effects	Hypotension Tachycardia Headache Dizziness Syncope Rash	
Nursing considerations	Take sublingual tablets under tongue or in buccal pouch; tablet may sting Check expiration date on bottle Discard unused med after 6 months Take sustained-release tablets with water, don't chew them Administer topically over 6 × 6 inch area using applicator, cover with plastic wrap, rotate sites Administer transdermal to skin free of hair; do not apply to distal extremities; remove before defibrillation or cardioversion Administer transmucosal tablets between lip and gum above the incisors or between cheek and gum; do not swallow or chew Administer translingual spray into oral mucosa; do not inhale Withdraw medication gradually over 4-6 wks Provide rest periods Teach to take medication when chest pain anticipated May take q 5 min × 3 doses Beta-adrenergic blockers and calcium-channel blockers also used for angina	

NONSTEROIDAL ANTI-INFLAMMATORY MEDICATIONS (NSAIDS)		
MEDICATION	ADVERSE EFFECTS	NURSING CONSIDERATIONS
Ibuprofen	GI upset—nausea, vomiting, diarrhea, constipation Skin eruption, dizziness, headache, fluid retention	Use cautiously with aspirin allergy Give with milk
Indomethacin	Peptic ulcer, ulcerative colitis Headache, dizziness Bone marrow depression	Observe for bleeding tendencies Monitor I and O
Naproxen	Headache, dizziness, epigastric distress Myocardial infaction	Administer with food Optimal therapeutic response is seen after 2 weeks of treatment Use cautiously in client with history of aspirin allergy

NONSTEROIDAL ANTI-INFLAMMATORY MEDICATIONS (NSAIDS) *(CONTINUED)*		
MEDICATION	**ADVERSE EFFECTS**	**NURSING CONSIDERATIONS**
Celecoxib	Fatigue Anxiety, depression, nervousness Nausea, vomiting, anorexia Dry mouth, constipation	COX-2 inhibitor Increasing doses do not appear to increase effectiveness Do not take if allergic to sulfonamides, ASA, or NSAIDs
Ketorolac	Peptic ulcer disease GI bleeding, prolonged bleeding Renal impairment	Dosage is decreased in clients greater than 65 years or with impaired renal function Duration of treatment is less than 5 days
Actions	NSAIDs inhibit prostaglandins COX-2 inhibitors block the enzyme responsible for inflammation without blocking the COX-1 enzyme ASA has antiplatelet activity	
Indications	Pain, fever, arthritis, dysmenorrhea ASA: transient ischemic attacks, prophylaxis of MI, ischemic stroke, angina Ibuprofen: gout, dental pain, musculoskeletal disorders	
Adverse effects	Headache Eye changes Dizziness Somnolence GI disturbances Constipation Bleeding Rash	
Nursing considerations	Take with food or after meals Periodic ophthalmologic exam Monitor liver and renal function Avoid OTC drugs; may contain similar medications Also have analgesic and antipyretic actions Post-op clients with adequate pain relief have fewer complications and a shorter recovery Pain is the fifth vital sign and needs to be assessed with others	

OPIOD ANALGESIC MEDICATIONS		
MEDICATION	**ADVERSE EFFECTS**	**NURSING CONSIDERATIONS**
Morphine sulfate	Dizziness, weakness Sedation or paradoxic excitement Nausea, flushing, and sweating Respiratory depression, decreased cough reflex Constipation, miosis, hypotension	Give in smallest effective dose Observe for development of dependence Encourage respiratory exercises Use cautiously to prevent respiratory depression Monitor vital signs Monitor I and O, bowel patterns Used for cardiac clients—reduces preload and afterload pressures, decreasing cardiac workload
Codeine	Same as morphine High dose may cause restlessness and excitement Constipation	Less potent and less dependence potential compared with morphine
Methadone	Same as morphine	Observe for dependence, respiratory depression Encourage fluids and high-bulk foods
Hydromorphone	Sedation, hypotension Urine retention	Keep narcotic antagonist (naloxone) available Monitor bowel function
Oxycodone and acetaminophen Oxycodone and aspirin	Lightheadedness, dizziness, sedation, nausea Constipation, pruritus Increased risk bleeding (oxycodone and aspirin)	Administer with milk after meals Commonly prescribed as oxycodone/acetaminophen or asprin, an acetaminophen and oxycodone combination
Hydrocodone/ Acetaminophen	Confusion Sedation Hypotension Constipation	Use with extreme caution with MAO inhibitors Additive CNS depression with alcohol, antihistamines, and sedative/hypnotics

OPIOD ANALGESIC MEDICATIONS *(CONTINUED)*		
MEDICATION	**ADVERSE EFFECTS**	**NURSING CONSIDERATIONS**
Action	Produces analgesia, euphoria, sedation; acts on CNS receptor cells	
Indications	Moderate-to-severe pain Chronic pain Preoperative medication	
Adverse effects	Dizziness Sedation Respiratory depression Cardiac arrest Hypotension	

Nursing considerations	Provide narcotic antagonist if needed
	    Turn, cough, deep breathe
	    Safety precautions (side rails, assist when walking)
	    Avoid alcohol, antihistamines, sedative, tranquilizers, OTC drugs
	    Avoid activities requiring mental alertness	

PAGET'S DISEASE MEDICATIONS		
MEDICATION	**ADVERSE EFFECTS**	**NURSING CONSIDERATIONS**
Calcitonin	Nausea, vomiting, flushing of face Increased urinary frequency	Retards bone resorption Decreases release of calcium from bone Relieves pain Observe for symptoms of tetany Give at hs
Etidronate disodium	Diarrhea	Prevents rapid bone turnover Don't give with food, milk, or antacids (reduces absorption) Monitor renal function
Mithramycin	GI upset Bone marrow depression Facial flushing	Cytotoxic Antibiotic Monitor BUN, liver, and renal function tests, platelet count and PT Check for signs of infection or bleeding
Action	Inhibits osteocytic activity	
Indications	Paget's disease	
Adverse effects	Decreased serum calcium Facial flushing	
Nursing considerations	Monitor serum calcium levels Facial flushing and warmth last 1 hour	

THROMBOLYTIC MEDICATIONS		
MEDICATION	ADVERSE EFFECTS	NURSING CONSIDERATIONS (SPECIFIC)
Reteplase Alteplase Tissue plasminogen activator	Bleeding	Tissue plasminogen activator is a naturally occurring enzyme Low allergenic risk but high cost
Anistreplase Streptokinase	Bleeding	Because streptokinase is made from a bacterium, client can have an allergic reaction. Not used if client had recent *Streptococcus* infection or received Streptase in past year
Action	Reteplase and Alteplase break down plasminogen into plasmin, which dissolves the fibrin network of a clot Anistreplase and Streptokinase bind with plasminogen to form a complex that digests fibrin	
Indications	MIs within the first 6 hours after symptoms, limited arterial thrombosis, thrombotic strokes, occluded shunts	
Nursing considerations (general)	Check for signs of bleeding; minimize number of punctures for inserting IVs; avoid IM injections; apply pressure at least twice as long as usual after any puncture	

VITAMINS		
MEDICATION	ADVERSE EFFECTS	NURSING CONSIDERATIONS
Cyanocobalamin (Vitamin B_{12})	Anaphylaxis Urticaria	Treatment of vitamin B_{12} deficiency, pernicious anemia, hemorrhage, renal and hepatic diseases Monitor reticulocyte count, iron, and folate levels Don't mix with other solutions in syringe Monitor K^+ levels Clients with pernicious anemia need monthly injections
Folic acid	Bronchospasm Malaise	Treatment of anemia, liver disease, alcoholism, intestinal obstruction, pregnancy Don't mix with other meds in syringe
Action	Coenzymes that speed up metabolic processes	
Indications	Vitamin deficiencies	
Adverse effects	Some vitamins are toxic at high levels	
Nursing considerations	Avoid exceeding RDA (recommended daily allowance)	

WOMEN'S HEALTH MEDICATIONS		
MEDICATION	**ADVERSE EFFECTS**	**NURSING CONSIDERATIONS**
Contraceptives, systemic Example: Ethinyl Estradiol/norgestrel	Headache Dizziness Nausea Breakthrough bleeding, spotting	Used to prevent pregnancy Use condoms against sexually transmitted diseases Take pill at same time every day No smoking
Contraceptives, systemic Levonorgestrel	Breakthrough bleeding, spotting	Prevention of pregnancy for 5 years as a contraceptive implant; emergency contraceptive in oral form when given within 72 hours of unprotected intercourse
Estrogens Estradiol Estrogens conjugated	Nausea Gynecomastia Contact lens intolerance	Treatment of menopausal symptoms, some cancers Prevention of osteoporosis Client should contact health care provider if breast lumps, vaginal bleeding, edema, jaundice, dark urine, clay-colored stools, dyspnea, blurred vision, numbness or stiffness in leg, chest pain
Progestins Medroxyprogestrone acetate	Nausea Contact lens intolerance	Management of abnormal uterine bleeding; prevent endometrial changes of estrogen replacement therapy, some cancers
Actions	Female hormones	
Indications	Contraceptives Treatment of menopausal symptoms Prevention of osteoporosis	
Adverse effects	Nausea Breakthrough bleeding Headache	
Nursing considerations	Client should know when to take medication and what to do for skipped doses Client should know when to contact prescribing health care provider	
Herbal	Black cohosh—relieves hot flashes; may increase hypotensive effect of antihypertensives; do not take for more than 6 months	

MEDICATION INTERACTIONS WITH GRAPEFRUIT JUICE (INCREASED SERUM DRUG LEVELS)	
Calcium channel blockers: amlodipine, diltiazem, felodipine, nicardipine, nifedipine, nimodipine, nisoldipine, verapamil	
Statins Caffeine	Carbamazepine Buspirone Midazolam
SSRIs: fluoxetine, fluvoxamine, sertraline Dextromethorphan Sirolimus	Sildenafil Praziquantel Tacrolimus

MEN'S HEALTH MEDICATIONS		
MEDICATION	ADVERSE EFFECTS	NURSING CONSIDERATIONS
Alpha₁-adrenergic blockers		
Terazosin	Dizziness Headache Weakness Nasal congestion Orthostatic hypotension	Used to decrease urinary urgency, hesitancy, nocturia in prostatic hyperplasia Caution to change position slowly Avoid alcohol, CNS depressant, hot showers due to orthostatic hypotension Requires titration Administer at bedtime due to risk orthostatic hypotension Effects may not be noted for 4 weeks
Tamsulosin	Dizziness Headache	Used to decrease urinary urgency, hesitancy, nocturia in prostatic hyperplasia Caution to change position slowly Administer 30 min. after same meal each day
5-alpha-reductase inhibitor		
Finasteride	Decreased libido Impotence	Used to treat benign prostatic hyperplasia by slowing prostatic growth May decrease serum PSA levels 6-12 months therapy required to determine if medication effective May cause harm to male fetus. Pregnant women should not be exposed to semen of partner taking finasteride or they should not handle crushed medication Monitor liver function tests
Dutasteride	Decreased libido Impotence	Used to treat benign prostatic hyperplasia by slowing prostatic growth May cause harm to male fetus. Pregnant women should not be exposed to semen of partner taking finasteride or they should not handle crushed medication Monitor liver function
Anti-impotence Sildenafil Vardenafil Tadalafil	Headache Flushing Dyspepsia Nasal congestion Mild visual disturbance	Enhances blood flow to the corpus cavernosum to ensure erection to allow sexual intercourse Should not take with nitrates in any form due to dramatic decrease in blood pressure Usually taken 1 hour before sexual activity (sildenafil, vardenafil) Tadalafil has longer duration of action (up to 36 hours) Should not take more than one time per day Notify health care provider if erection lasts longer than 4 hours
Saw palmetto	Urinary antiseptic used to treat PBH; may cause false-negative PSA test result	

HERBAL SUPPLEMENTS		
SUPPLEMENT	ADVERSE EFFECTS/ CONTRAINDICATIONS	NURSING CONSIDERATIONS
Immune System		
Echinacea Immunostimulant, anti-inflammatory, antiviral, antibacterial Used to prevent and treat colds, flu, wound healing, urinary tract infections	Immune suppression, tingling sensation and/ or unpleasant taste on tongue, nausea, vomiting, allergic reactions	Decreases effectiveness of immunosuppressants Contraindicated in autoimmune diseases Avoid if allergic to ragweed, members of daisy family of plants
Garlic Antimicrobial, antilipidemic, antithrombotic, antitumor, anti-inflammatory Used to reduce cholesterol, prevent atherosclerosis, cancer, stroke, and MI; decrease blood pressure prevent and treat colds and flu	Flatulence, heartburn, halitosis, irritation of mouth, esophagus, stomach, allergic reaction Contraindicated with peptic ulcer, reflux	May potentiate anticoagulant and antiplatelets, antihyperlipidemics, antihypertensives, antidiabetic medications, and herbs with these effects May decrease efficacy of cyclosporine, hormonal contraceptives Avoid if allergic to members of the lily family of plants
Ginseng Stimulant and tonic to immune and nervous systems Used to increase stamina, as aphrodisiac, adjunct chemotherapy and radiation therapy	Headache, insomnia, nervousness, palpitations, excitation, diarrhea, vaginal bleeding May cause headache, tremors, irritability, manic episodes if combined with MAOIs or caffeine	May falsely elevate digoxin levels; observe for signs usually associated with high digoxin levels May antagonize Coumadin Potentiates antidiabetic medications, steroids, estrogens Caution with cardiovascular disease, hypotension, hypertension, steroid therapy
Female Reproductive System		
Evening Primrose Oil Anti-inflammatory, sedative, astringent Used for premenstrual and menopausal problems, rheumatoid arthritis, elevated serum cholesterol, hypertension, eczema, diabetic neuropathy	Headache, rash, nausea, seizures, inflammation Contraindicated for clients with epilepsy, schizophrenia	May potentiate antiplatelet and anticoagulant meds Increases risk for seizures when taken with phenothiazines, antidepressants
Musculoskeletal System		
Chondroitin Collagen synthesis Used for arthritis for cartilage synthesis (with glucosamine)	Dyspepsia, nausea	May potentiate effects of anticoagulants
Glucosamine Collagen synthesis Used for arthritis for cartilage synthesis (with chondroitin)	Dyspepsia, nausea	May impede insulin secretion or increase resistance

HERBAL SUPPLEMENTS (CONTINUED)		
SUPPLEMENT	ADVERSE EFFECTS/ CONTRAINDICATIONS	NURSING CONSIDERATIONS
Neurological System		
Capsicum/Cayenne Pepper Analgesia, improves blood circulation Used for arthritis, bowel disorders, nerve pain, PAD, chronic laryngitis, personal self-defense spray	GI discomfort, burning pain in eyes, nose, mouth, blepharospasm and swelling in eyes, skin tissue irritation, cough, bronchospasm Avoid if allergic to ragweed or to chili pepper	May decrease effectiveness of antihypertensives, increases risk of cough with ACE inhibitors May potentiate antiplatelet and anticoagulant meds and herbs May cause hypertensive crisis with MAOIs Increases theophylline absorption
Feverfew Analgesic, antipyretic Used for migraine prophylaxis, fever, menstrual problems, arthritis	Mouth ulcers, heartburn, indigestion, dizziness, tachycardia, allergic reactions	Potentiates antiplatelet and anticoagulant meds Do not stop abruptly—causes moderate to severe pain with joint and muscle stiffness Caution if allergic to daisy family of plants
Gastrointestinal System		
Flaxseed Laxative, anticholesteremic Used for constipation, decrease cholesterol, prevent atherosclerosis, colon disorders	Diarrhea, flatulence, nausea Contraindicated if client has strictures or acute GI inflammation	May decrease absorption of oral meds—do not take within 2 hrs Immature flax seeds can be very toxic Increase fluids to minimize flatulence
Ginger Antiemetic, antioxidant, digestive aid, anti- inflammatory Used for nausea, vomiting, indigestion, gas, lack of appetite	Minor heartburn, dermatitis Contraindicated with gallstones	May potentiate antiplatelet and anticoagulant meds, antidiabetic meds, herbs that increase bleeding times
Licorice Demulcent (soothes), expectorant, anti- inflammatory Used for coughs, colds, stomach pains, ulcers	Hypokalemia, headache, edema, lethargy, hypertension, heart failure (with overdose), cardiac arrest Contraindicated in renal or liver disease, heart disease, hypertension; caution with hormonal contraceptives	Decreases effect of spironolactone Avoid use with digoxin, loop diuretics, corticos-teroids
Genitourinary System		
Saw Palmetto Mild diuretic, urinary antiseptic Used for BPH, increasing sexual vigor, cystitis	Constipation, diarrhea, nausea, decreased libido, back pain	May interact with hormonal medications such as HRT and oral contraceptives May cause a false negative PSA test result
Psychiatric		
Chamomile Sedative/hypnotic, anti- inflammatory, antispasmodic, anti-infective Used for stress, anxiety, insomnia, GI disorders	Allergic reactions, contact dermatitis, vomiting, depression	May potentiate sedatives and anticoagulants Avoid if allergic to ragweed, members of daisy family of plants
Kava Anti-anxiety, sedative/hypnotic, muscle relaxant Used for anxiety, insomnia, seizure disorders	Hepatotoxicity, psychological dependence, mild euphoria, fatigue, sedation, suicidal thoughts, visual problems, scaly skin reaction Contraindicated in Parkinson's, history of stroke, endogenous depression	May potentiate sedative effects of other sedating medications (benzodiazepines, barbiturates), anticonvulsants, and herbs (chamomile, valerian)

HERBAL SUPPLEMENTS *(CONTINUED)*		
SUPPLEMENT	ADVERSE EFFECTS/ CONTRAINDICATIONS	NURSING CONSIDERATIONS
Melatonin Hormone from pineal gland Used for insomnia, jet lag	Headache, confusion, sedation, tachycardia	Potentiates CNS depressants May decrease effectiveness of immunosup-pressants, nifedipine
St. John's Wort Antidepressant, sedative effects, antiviral, antimicrobial Used for mild to moderate depression, sleep disorders, skin and wound healing	Photosensitivity, fatigue, allergic reactions, dry mouth, dizziness, restlessness, nausea Contraindicated for major depression, transplant recipients, clients taking SSRIs (increases risk of serotonin syndrome), MAOIs (increases risk of hypertensive crisis), hormonal contraceptives	Usually decreases effectiveness of (digoxin, antineoplastics, antiviral AIDS drugs, anti-rejection drugs, theophylline, warfarin, hormonal contraceptives May potentiate drugs and herbs with sedative effects Should avoid tyramine in diet, OTC medications
Valerian Sedative/hypnotic, antispasmodic Used for insomnia, restlessness, anxiety	Headache, blurred vision, nausea, excitability Contraindicated in liver disease may be hepatotoxic	May potentiate other CNS depressant medications, antihistamincs, and sedating herbs
Cardiovascular System		
Gingko Enhances cerebral and peripheral blood circulation; antidepressive Used for dementia, short-term memory loss, vertigo, PADs, depression, sexual dysfunction (including from SSRIs)	Headache, GI upset, contact dermatitis, dizziness	May potentiate antiplatelet and anticoagulant meds, ASA, NSAIDS, and herbs, which increase bleeding time May potentiate MAOIs May decrease effectiveness of anticonvulsants
Hawthorn Antianginal, antiarrhythmic, vasodilator, antihypertensive, antilipidemic Used for mild to moderate heart failure, hypertension, cholesterol reduction	Nausea, fatigue, sweating	May potentiate or interfere with wide range of cardiovascular medications used for CHF, angina, arrhythmias, hypertension, vasodilation Potentiates digoxin Potentiates CNS depressants Avoid if allergic to members of the rose family of plants
Respiratory System		
Eucalyptus Decongestant, anti-inflammatory, antimicrobial, antifungal Used for coughs, bronchitis, nasal congestion, sore muscles, wounds	Nausea, vomiting, epigastric burning, dizziness, muscle weakness, seizures Contraindicated with liver disease, inflammation of intestinal tract	Potentiates antidiabetic medications and possibly other herbs that cause hypoglycemia May increase metabolism of any drugs metabolized in liver

Volume Equivalents

1 fluid ounce	= 2 tablespoons
1 tablespoon	= 15 milliliters
	= 3 teaspoons
1 teaspoon	= 5 milliliters
1 cup	= 240 milliliters
	= 8 fluid ounces

Mass Equivalents

1 kilogram = 2.2 pounds

Temperature Conversion

$$\left(\text{Celsius degrees} \times \frac{9}{5}\right) + 32 = \text{Fahrenheit degrees}$$

$$\left(\text{Fahrenheit degrees} - 32\right) \times \frac{5}{9} = \text{Celsius degrees}$$

Common Conversions

1 gr	= 60 mg
1 tsp	= 5 mL
1 tbsp	= 15 mL
1 oz	= 30 mL
1 kg	= 2.2 lbs

$$F = C\frac{9}{5} + 32$$

$$C = F - 32\frac{5}{9}$$

ADVERSE EFFECTS OF MEDICATIONS

▶ **ANAPHYLAXIS**

A. Assessment

1. Hives, rash
2. Difficulty breathing
3. Decreased BP, increased pulse, increased respirations
4. Dilated pupils
5. Diaphoresis
6. "Panicked" feeling

B. Nursing considerations

1. Epinephrine 0.3 ml of 1:1,000 solution IM
2. Massage site to speed absorption
3. May repeat dose in 15–20 min
4. Wear Medic-Alert identification
5. Carry emergency epinephrine

▶ **DELAYED ALLERGIC REACTION**

A. Assessment

1. Rash, hives
2. Swollen joints

B. Nursing considerations

1. Discontinue medication
2. Notify health care provider
3. Skin care
4. Comfort measures
5. Antihistamines, topical
6. Corticosteriods

▶ **DERMATOLOGICAL REACTIONS**

A. Assessment

1. Hives, rashes, lesions
2. Exfoliative dermatitis (rash, fever, enlarged lymph nodes, enlarged liver)
3. Erythema multiform excudativum (Stevens-Johnson syndrome—dark red papules that don't itch or hurt)

B. Nursing considerations

1. Frequent skin care
2. Avoid rubbing, tight clothing, harsh soaps, perfumed lotions
3. Antihistamines
4. Topical corticosteroids

▶ STOMATITIS

A. Assessment

1. Swollen gums (gingivitis)
2. Swollen, red tongue (glossitis)
3. Difficulty swallowing
4. Bad breath
5. Pain in mouth and throat

B. Nursing considerations

1. Frequent mouth care with nonirritating (nonalcoholic) solution
2. Frequent, small feedings
3. Antifungal meds
4. Local anesthetics

▶ SUPERINFECTIONS

A. Assessment

1. Fever
2. Diarrhea
3. Black hairy tongue
4. Glossitis
5. Mucous membrane lesions
6. Vaginal itching and discharge

B. Nursing considerations

1. Frequent mouth care
2. Good skin care
3. Small, frequent feedings
4. Antifungal meds

▶ BONE MARROW DEPRESSION

A. Assessment

1. Fever
2. Chills
3. Sore throat
4. Weakness
5. Back pain
6. Dark urine
7. Anemia (low Hct)
8. Thrombocytopenia (low platelet count)
9. Leukopenia (low WBC)

B. Nursing considerations

1. Monitor CBC
2. Rest

3. Protection from infections

4. Avoid activities that may cause injury

▶ LIVER IMPAIRMENT

A. Assessment

1. Fever

2. Malaise

3. Nausea, vomiting

4. Jaundice

5. Light stools, dark urine

6. Abdominal pain

7. Elevated AST, ALT

8. Elevated bilirubin

9. Altered PTT

B. Nursing considerations

1. Small, frequent feedings

2. Good skin care

3. Comfort measures

4. Cool environment

5. Rest

▶ RENAL IMPAIRMENT

A. Assessment

1. Elevated BUN, creatinine

2. Decreased Hct

3. Altered electrolytes (K^+, Na^+)

4. Fatigue

5. Edema

6. Irritability

7. Skin care

B. Nursing considerations

1. Diet and fluid restrictions

2. Good skin care

3. Electrolyte replacement

4. Rest

5. Dialysis

▶ OCULAR IMPAIRMENT

A. Assessment

1. Blurred vision

2. Color vision changes

3. Blindness

B. Nursing considerations
1. Monitor vision carefully
2. Monitor lighting and exposure to light

▶ AUDITORY IMPAIRMENT

A. Assessment
1. Dizziness
2. Ringing in ears
3. Loss of balance
4. Loss of hearing

B. Nursing considerations
1. Monitor hearing ability
2. Safety measures to prevent injury (falls)

▶ CNS IMPAIRMENT

A. Assessment
1. Confusion, delirium
2. Insomnia
3. Drowsiness
4. Hallucinations

B. Nursing considerations
1. Safety measures to prevent injury
2. Avoid activities that require alertness (driving a car)
3. Orient to surroundings

▶ ANTICHOLINERGIC EFFECTS

A. Assessment
1. Dry mouth
2. Altered taste perception
3. Dysphagia
4. Heartburn
5. Urinary retention
6. Impotence
7. Blurred vision
8. Nasal congestion

B. Nursing considerations
1. Sugarless lozenges
2. Good mouth care
3. Void before taking medication
4. Safety measures for vision changes

▶ PARKINSON-LIKE EFFECTS

A. Assessments

1. Akinesia

2. Tremors

3. Drooling

4. Changes in gait

5. Rigidity

6. Akathisia (extreme restlessness)

7. Dyskinesia (spasms)

B. Nursing considerations

1. Anticholinergic meds

2. Antiparkinson meds

3. Safety measures for gait changes

Chapter 4

PHYSIOLOGICAL INTEGRITY: REDUCTION OF RISK POTENTIAL

Units

1. **Sensory and Perceptual Alterations**

2. **Alterations in Body Systems**

3. **Perioperative Care**

4. **Diagnostic Tests**

5. **Therapeutic Procedures**

▶ **IMPAIRED VISION**

A. Assessment

1. Redness, burning, pain in eyes

2. Edema

3. Increased lacrimation and exudate

4. Headache, squinting

5. Nausea and vomiting

6. Altered growth and development

7. Visual disturbances

8. Altered visual function tests (see Table 1)

Table 1 VISUAL FUNCTION TESTS		
TEST	**PROCEDURE**	**CLIENT PREPARATION**
Tonometry– measures intraocular pressure	Cornea is anesthetized Tonometer registers degree of indentation on cornea when pressure is applied Pressure increased in glaucoma	Client will be recumbent Remove contact lenses Advise not to squint, cough, or hold breath during procedure
Visual fields– measurement of range of vision (perimetry)	Client is seated a measured distance from chart of concentric circles Client asked to fix eyes on a point on a chart at center of circle Client instructed to indicate when he/she first sees pointer; this point is recorded as a point in field of vision This procedure is repeated around 360° of a circle Normal visual fields for each eye are approximately a 50° angle superiorly, 90° laterally, 70° inferiorly, and 60° medially	None
Snellen test– test of visual acuity	Client stands 20 feet from chart of letters One eye is covered at a time Client reads chart to smallest letter visible Test results indicate comparison of distance at which this client reads to what normal eye sees at 20 feet	None

B. Diagnose

    1. Disorders of accommodation (see Table 2)

    2. Burns of the eye (see Table 3)

    3. Eye trauma (see Table 4)

    4. Eye infections/inflammation (see Table 5)

Table 2 DISORDERS OF ACCOMMODATION	
TYPES	NURSING CONSIDERATIONS
Myopia (nearsightedness)—light rays refract at a point in front of the retina	Corrective lenses
Hyperopia (farsightedness)—light rays refract behind the retina	Corrective lenses
Presbyopia with aging	Commonly occurs after age 35 Corrective lenses
Astigmatism—uneven curvature of cornea causing blurring of vision	Corrective lenses

Table 3 BURNS OF THE EYE	
TYPES	NURSING CONSIDERATIONS
Chemical Acids, cleansers, insecticides	Eye irrigation with copious amounts of water for 15–20 minutes
Radiation Sun, lightening, eclipses	Prevention—use of eye shields
Thermal Hot metals, liquids, other occupational hazards	Use of goggles to protect the cornea; patching; analgesics

Table 4 EYE TRAUMA	
TYPES	NURSING CONSIDERATIONS
Nonpenetrating—abrasions	Eye patch for 24 hours
Nonpenetrating—contusions	Cold compresses, analgesics
Penetrating—pointed or sharp objects	Cover with patch; refer to surgeon

C. Plan/Implementation

    1. Prevent eye injuries

        a. Provide safe toys

        b. Use eye protectors when working with chemicals, tools

        c. Use eye protectors during sports

        d. Protect eyes from ultraviolet light

2. Care of the blind client

   a. Enhance communication

      1) Address client by name

      2) Always introduce self

      3) State reason for being there

      4) Inform client when leaving the room

Table 5 EYE INFECTION/INFLAMMATION		
TYPE OF INFECTION	CAUSE	NURSING CONSIDERATIONS
Conjunctivitis (pinkeye)	Bacteria Virus Allergies	Warm, moist compresses Topical antibiotics Hydrocortisone ophthalmic ointment
Stye	*Staphylococcal* organism	Warm compresses Antibiotics Incision and drainage
Chalazion (inflammatory cyst)	Duct obstruction	Incision and drainage
Keratitis (inflammation of cornea)	Virus Spread of systemic disease	Antibiotics Hot compresses Steroids, except with herpes simplex
Uveitis (inflammation of iris, ciliary body, choroid)	Local or systemic infection	Warm compresses Dark glasses Antibiotics, analgesics, sedatives

   b. Provide sense of safety and security

      1) Explain all procedures in detail

      2) Keep furniture arrangement consistent

      3) Provide hand rail

      4) Doors should never be half open

      5) Have client follow attendant when walking by lightly touching attendant's elbow (1/2 step ahead)

      6) Instruct client in use of lightweight walking stick when walking alone

   c. Foster sense of independence

      1) Provide assistance only when needed

      2) Identify food and location on plate or tray

      3) Encourage recreational and leisure time activities

3. Care of artificial eye

   a. Remove daily for cleansing

   b. Cleanse with mild detergent and water

   c. Dry and store in water or contact-lens soaking solution

   d. Remove before general surgery

e. Insertion method

1) Raise upper lid and slip eye beneath it

2) Release lid

3) Support lower lid and draw it over the lower edge of eye

f. Removal method

1) Draw lower lid downward

2) Slip eye forward over lower lid and remove

4. Instill eye drops

D. Evaluation

1. Has client safety been maintained?

2. Is the client able to instill eye drops using correct technique?

▶ RETINOPATHY OF PREMATURITY (ROP)

A. Assessment

1. Demarcation line forms (separates avascular retina anteriorly with vascularized retina posteriorly)

2. Ridge forms

3. Retinal detachment

B. Diagnose

1. Cause of blindness in premature infants

2. High concentrations of oxygen cause the premature infant's retinal vessels to constrict, causing blindness

3. Sometimes occurs when oxygen concentrations are greater than 40%, and when used for longer than 48 to 72 hours in infants

C. Plan/Implementation

1. Ensure that all infants born before 36 weeks or less than 2,000 g at birth have eye exam by experts

2. Use minimum amount of oxygen

3. Monitor pO_2 continuously

4. Maintain SaO_2 level within normal limits (range 95–100 mm Hg)

5. Administer vitamin E as ordered—thought to affect tissue response to oxygen (therapy is controversial)

6. Decrease environmental stimuli and continuous direct lighting

D. Evaluation

1. Have complications of oxygen administration been avoided in the premature infant?

2. Has the infant's eyesight been maintained?

▶ STRABISMUS

A. Assessment

1. Visible deviation of eye

2. Diplopia

3. Child tilts head or squints to focus

B. Diagnose

    1. Eyes do not function as a unit

    2. Imbalance of the extraocular muscles

C. Plan/Implementation

    1. Nonsurgical intervention begins no later than age 6

    2. Occlusion of unaffected eye to strengthen weaker eye

    3. Corrective lenses combined with other therapy to improve acuity

    4. Orthoptic exercises designed to strengthen eye muscles

    5. Surgery on rectus muscles of eye

D. Evaluation

    1. Has normal vision been restored?

    2. Is child compliant with exercise regime?

▶ DETACHED RETINA

A. Assessment

    1. Flashes of light

    2. Blurred or "sooty" vision, "floaters"

    3. Sensation of particles moving in line of vision

    4. Delineated areas of vision blank

    5. A feeling of a curtain coming up or down

    6. Loss of vision

    7. Confusion, apprehension

B. Diagnose

    1. Separation of the retina from the choroid

    2. Cause

        a. Trauma

        b. Aging process

        c. Diabetes

        d. Tumors

C. Plan/Implementation

    1. Bedrest—do not bend forward, avoid excessive movements

    2. Affected eye or both eyes may be patched to decrease movement of eye (as ordered by health care provider)

    3. Specific positioning—area of detachment should be in the dependent position

    4. Take precautions to avoid bumping head, moving eyes rapidly, or rapidly jerking the head

    5. Surgery to reattach retina to choroid; gas or air bubble used to apply pressure to retina

    6. No hair-washing for 1 week

    7. Administer sedatives and tranquilizers

    8. Avoid strenuous activity for 3 months

9. Care of client undergoing eye surgery
   a. Preoperative care
      1) Assess visual acuity
      2) Prepare periorbital area
      3) Orient to surroundings
      4) Preoperative teaching—prepare for postoperative course
      5) Teach postop need to avoid straining at stool, stooping
   b. Postoperative care
      1) Observe for complications—hemorrhage, sharp pain, infection
      2) Avoid sneezing, coughing, straining at stool, bending down
      3) Protect from injury; restrict activity
      4) Keep signal bell within reach
      5) Administer medications as ordered: antiemetics for nausea/vomiting, sedatives for restlessness
      6) Eye shield worn for protective purposes
      7) Discharge teaching—avoid stooping or straining at stool; use proper body mechanics

D. Evaluation
   1. Has normal vision been restored?
   2. Have complications been prevented?

▶ CATARACTS

A. Assessment
   1. Objects appear distorted and blurred; decreased color perception
   2. Annoying glare; double vision
   3. Pupil changes from black to gray to milky white

B. Diagnose
   1. Partial or total opacity of the normally transparent crystalline lens
   2. Cause
      a. Congenital
      b. Trauma
      c. Aging process
      d. Associated with diabetes mellitus, intraocular surgery
      e. Drugs—steroid therapy
      f. Exposure to radioactivity

C. Plan/Implementation
   1. Surgical management—laser surgery
      a. Extracapsular extraction—cut through the anterior capsule to expose the opaque lens material, most common procedure
      b. Intracapsular extraction—removal of entire lens and capsule; easier for health care provider to do; places client at greater risk for retinal detachment and loss of structure for intraoccular lens implant
      c. Lens implantation

    d. Observe for postoperative complications

        1) Hemorrhage indicated by sudden sharp pain

        2) Increased intraocular pressure

        3) Infection—yellow or green drainage

        4) Slipped suture(s)

        5) If lens implant—pupil should remain constricted; if aphakic (without lens) pupil remains dilated

    e. Avoid straining; no heavy lifting

    f. Bend from the knees to pick things up

    g. Instruct in instillation of eye drops to affected eye, use of night shields

    h. Usually suggest to sleep on unaffected side (decreases pain and swelling when elevated)

    i. Protect eye from bright lights and water

    j. Adjustments needed in perception if aphakic

    k. Report increased pain, change in vision, increased floaters

D. Evaluation

    1. Has vision been restored?

    2. Have complications been prevented?

▶ GLAUCOMA

A. Assessment

    1. Cloudy, blurry vision or loss of vision

    2. Artificial lights appear to have rainbows or halos around them

    3. Decreased peripheral vision

    4. Pain, headache

    5. Nausea, vomiting

B. Diagnose

    1. Abnormal increase in intraocular pressure leading to visual disability and blindness; obstruction of outflow of aqueous humor

    2. Types

        a. Angle-closure (closed-angle) glaucoma—sudden onset, emergency

        b. Open-angle (primary glaucoma)—blockage of aqueous humor flow

    3. Causes

        a. Closed-angle glaucoma—associated with emotional disturbances, allergy, and vasomotor disturbances

        b. Open-angle glaucoma—associated with trauma, tumor, hemorrhage, iritis, and aging

    4. Potential nursing diagnosis

        a. Disturbed sensory perception

C. Plan/Implementation

    1. Medications: prostaglandin agonists, adrenergic agonists, beta-adrenergic blockers, cholinergic agonists, carbonic anhydrase inhibitors

    2. Surgery—laser trabeculoplasty

3. Avoid tight clothing (e.g., collars)

4. Reduce external stimuli

5. Avoid heavy lifting, straining at stool

6. Avoid use of mydriatics (e.g., Atropine)

7. Educate public to five danger signs of glaucoma

   a. Brow arching

   b. Halos around lights

   c. Blurry vision

   d. Diminished peripheral vision

   e. Headache or eye pain

D. Evaluation

1. Has vision been restored?

2. Have complications been prevented?

▶ HEARING LOSS

A. Conductive loss

1. Assessment

   a. Pain, fever, headache

   b. Discharge

   c. Altered growth and development

   d. Personality changes, e.g., irritability, depression, suspiciousness, withdrawal

2. Analysis

   a. Disorder in auditory canal, eardrum, or ossicles

   b. Causes

      1) Infection

      2) Inflammation

      3) Foreign body

      4) Trauma

      5) Ear wax

   c. Complications—meningitis resulting from initial infection

   d. Diagnostics

      1) Audiogram—quantitative (degree of loss)

      2) Tuning fork—qualitative (type of loss)

3. Plan/Implementation

   a. Heat

   b. Antibiotics

   c. Hearing aid

   d. Ear irrigations

      1) Tilt head toward side of affected ear; gently direct stream of fluid against sides of canal

      2) After procedure, instruct client to lie on affected side to facilitate drainage

      3) Contraindicated if there is evidence of swelling or tenderness

e. Ear drops

1) Position the affected ear uppermost

2) Pull outer ear upward and backward for adult (3 years of age and older)

3) Pull outer ear downward and backward for child (under 3 years of age)

4) Place drops so they run down the wall of ear canal

5) Have client lie on unaffected ear to encourage absorption

f. Surgery

1) Preoperative care

a) Baseline hearing assessment

b) Assessment of preoperative symptoms

c) Preparation depends on nature of incision

d) Encourage client to wash hair prior to surgery

e) Teaching—expect postoperative hearing loss; discuss need for special position of operative ear as ordered

2) Postoperative care

a) Reinforce dressing, don't change

b) Avoid noseblowing, sneezing, and coughing

c) Observe for possible complications

i) Facial nerve damage—may be transient

ii) Infection

iii) Vertigo, tinnitus

d) Do not apply any pressure if surgery is on internal ear-notify health care provider immediately

e) Administer medications

f) Provide for client safety

g) Position on unaffected side (decreases swelling and pain of surgical site)

3) Discharge teaching—avoid getting water in ear, flying, drafts, crowds, people with respiratory infections

4. Evaluation

a. Have complications been prevented?

b. Have efforts been made to minimize hearing loss?

B. Perceptive (sensorineural) loss

1. Assessment

a. Pain, fever, headache

b. Discharge

c. Altered growth and development

d. Personality changes, e.g., irritability, depression, suspiciousness, withdrawal

2. Analysis

a. Due to disorder of the organ of Corti or the auditory nerve

    b. Causes

        1) Congenital—maternal exposure to communicable disease

        2) Infection, drug toxicity

        3) Trauma

        4) Labyrinth dysfunction—Ménière's disease

    c. Complications

        1) Vertigo

        2) Tinnitus

        3) Vomiting

3. Plan/Implementation

    a. Care of the deaf/hard of hearing client

        1) Enhance communication

            a) Position self directly in front of client

            b) Well-lit, quiet room

            c) Get client's attention

            d) Move close to better ear, if appropriate

            e) Speak clearly and slowly; do not shout

            f) Keep hands and other objects away from mouth when speaking

            g) Have client repeat statements

            h) Use appropriate hand motions

            i) Write messages down if client able to read

        2) Health teaching

            a) Provide health care resources

            b) Encourages use of visual cues

            c) Advise that auditory cues (such as smoke alarms) may not be feasible

    b. Surgery

4. Evaluation

    a. Has hearing loss been reversed/minimized?

    b. Has client adjusted to change in hearing?

▶ ACUTE OTITIS MEDIA

A. Assessment

1. Fever, chills

2. Headache

3. Ringing in ears

4. Deafness

5. Sharp pain

6. Head rolling, crying, ear-tugging (child)

7. Nausea, vomiting

8. Red, bulging, tympanic membrane

B. Diagnose

1. Definition—infection of middle ear

2. Cause—pathogenic organisms, (i.e., bacteria and viruses)

3. Complications

   a. Chronic otitis media—children more susceptible because of short eustachian tube

   b. Residual deafness

   c. Perforation of tympanic membrane

   d. Cholesteatoma growth

   e. Mastoiditis or meningitis

C. Plan/Implementation

1. Administer medication as ordered

   a. Antibiotics—organism-specific

   b. Antihistamines for allergies

   c. Nasal decongestants

2. Report persistent symptoms to health care provider

3. Ventilatory tubes—inserted in eustachian tube for continuous ventilation

4. Myringotomy—tympanic membrane incision to relieve pressure and release purulent fluid; no water can be allowed to enter the ear

5. Tympanoplasty—surgical reconstruction of ossicles and tympanic membrane

6. Bedrest if temperature is elevated

7. Position on side of involved ear to promote drainage

D. Evaluation

1. Has permanent hearing loss been prevented?

2. Have complications been prevented?

▶ MÉNIÈRE'S DISEASE

A. Assessment

1. Nausea and vomiting

2. Incapacitating vertigo, tinnitus

3. Feeling of pressure/fullness in the ear

4. Fluctuating, progressive decreased hearing on involved side

5. Nystagmus, headache

B. Diagnose

1. Dilation of the membrane of the labyrinth

2. Recurrent attacks of vertigo with sensorineural hearing loss

3. Attacks recur several times a week; periods of remission may last several years

4. Diagnostic tests—Weber and Rinne test, CT

5. Complication—hearing loss

C. Plan/Implementation

1. Drug therapy

   a. Antihistamines in acute phase (epinephrine, diphenhydramine)

   b. Antiemetics (e.g., prochlorperazine)

   c. Antivertigo medications (e.g., meclizine, diazepam)

   d. Diuretics (e.g., hydrochlorothiazide, triamterene)

2. Bedrest during acute phase

3. Provide protection when ambulatory

4. Low-sodium diet (2,000 mg/day); avoid caffeine, nicotine, alcohol

5. Decompression of endolymphatic sac with Teflon shunt (method of choice)

6. Total labyrinthectomy—last resort due to possible complication of Bell's palsy

7. Client education

   a. Need to slow down body movements—jerking or sudden movements may precipitate attack

   b. Need to lie down when an attack occurs

   c. If driving, pull over and stop car

8. Occupational counseling—if occupation involves operating machinery

D. Evaluation

1. Does client use strategies to prevent injury secondary to dizziness, vertigo?

2. Does client demonstrate knowledge of medications?

▶ CRANIAL NERVE DISORDERS

A. Assessment (see Table 6)

B. Diagnose (see Table 6)

C. Plan/Implementation (see Table 6)

D. Evaluate

  1. Has client adjusted to altered body image?

Table 6 CRANIAL NERVE DISORDERS			
	TRIGEMINAL NEURALGIA (TIC DOULOUREUX)	**BELL'S PALSY (FACIAL PARALYSIS)**	**ACOUSTIC NEUROMA**
Assessment	Stabbing or burning facial pain—excruciating, unpredictable, paroxysmal Twitching, grimacing of facial muscles	Inability to close eye Decreased corneal reflex Increased lacrimation Speech difficulty Loss of taste Distortion of one side of face	Deafness—partial, initially Dizziness
Analysis	Type of neuralgia involving one or more branches of the fifth cranial nerve Causes—infections of sinuses, teeth, mouth, or irritation of nerve from pressure	Peripheral involvement of the seventh cranial nerve Predisposing factors—vascular ischemia, viral disease, edema, inflammatory reactions	Benign tumor of the eighth cranial nerve
Nursing considerations	Identify and avoid stimuli that exacerbate the attacks Administer medications—carbamazepine and analgesics Treatment—carbamazepine, alcohol injection to nerve, resection of the nerve, microvascular decompression Avoid rubbing eye Chew on opposite side of mouth	Protect head from cold or drafts Administer analgesics Assist with electric stimulation Teach isometric exercises for facial muscles (blow and suck from a straw); massage, warm packs Provide emotional support for altered body image Prevent corneal abrasions (artificial tears) Treatment—electrical stimulation, analgesics, steroid therapy, antiviral medications Recovery takes 3–5 weeks	Pre- and postoperative care for posterior fossa craniotomy Comfort measures—assist with turning of head and neck Treatment—surgical excision of tumor

▶ GUILLAN-BARRÉ SYNDROME

A. Assessment

  1. Paresthesias, pain often occurring in glove-and-stocking distribution; pain

  2. Motor losses symmetrical, usually beginning in lower extremities, then extend upward to include trunk, upper extremities, cranial nerves, and vasomotor function; deep tendon reflexes disappear; respiratory muscle compromise

3. Excessive or inadequate autonomic dysfunction

   a. Hypotension, tachycardia

   b. Vasomotor flushing

   c. Paralytic ileus

   d. Profuse sweating

4. Plateau period—progresses to peak severity between 2–4 weeks; average 10 days

5. Recovery period—several months to a year; 10% residual disability

B. Diagnose

1. Progressive inflammatory autoimmune response occurring in peripheral nervous system, resulting in compression of nerve roots and peripheral nerves; demyelination occurs and slows or alters nerve conduction

2. Possible causes

   a. Infective, viral

   b. Autoimmune response

   c. May follow immunizations

3. Course

   a. Acute, rapidly ascending sensory and motor deficit that may stop at any level of the CNS

   b. Protracted, develops slowly, regresses slowly

   c. Prolonged course with phases of deterioration and partial remission

C. Plan/Implementation

1. Intervention is symptomatic

2. Steroids in acute phase

3. Plasmapheresis, IV immunoglobulins, adrenocorticotropic hormone, corticosteroids

4. Mechanical ventilation, elevate head of bed, suctioning

5. Prevent hazards of immobility

6. Maintain adequate nutrition, hydration

7. Physical therapy, range of motion

8. Pain-reducing measures

9. Eye care

10. Prevention of complications—URI, aspiration, constipation, urinary retention

11. Psychosocial support to deal with fear, anxiety, and altered body image

D. Evaluation

1. Has client recovered without major complications?

2. Has client comfort been maintained?

▶ MENINGITIS

A. Assessment

1. Headache, fever, photophobia

2. Signs of meningeal irritation

    a. Nuchal rigidity—stiff neck

    b. Kernig's sign—when hip flexed to 90°, complete extension of the knee is restricted and painful

    c. Brudzinski's sign—attempts to flex the neck will produce flexion at knee and thigh

    d. Opisthotonic position—extensor rigidity with legs hyperextended and forming an arc with the trunk

3. Changes in level of consciousness

4. Seizures

5. Symptoms in infants

    a. Refuse feedings, vomiting, diarrhea

    b. Bulging fontanelles

    c. Vacant stare, high-pitched cry

B. Diagnose

1. Causes

    a. Infection (viral, bacterial, fungal)

    b. Neurosurgical procedures, basilar-skull fractures

    c. Otitis media, mastoiditis

C. Plan/Implementation

1. IV antibiotic therapy—penicillin, cephalosporin, vancomycin

2. Monitor ABG, arterial pressures, body weight, serum electrolytes, urine volume, specific gravity, osmolality

3. Droplet precautions for *Haemophilus influenzae* type b and *Neisseria meningitidis*

4. Prevention

    a. Vaccine 65+ years old with chronic diseases; revaccination in 5 years

    b. Hib vaccine for infants

D. Evaluation

1. Is client able to maintain optimal neurological function?

2. Have complications been prevented?

▶ MIGRAINE HEADACHE

A. Assessment

1. Prodromal—depression, irritability, feeling cold, food cravings, anorexia, change in activity level, increased urination

2. Aura—light flashes and bright spots, numbness and tingling (lips, face, hands), mild confusion, drowsiness, dizziness, diploplia

3. Headache—throbbing (often unilateral), photophobia, nausea, vomiting, 4 to 72 hours

4. Recovery—pain gradually subsides, muscle aches in neck and scalp, sleep for extended period

B. Diagnose

1. Episodic events or acute attacks

2. Seen more often in women before menses

3. Familial disorders due to inherited vascular response to different chemicals

4. Precipitating factors—stress, menstrual cycles, bright lights, depression, sleep deprivation, fatigue, foods containing tyramine, monosodium glutamate, nitrites, or milk products (aged cheese, processed foods)

C. Plan/Implementation

1. Prevention and treatment

   a. Medications

      1) Beta blockers

      2) Triptan preparations—activate serotonin receptors

      3) Acetaminophen, NSAIDS

      4) Topiramate

      5) Ergotamines—dihydroergotamine ; take at beginning of headache

   b. Modify trigger factors

2. Implementation

   a. Avoid triggers

   b. Comfort measures

   c. Quiet dark environment

   d. Elevate head of bed 30°

3. Complementary/Alternate therapy

   a. Riboflavin (vitamin B_2) supplement

      1) 400 mg daily may reduce the number and duration but not the severity of the headaches

      2) Take as an individual supplement

   b. Massage, meditation, relaxation techniques

▶ HUNTINGTON'S DISEASE

A. Assessment

1. Depression and temper outbursts

2. Choreiform movements

   a. Slight to severe restlessness

   b. Facial grimacing

   c. Arm movements

   d. Irregular leg movements

   e. Twisting, turning, struggling

   f. Tongue movements

   g. Person is in constant motion by end of diseased progression

   3. Personality changes
      a. Irritabilty
      b. Paranoia, demanding, memory loss, decreased intellectual function
      c. Dementia
      d. Psychosis seen at end stage

B. Diagnose
   1. Rare, familial, progressive, degenerative disease that is passed from generation to generation (dominant inheritance)

C. Plan/Implementation
   1. Drug therapy—intended to reduce movement and subdue behavior changes
      a. Chlordiazepoxidehydrochloride
      b. Haloperidol
      c. Chlorpromazine
   2. Supportive, symptomatic
   3. Genetic counseling for all family members

D. Evaluation
   1. Has family undergone genetic counseling?
   2. Has client comfort been maintained?

▶ **ALTERATIONS IN GLUCOSE METABOLISM**

A. Assessment

1. Polyuria, polydipsia, polyphagia

2. Weight change

B. Diagnose

1. Diabetes mellitus is a genetically heterogeneous group of disorders that is characterized by glucose intolerance

2. Types (see Table 1)

Table 1 ALTERATIONS IN GLUCOSE METABOLISM	
TYPE	**NURSING CONSIDERATIONS**
Type 1 diabetes	Acute onset before age 30
	Insulin-producing pancreatic beta cells destroyed by autoimmune process
	Requires insulin injection
	Ketosis prone
Type 2 diabetes	Usually older than 30 and obese
	Decreased sensitivity to insulin (insulin resistance) or decreased insulin production
	Ketosis rare
	Treated with diet and exercise
	Supplemented with oral hypoglycemic medications
Others: Gestational diabetes Impaired fasting glucose	Onset during pregnancy, second or third trimester
	High-risk pregnancy
	Fasting plasma glucose of greater than or equal to 100 mg/dL (5.6 mmol/L) and less than 126 mg/dL (7mmol/L); risk factor for future diabetes risk

3. Risk factors for type 2 diabetes

   a. Parents or siblings with diabetes

   b. Obesity (20% or more above ideal body weight)

   c. African American, Hispanic, Native American, or Asian American

   d. Older than 45 years

   e. Previously impaired fasting glucose

   f. Hypertension

   g. HDL cholesterol levels less than or equal to 35 mg/dL; triglyceride levels greater than or equal to 250 mg/dL

   h. History of gestational diabetes or delivery of baby greater than 9 lb

4. Diagnostic tests

   a. Blood glucose monitoring—presence of sugar in the urine is a sign of diabetes and calls for an immediate blood glucose test; normal range in fasting blood is 60–110 mg/dL(3.3–6.1 mmol/L)

   b. Urine ketones indicate that diabetic control has deteriorated; body has started to break down stored fat for energy

   c. Glycosylated hemoglobin (HbA1c)—blood sample can be taken without fasting; normal 4–6%

   d. Special considerations—medications, illness, and stress will affect testing

C. Plan/Implementation

   1. Nutrition management

      a. Provide all essential food constituents—lower lipid levels if elevated

      b. Achieve and maintain ideal weight

      c. Meet energy needs

      d. Achieve normal-range glucose levels

      e. Methods

         1) Food exchange—foods on list in specified amounts contain equal number of calories and grams of protein, fat, and carbohydrate (see Table 2)

         2) Carbohydrate counting

         3) Food guide pyramid

         4) Glycemic index

Table 2 DIABETIC EXCHANGE LIST	
EXCHANGE	**EXAMPLE**
Bread/starch	1 slice of bread 1/2 cup pasta
Vegetable	1 cup raw leafy vegetables 1/2 cup cooked vegetables
Milk	1 cup yogurt 2 oz processed cheese
Meat, poultry, eggs, fish	2–3 oz cooked meat, fish, poultry 2 eggs
Fruit	1/2 cup cooked fruit 1 medium apple
Fat	1 tsp mayonnaise
Free items	Mustard, pickle, herbs

   2. Insulin management

      a. Insulin lowers blood glucose by facilitating uptake and the use of glucose by muscle and fat cells; decreases the release of glucose from the liver

      b. Mixing insulins—draw up regular insulin first

   c. Site selection—abdomen, posterior arms, anterior thighs, hips; rotate sites

   d. Self-injection—use disposable syringe once and discard into hard plastic container with tight-fitting top

   e. "Sick day rules"

      1) Take insulin or oral agent as ordered

      2) Check blood glucose and urine ketones every 3–4 hours

      3) Report altered levels to health care provider

      4) If unable to follow normal meal plan, substitute soft foods (soup, custard, gelatin) 6–8 times per day

      5) If vomiting, diarrhea, or fever, report to health care provider and take liquids (cola, broth, Gatorade) every 0.5–1 hour

3. Oral hypoglycemic medications—improve both tissue responsiveness to insulin and/or the ability of the pancreatic cells to secrete insulin

4. Self-monitoring of blood glucose (SMBG)

   a. Check client's eyesight to make sure he/she can see directions and read results

   b. Calibrate monitor as instructed by manufacturer

   c. Check expiration date on test strips

   d. If taking insulin, check 2–4 times daily

   e. If not receiving insulin, check 2–3 times per week

   f. Keep log book of results

   g. Testing should be done at peak action time of medication

5. Skin and foot care

   a. Inspect feet daily (use mirror if client is elderly or has decreased joint mobility)

   b. Wear well-fitting shoes; break in new shoes slowly (wear 1–2 hours initially with gradual increase in time)

   c. Don't walk barefoot or use heating pad on feet

   d. Cut toenails straight across without rounding corners

6. Exercise

   a. Use proper foot care

   b. Don't exercise in extreme temperatures

   c. Don't exercise when control of diabetes is poor

7. Complications

   a. Hypoglycemia (insulin reaction) (see Table 3)

   b. Hyperglycemia (diabetic ketoacidosis) (see Table 3)

   c. HHNKS (hyperglycemic hyperosmolar nonketotic syndrome; see Table 3)

   d. Diabetic retinopathy

   e. Coronary artery disease

   f. Cerebrovascular disease

Table 3 GLUCOSE IMBALANCES			
	HYPOGLYCEMIA (INSULIN REACTION)	HYPERGLYCEMIA (DIABETIC KETOACIDOSIS)	HHNKS (HYPERGLYCEMIA HYPEROSMOLAR NONKETOTIC SYNDROME)
Assessment	Blood sugar less than 50–60 mg/dL (2.8–3.3 mmol/L) Irritability, confusion, tremors, blurring of vision, coma, seizures Hypotension, tachycardia Skin cool and clammy, diaphoresis	Blood sugar 300–800 mg/dL (16.7–44.4 mmol/L) Headache, drowsiness, weakness stupor, coma Hypotension, tachycardia Skin warm and dry, dry mucous membranes, elevated temperature Polyuria progressing to oliguria, polydipsia, polyphagia Kussmaul's respirations (rapid and deep) Fruity odor to breath	Glucose levels greater than 800 mg/dL (44.4 mmol/L) Occurs in adults greater than 50 year old Occurs in Type 2 (NIDDM) diabetics Ketosis and acidosis do not occur Hypotension Dry mucous membranes, poor skin turgor Tachycardia Alteration in sense of awareness, seizures, hemiparesis
Plan/Implementation	Liquids containing sugar if conscious; skim milk is ideal if tolerated Dextrose 50% IV if unconscious, glucagon 1 mg IM, SQ Follow with additional carbohydrate in 15 minutes Determine and treat cause Client education	Major complication is fluid volume deficit 1 L of 0.9% NaCl per hour during first 2–3 hrs followed by 0.45% NaCl 200–500 ml/h; then D_5W or D_5 1/2 NS Regular IV insulin 5 units/h Potassium replacement EKG q 2–4 h Check K^+ q 2–4 h Assess level of consciousness, urine output, temperature hourly Assess vital signs q 15 minutes until stable Assess CVP q 30 minutes Check blood glucose levels hourly	Normal saline or 0.45% NaCl Regular insulin Potassium as soon as urine output is satisfactory Determine and treat cause Client education Exercise regimen
Cause	Too much insulin or oral hypoglycemia agent Inadequate food Excessive physical activity	Decreased or missed insulin Illness or infection Untreated diabetes	Acute illness Medications (thiazides) Treatments (dialysis)

▶ ALTERATIONS IN PROTEIN METABOLISM

A. Assessment (see Table 4)

B. Diagnose—potential nursing diagnoses

   1. Nutrition: less than body requirements, altered

   2. Knowledge deficit regarding dietary restrictions

C. Plan/Implementation (see Table 4)

D. Evaluation

   1. Have complications been prevented?

   2. Are parents knowledgeable about nutritional need of infant?

Table 4 ALTERATIONS IN PROTEIN METABOLISM		
DISORDER	**ASSESSMENT**	**NURSING CONSIDERATIONS**
Phenylketonuria (PKU)—inborn error of phenylalanine utilization	High blood phenylalanine that leads to intellectual delay	Specially prepared milk substitutes for infants (Lofenalac) Low-protein diet for children (no meat, dairy products, eggs, NutraSweet)
Gout—inborn error of purine metabolism	High uric acid level that leads to progressive joint deterioration	Low-purine diet (no fish or organ meats)
Celiac disease—(sprue) inborn error of wheat and rye metabolism	Intestinal malabsorption that leads to malnutrition Diarrhea Failure to thrive	Gluten-free diet (no wheat, oats, rye, barley)
Renal failure	Increased protein and albumin losses in urine that leads to protein deficiency	High-calorie, low-protein diet, as allowed by kidney function
Protein allergy	Diarrhea that leads to malnutrition and water loss	Change dietary protein source

▶ ALTERATIONS IN FAT METABOLISM

A. Assessment (see Table 5)

B. Diagnose—potential nursing diagnoses

   1. Nutrition: less than body requirements, altered

   2. Knowledge deficit regarding dietary restriction

C. Plan/Implementation (see Table 5)

D. Evaluation

   1. Have client's nutritional needs been met?

   2. Is client knowledgeable about dietary modifications?

Table 5 ALTERATIONS IN FAT METABOLISM		
DISORDER	**ASSESSMENT**	**NURSING CONSIDERATIONS**
Hepatobiliary disease	Decreased bile leads to fat malabsorption	Low-fat, high-protein diet Vitamins
Cystic fibrosis	Absence of pancreatic enzymes leads to malabsorption of fat (and fat-soluble vitamins), weight loss Infection and lung disease lead to increased need for calories and protein	Pancreatic enzyme replacement (cotazym pancreas) before or with meals High-protein diet High-calorie diet in advanced stages
Atherosclerosis (thickening and hardening of the arteries)	Associated with high blood cholesterol and triglyceride levels Risk factors—diet, high blood pressure, diabetes, stress, sedentary lifestyle, and smoking	Low-saturated fat diet Cholesterol-lowering medications given before meals

▶ INFECTIONS OF THE GI TRACT

A. Assessment

1. Headache

2. Abdominal discomfort, anorexia

3. Watery diarrhea, nausea, vomiting

4. Low-grade fever

B. Diagnose

1. Acute illness caused by ingested food contaminated by toxins or parasites

2. Types (see Table 6)

Table 6 COMMON INFECTIONS OF THE GASTROINTESTINAL TRACT		
PARASITE OR BACTERIUM	**SOURCE**	**NURSING CONSIDERATIONS**
Enterotoxigenic *E. coli*	Undercooked beef	Causes rapid, severe dehydration; cook beef until meat no longer pink and juices run clear
Salmonella	Poultry, eggs	Causes gastroenteritis, systemic infection
Campylobacter	Poultry, beef, pork	Cook and store food at appropriate temperatures
Giardia lamblia	Protozoan, contaminated water	Treated with metronidazole, good personal hygiene
Shigella	Fecal contamination	Affects pediatric population, antimicrobial therapy

C. Plan/Implementation

1. Prevention

   a. Good sanitation

   b. Good hygiene measures, e.g., handwashing

   c. Proper food preparation, e.g., thorough cooking; heat canned foods 10–20 minutes and inspect cans for gas bubbles

2. Nursing considerations

   a. Maintain fluid and electrolytes

   b. Monitor vital signs

   c. Medications: antibiotics, antispasmodics, antiemetics

   d. Teach importance of good handwashing and cleaning of utensils when preparing food

D. Evaluation

1. Have client's symptoms resolved?

2. Are the stool cultures negative?

▶ HIATAL HERNIA

A. Assessment

1. Heartburn

2. Regurgitation

3. Dyspepsia

B. Diagnose

1. Opening in diaphragm through which the esophagus passes becomes enlarged, part of the upper stomach comes up into the lower portion of the thorax

C. Plan/Implementation

1. Administer medications

    a. H_2 receptor blockers (e.g., cimetadine, ranitidine)

    b. Antacids (e.g., aluminum hydroxide, magnesium hydroxide)

    c. Cytoprotective medications (e.g., sucralfate)

    d. Proton pump inhibitors (pantoprazole)

2. Surgery to tighten cardiac sphincter (fundoplication)

3. Small, frequent feedings

4. Do not lie down for at least 1 hour after meals; elevate head of bed 4–8 inches when sleeping

5. Do not eat before going to bed to prevent reflux of food

D. Evaluation

1. Has client comfort been maintained?

2. Is client knowledgeable about ways to prevent symptoms?

▶ PYLORIC STENOSIS

A. Assessment

1. Vomiting (projectile in infants)

2. Epigastric fullness

3. Irritability (in infants)

4. Infant always hungry

5. Infant fails to gain weight

6. Palpable olive-shaped tumor in epigastrium (infants)

7. Peristaltic waves

B. Diagnose

1. In adults, narrowing or obstruction of the pyloric sphincter caused by scarring from healing ulcers; in infants, obstruction caused by hypertrophy and hyperplasia of pylorus

2. Inflammation and edema can reduce the size of the opening until there is complete obstruction

3. Infants usually don't show symptoms until the second to fourth week after birth; then regurgitation develops into projectile vomiting; most frequently seen in male, white, full-term infants

4. Obstruction in adults usually caused by peptic ulcer

5. Surgical intervention

    a. Pyloromyotomy (infants)—incision through circular muscles of the pylorus

    b. Vagotomy and antrectomy—removal of gastrin-secreting portion of the stomach and severing of vagus nerves

    c. Vagotomy and pyloroplasty or gastroenterostomy—establishes gastric drainage, involves severing of vagus nerves

C. Plan/Implementation

1. Preoperative

   a. Prevent regurgitation and vomiting

      1) IV fluids

      2) Check skin turgor, fontanelles, urinary output

      3) Measure vomitus

      4) Correct fluid and electrolyte abnormalities—alkalosis, hypokalemia

      5) Gastric decompression with NG tube

      6) Monitor for complications—alkalosis, hypokalemia, dehydration, and shock

      7) Support parents

         a) Allow verbalization of parents' anxieties

         b) Instruct parents on expected progress and behavior

2. Postoperative

   a. Keep incision site clean and dry

   b. Provide parenteral fluids at ordered rate

   c. Monitor warmth

   d. Small, frequent feedings of glucose water or electrolyte solution 4–6 hours postoperatively

   e. If clear fluids retained start formula 24 hours postop

   f. Teach parents to fold diaper so it doesn't touch incision

D. Evaluation

1. Has client's fluid and electrolyte balance been maintained?

2. Have complications been prevented?

▶ GASTRITIS

A. Assessment

1. Uncomfortable feeling in abdomen

2. Headache

3. Anorexia, nausea, vomiting (possibly bloody)

4. Hiccupping

B. Diagnose

1. Inflammation of stomach that may be acute or chronic

C. Plan/Implementation

1. NPO slowly progressing to bland diet

2. Antacids often relieve pain

3. Referral to appropriate agency if alcohol abuse is verified

D. Evaluation

1. Has client comfort been maintained?

2. Have proper referrals been made?

▶ GI ULCER

A. Assessment (see Table 7)

B. Diagnose

1. Excavation formed in the mucosal wall, caused by erosion that may extend to muscle layers or through the muscle to the peritoneum (see Figure 1)

2. *H. pylori* frequently present

3. Familial tendency

Table 7 DUODENAL VERSUS GASTRIC ULCER		
	CHRONIC DUODENAL ULCER	CHRONIC GASTRIC ULCER
Age	30–60 years	50 years and older
Sex	Male-female ratio: 3:1	Male-female ratio: 1:1
Risk factors	Blood group type O, COPD, chronic renal failure, alcohol, smoking, cirrhosis, stress	Gastritis, alcohol, smoking, NSAIDs, stress
Gastric secretion	Hypersecretion	Normal to hyposecretion
Pain	2–3 hours after meal; nighttime, often in early sleeping hours Food intake relieves pain	1/2 to 1 hour after meal or when fasting Relieved by vomiting Ingestion of food does not help
Vomiting	Rare	Frequent
Hemorrhage	Less likely	More likely
Malignancy	Rare	Occasionally

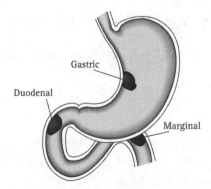

Figure 1. Sites for Ulcers

C. Plan/Implementation

1. Avoid oversecretion and hypermotility in the gastrointestinal tract

2. Dietary modification

   a. Eat 3 meals per day; small frequent feedings not necessary if taking antacids or histamine blocker

   b. Avoid extremes in temperature

    c. Avoid coffee, alcohol, and caffeinated beverages

    d. Avoid milk and cream

3. Reduce stress

4. Stop smoking—inhibits ulcer repair

5. Medications

    a. Antacids (e.g., magnesium and aluminum hydroxide); administer 1 hour before or after meals

    b. Histamine receptor site antagonist (e.g., cimetidine, ranitidine); take with meals

    c. Anticholinergics (e.g., propantheline); give 30 minutes before meals

    d. Cytoprotective medications (e.g., sucralfate); give 1 hour before meals

    e. Proton pump inhibitors (e.g., omeprazole)

6. Surgical intervention (see Figure 2: Common Surgeries for Ulcers)

    a. Diagnostic workup—upper-GI series, endoscopy, CT scan

    b. Gastrectomy—removal of stomach and attachment to upper portion of duodenum

    c. Vagotomy—cutting the vagus nerve (decreases HCl secretion)

    d. Billroth I—partial removal (distal one-third to one-half) of stomach, anastomosis with duodenum

    e. Billroth II—removal of distal segment of stomach and antrum, anastomosis with jejunum

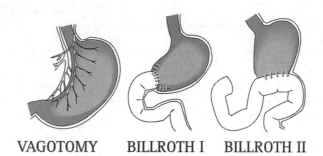

VAGOTOMY   BILLROTH I   BILLROTH II

Figure 2. Common Surgeries for Ulcers

7. Postoperative

    a. Assess vital signs

    b. Inspect dressings

    c. Provide gastric decompression as ordered

    d. Vitamin B_{12} via parenteral route (required for life); iron supplements

    e. Encourage deep breathing

    f. Observe for peristalsis

        1) Levin tube—single-lumen tube at low suction

        2) Salem sump—double-lumen for drainage

            a) Prevent irritation to nostril

            b) Lubricate tube around nares with water-soluble jelly

            c) Control excessive nasal secretions

            d) Observe nasogastric drainage for volume and blood

3) Listen for bowel sounds

4) Record passage of flatus or stool

g. Teach preventive measures for "dumping syndrome" (rapid passage of food from stomach causing diaphoresis, diarrhea, hypotension)

1) Restrict fluids with meals, drink 1 hour ac or 1 hour pc

2) Eat in semi-recumbent position

3) Lie down 20–30 minutes after eating

4) Eat smaller, frequent meals

5) Complex carbohydrates, avoid simple sugars

6) Antispasmotics

D. Evaluation

1. Have client's nutritional needs been met?

2. Is client knowledgeable about measures to prevent complications postoperatively?

▶ ESOPHAGEAL ATRESIA AND TRACHEOESOPHAGEAL FISTULA

A. Assessment

1. Excessive saliva, drooling

2. Stomach distention

3. Choking, coughing, sneezing

4. Cyanosis

B. Diagnose

1. Failure of esophagus to develop as a continuous tube (see Figure 3)

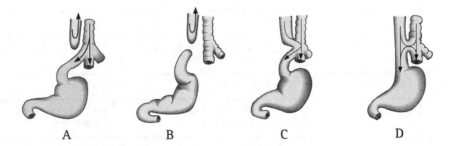

Figure 3. Tracheoesophageal Fistula

2. Often occurs with anomalies of heart or the genitourinary or musculoskeletal system

C. Plan/Implementation

1. Surgical repair

a. Preoperative

1) Position supine or prone with head of bed elevated on incline plane at least 30 degrees

2) IV fluids and antibiotics through umbilical artery catheter

3) Maintain patent airway

  b. Postoperative

  1) Care for incision site—observe for inflammation

  2) Prevent pulmonary complications—suction and position

  3) IV fluids and antibiotics

  4) PN until gastrostomy or oral feedings tolerated

D. Evaluation

  1. Has defect been repaired?

  2. Have infant's nutritional needs been met?

► CROHN'S DISEASE (REGIONAL ENTERITIS, ILEITIS, OR ENTEROCOLITIS) ULCERATIVE COLITIS

A. Assessment (see Table 8)

B. Diagnose

  1. Crohn's disease—inflammatory condition of any area of large or small intestine, usually ileum and ascending colon

  2. Ulcerative colitis—inflammatory condition of the colon characterized by eroded areas of the mucous membrane and tissues beneath it

Table 8 CROHN'S DISEASE VERSUS ULCERATIVE COLITIS		
	CROHN'S DISEASE REGIONAL ENTERITIS	ULCERATIVE COLITIS
Assessment		
Usual age of onset	20–30 and 50–80 years	Young adult to middle age (30–50)
Fatty stool (steatorrhea)	Frequent	Absent
Malignancy results	Rare	10–15%
Rectal bleeding	Occasional: mucus, pus, fat in stool	Common; blood, pus, mucus in stool
Abdominal pain	After meals	Predefecation
Diarrhea	Diarrhea rare; 5–6 unformed stools per day	10–20 liquid stools per day; often bloody
Nutritional deficit, weight loss, anemia, dehydration	Common	Common
Fever	Present	Present
Anal abscess	Common	Common
Fistula and anorectal fissure fistula	Common	Rare
Diagnose		
Level of involvement	Ileum, right colon	Rectum, left colon
Inflammation	Noncontinuous segment	Continuous segment

Table 8 CROHN'S DISEASE VERSUS ULCERATIVE COLITIS *(CONTINUED)*		
	CROHN'S DISEASE REGIONAL ENTERITIS	ULCERATIVE COLITIS
Course of disease	Prolonged, variable Complications–bowel abscess, fistula formation, intestinal obstruction	Remissions and relapses Complications–hemorrhage, abscess formation, arthritis, uveitis
Nursing considerations	High-protein, high-calorie, low-fat, and low-fiber diet May require PN to rest bowel Analgesics, anticholinergics, sulfonamides (Gantrisin), corticosteriods, antidiarrheals, and antiperistaltics Maintain fluid/electrolyte balance Monitor electrolytes Promote rest, relieve anxiety Ileostomy in severe cases	

C. Plan/Implementation

1. Diet—high-protein, high-calorie, low-fat, and fiber; PN used for bowel rest
2. Medications—analgesics, anticholinergics, antibiotics, corticosteroids to reduce inflammation; immune modulators, salicylate-containing compounds
3. Maintain fluid, electrolyte balance; provide PN if bowel rest is needed
4. Ileostomy

D. Evaluation

1. Is client able to care for ileostomy?
2. Did client adjust to the change in body image?

▶ APPENDICITIS

A. Assessment

1. Periumbilical abdominal pain shifts to right lower quadrant at McBurney's point (located between umbilicus and the right iliac crest)
2. Anorexia, nausea, vomiting
3. Localized tenderness
4. Muscle guarding
5. Low-grade fever

B. Diagnose

1. Highest incidence 11–30 years of age
2. Differential CBC count; WBC 15,000 to 20,000 cells/mm^3

C. Plan/Implementation

1. No heating pads, enemas, or laxatives preop
2. Maintain NPO status until blood laboratory reports received, IV fluids to prevent dehydration
3. No analgesics until cause of pain is determined
4. Ice bag to abdomen to alleviate pain

5. Observe for signs and symptoms of peritonitis

6. Surgical removal of appendix (appendectomy)

   a. Normal postop care

   b. Fowler's position to relieve abdominal pain and ease breathing

7. Sudden cessation of pain—perforation emergency

8. Antibiotic therapy

D. Evaluation

1. Is client comfort maintained after surgery?

2. Is client able to resume normal activities?

▶ DIVERTICULAR DISEASE

A. Assessment

1. Cramping pain in left lower quadrant of abdomen relieved by passage of stool or flatus

2. Fever, increased WBC

3. Constipation alternating with diarrhea

B. Diagnose

1. Infection, inflammation, or obstruction of diverticula (sacs or pouches in the intestinal wall) cause the client to become symptomatic

2. Associated with deficiency in dietary fiber

C. Plan/Implementation

1. Uncomplicated

   a. Antispasmodics, anticholinergic (e.g., dicyclomine)

   b. Bulk laxatives

   c. High-fiber diet; avoid food with seeds

   d. Increase fluids

2. Acute

   a. Bedrest

   b. NPO progressing to oral fluids to semi-solids

   c. IV fluids

   d. NG tube

   e. Antibiotics

   f. Surgery–drain abscess, resect obstruction

D. Evaluation

1. Has client comfort been maintained?

2. Is client compliant with medication regimen?

▶ PERITONITIS

A. Assessment

1. Abdominal pain, possibly severe

2. Abdominal rigidity and distension, rebound tenderness

3. Nausea, vomiting

4. Ascites

5. Increased temperature, leukocytosis

6. Paralytic ileus

7. Symptoms may be masked in elderly persons or those receiving corticosteroids

B. Diagnose

1. Inflammation of part or all of the parietal and visceral surfaces of the abdominal cavity

2. Causes

   a. Ruptured appendix, ectopic pregnancy

   b. Perforated ulcer, bowel, or bladder

   c. Traumatic injury

   d. Blood-borne organisms

C. Plan/Implementation

1. Preoperative care

   a. Monitor vital signs, I and O

   b. Antibiotics and IV fluids

   c. Gastric decompression; monitor NG drainage

   d. NPO

   e. Reestablish fluid/electrolyte balance, monitor serum electrolytes

   f. Analgesics

2. Postoperative care

   a. NPO

   b. NG tube

   c. Semi-Fowler's position

   d. IV fluids with electrolyte replacement

   e. Antibiotics

   f. PN

D. Evaluation

1. Are the client's vital signs stable?

2. Has the client's fluid and electrolyte balance been maintained?

▶ HIRSCHSPRUNG'S DISEASE

A. Assessment

1. Newborn—failure to pass meconium, refusal to suck, abdominal distention

2. Child—failure to gain weight, delayed growth, constipation alternating with diarrhea, foul-smelling stools, abdominal distension, visible peristalsis

B. Diagnose

1. A ganglionic disease of the intestinal tract; inadequate motility causes mechanical obstruction of intestine

2. Diagnostic tests—radiographic contrast studies

C. Plan/Implementation

1. Help parents adjust to congenital defect in child

2. Foster infant/parent bonding

3. Prepare for surgery

    a. Enemas

    b. Low-fiber, high-calorie, high-protein diet

    c. PN if needed

    d. Oral antibiotics

    e. Measure abdominal girth at level of umbilicus

4. Postoperative care

    a. Monitor fluid and electrolytes

    b. Maintain nutrition

    c. Let parents know colostomy is usually temporary, closed when child is 17–22 lb

D. Evaluation

1. Have the child and parents adjusted to the change in body image?

2. Are the parents knowledgeable about stoma care?

▶ INTUSSUSCEPTION

A. Assessment

1. Colicky abdominal pain

2. Causes child to scream and draw knees to abdomen

3. Vomiting

4. Currant jellylike stools containing blood and mucus

5. Tender, distended abdomen

6. May have palpable sausage-shaped mass in the upper right quadrant of the abdomen

7. Usual client is 3 months to 3 years old

B. Diagnose

1. Telescoping of one portion of the bowel into another (usually the ileum into the cecum and colon)

2. Results in intestinal obstruction, and blocked blood and lymph circulation

3. Diagnosis can often be made based on findings alone

C. Plan/Implementation

1. Non-surgical intervention

    a. Water-soluble contrast medium or air pressure to "push" the telescoped portion out

    b. Postprocedural care

        1) Assess vital signs

        2) Auscultate bowel sounds

        3) Observe for passage of water-soluble contrast medium

        4) Encourage parental rooming-in

2. Surgical intervention

    a. Manually reducing the telescoped portion of the bowel

    b. Removal of any damaged bowel portions

3. Preparation for surgery

    a. NPO

      b. CBC and urinalysis

      c. Sedation

      d. Correct hypovolemia and electrolyte imbalances

      e. Treat peritonitis, if present

      f. Nasogastric suctioning (decompression) may be needed

      g. Consent form signed

  4. Postoperative care

      a. Assess vital signs

      b. Inspect sutures and dressing

      c. Auscultate for return of bowel sounds

      d. Administer pain medications and antibiotics as ordered

      e. Progress diet with return of bowel sounds

  5. Evaluation

      a. Have the child and parents adjusted to the change in body image?

      b. Are the parents knowledgeable about care?

▶ ABDOMINAL HERNIAS

A. Assessment

  1. Lump at site of hernia may disappear in reclining position and reappear on standing/coughing/lifting

  2. Strangulated hernia—severe abdominal pain, nausea and vomiting, distention, intestinal obstruction

B. Diagnose

  1. Protrusion of an organ through the wall of the cavity in which it is normally contained

  2. Types

      a. Inguinal—protrusion of intestine through abdominal ring into inguinal canal

      b. Femoral—protrusion of intestine into femoral canal

      c. Umbilical—protrusion of intestine through umbilical ring

      d. Ventral or incisional—protrusion through site of an old surgical incision

      e. Reducible—the protruding structure can be replaced by manipulation into the abdominal cavity

      f. Irreducible or incarcerated—the protruding structure cannot be replaced by manipulation

      g. Strangulated—blood supply to the intestines is obstructed (emergency situation)

C. Plan/Implementation

  1. Preoperative care for herniorrhaphy

      a. Assess respiratory system for potential causes of increased intra-abdominal pressure—may cause interference with postop healing

      b. Surgery is postponed until respiratory conditions are controlled

      c. Truss—pad placed under hernia, held in place with belt

2. Postoperative care

    a. Relieve urinary retention

    b. Turning and deep breathing, but avoid coughing

    c. Provide scrotal support

    d. Provide ice packs for swollen scrotum

    e. Advise no pulling, pushing, heavy lifting for 6–8 weeks

    f. Inform client that sexual function is not affected

    g. Instruct client that ecchymosis will fade in a few days

D. Evaluation

1. Has normal bowel function been re-established?

2. Has client comfort been maintained?

▶ MECKEL'S DIVERTICULUM

A. Assessment

1. Symptoms seen by 2 years of age

2. Painless rectal bleeding, abdominal pain

3. Hematochezia (currant jelly–like stool)

4. Signs and symptoms of appendicitis if diverticulum becomes inflamed from infection

B. Diagnose

1. A congenital sac or pouch in the ileum

2. Contains gastric or pancreatic tissue that secretes acid

3. Most common GI malformation

C. Plan/Implementation

1. Preoperative care

    a. IV fluids

    b. Observe for rectal bleeding

    c. Bedrest

2. Postoperative care

    a. Surgical (if symptomatic)–removal of the diverticulum

    b. Prevent infection

    c. Maintain nutrition

D. Evaluation

1. Has client comfort been maintained?

2. Has the client's elimination been maintained?

▶ INTESTINAL OBSTRUCTION

A. Assessment

1. Nausea, vomiting

2. High-pitched bowel sounds above area of obstruction, decreased or absent bowel sounds below the area of obstruction

3. Abdominal pain and distention, pain often described as "colicky"

4. Obstipation (absence of stool and gas)

B. Diagnose

1. Mechanical obstruction—physical blockage of lumen of intestines, usually seen in the small intestine

   a. Hernia

   b. Tumors

   c. Adhesions

   d. Strictures due to radiation or congenital

   e. Intussusception (telescoping of bowel within itself)

   f. Volvulus (twisting of bowel)

2. Nonmechanical obstruction (paralytic ileus)—no mechanical blockage, absence of peristalsis

   a. Abdominal trauma/surgery

   b. Spinal injuries

   c. Peritonitis, acute appendicitis

   d. Wound dehiscence (breakdown)

C. Plan/Implementation

1. Intestinal decompression

   a. Insertion of a plastic or rubber tube into the stomach or intestine via the nose or mouth; the purpose may be diagnostic, preventive, or therapeutic; fluid or air may be removed

   b. Tubes

      1) Salem sump or Levin tubes (nasogastric)

      2) Miller-Abbot (intestinal)

      3) Cantor (intestinal)

2. NPO

3. Fluid/electrolyte replacement; monitor I and O and electrolyte levels

4. Assist with ADL

5. Good oral and skin care

6. Fowler's position to facilitate breathing

7. Bowel surgery

   a. Purpose—removal of diseased portion of bowel; creation of an outlet for passage of stool when there is an obstruction or need for "bowel rest"

   b. Types of surgeries

      1) Exploratory laparotomy; possible adhesion removal

      2) Resection and anastomosis—diseased portion of bowel is removed and remaining ends are joined together

      3) Abdominal perineal resection—abdominal incision through which the proximal end of the sigmoid colon is exteriorized through a permanent colostomy; the distal end of the sigmoid colon, rectum, and anus are removed through the perineal route

      4) Intestinal ostomies

D. Evaluation

1. Has intestinal obstruction been cleared?

2. Has normal bowel function returned?

▶ INTESTINAL OSTOMIES FOR FECAL DIVERSION

A. Assessment

1. Cancer of colon or rectum

2. Diverticulitis

3. Intestinal obstruction

B. Diagnose

1. Ostomy is opening into colon to allow passage of intestinal contents

2. Stoma is opening on abdomen where intestine is sutured to skin surface

3. Types (see Figure 4)

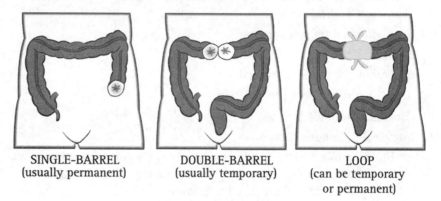

SINGLE-BARREL	DOUBLE-BARREL	LOOP
(usually permanent)	(usually temporary)	(can be temporary or permanent)

Figure 4. Types of Colostomies

4. Common intestinal ostomies (see Table 9)

5. Continent ileal reservoir (Koch pouch)—surgical creation of pouch of small intestine acts as an internal reservoir for fecal discharge, nipple value as outlet

C. Plan/Implementation

1. Preoperative care

   a. Psychological support and explanations

   b. Diet—high calorie, high protein, high carbohydrates, low-residue week before; NPO after midnight

   c. Place tube prior to surgery—NG or intestinal

   d. Activity—assist PRN, client will be weakened from extensive preparation procedures

   e. Elimination—laxatives, enemas evening before and morning of surgery

   f. Have enterostomal health care provider see client for optimum placement of stoma

   g. Medications—antibiotics (e.g., erythromycin) day before surgery

   h. Monitor for fluid/electrolyte imbalance

   i. Referral to enterostomal therapist and United Ostomy Association

2. Postoperative care

   a. NG or intestinal decompression until peristalsis returns; maintain NPO status

   b. Clear liquids progressing to solid, low-residue diet for first 6–8 weeks

    c. Monitor I and O and fluid/electrolyte balance

    d. Observe and record condition of stoma

        1) First few days appears beefy-red and swollen

        2) Gradually, swelling recedes and color is pink or red

        3) Notify health care provider immediately if stoma is dark blue, "blackish," or purple—indicates insufficient blood supply

    e. Observe and record description of any drainage from stoma

        1) Usually just mucus or serosanguineous for first 1–2 days

        2) Begins to function 3–6 days postop

    f. Promote positive adjustment to ostomy

        1) Encourage client to look at stoma

        2) Encourage early participation in ostomy care

        3) Reinforce positive aspects of colostomy

Table 9 COMMON INTESTINAL OSTOMIES FOR FECAL DIVERSION

	ILEOSTOMY	TRANSVERSE COLOSTOMY	DESCENDING OR SIGMOID COLOSTOMY
Part of intestine involved	End of ileum, rest of large intestine removed	Transverse colon (usually temporary)	Descending or sigmoid colon (usually permanent)
Ostomy returns	Liquid, semiliquid, soft	Soft to fairly firm; softer toward ileum	Descending—fairly firm stool; sigmoid—solid stool
Odor	Slightly odorous	Very foul-smelling	Usually foul-smelling
Drainage	Highly corrosive because of enzymes	Irritating	Less irritating
Appliance	Open-ended pouch worn at all times (fecal material drained, then appliance reclosed)	Pouch worn continually	Varies; with regular irrigation, sometimes no appliance is worn; if firm stool, many use closed pouch; if liquid, open-ended pouch
Nursing considerations	If continent ileal reservoir (Koch pouch) made in surgery, no appliance worn; contents removed q 4–6 hours via catheter Usually on low-residue diet; no meats, corn, nuts	Usually single-loop colostomy; inflamed bowel segment brought through abdominal wall; incision closed; opening made by cautery (painless) in loop for fecal drainage Diet usually not restricted after first 6 weeks	Typical for colon cancers Reinforce dressing postop Diet usually not restricted after first 6 weeks

3. Skin care

    a. Effect on skin depends on composition, quantity, consistency of drainage, medications, location of stoma, frequency in removal of appliance adhesive

    b. Principles of skin protection (see Figure 5)

        1) Pouch opening $1/8$ inch larger than stoma

        2) Use skin barrier under all tapes (water, paste, powder)

        3) Use skin barrier to protect skin immediately surrounding the stoma

        4) Cleanse skin gently and pat dry; do not rub

5) Pouch applied by pressing adhesive area to skin for 30 seconds

6) Change appliance immediately when seal breaks or when $^1/_3$ or $^1/_4$ full

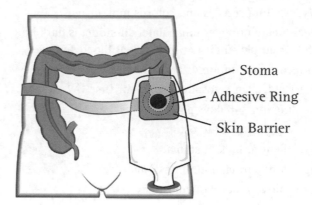

Stoma
Adhesive Ring
Skin Barrier

Figure 5. Colostomy Appliance

4. Colostomy irrigations for sigmoid colostomy

   a. Purpose—to stimulate emptying of colon of gas, mucus, feces at scheduled times to avoid need for appliance

   b. Usually begins 5–7 days postop

   c. When possible, should be sitting upright on toilet for procedure

   d. Performed after a meal, same time each day

   e. 500–1,500 mL of lukewarm water used for solution

   f. Special irrigating sleeve and cone are used

   g. Insert catheter 8 cm (3 inches)

   h. Hang irrigating container at shoulder height (18–20 inches above stoma)

   i. Clamp tubing if client reports cramps; allow client to rest before resuming procedure

   j. Water flows in over 5–10 minutes

   k. Allow 10–15 minutes for most of return

   l. Leave sleeve in place while client moves around for 30–45 minutes

   m. Clean with soap and water, pat dry

5. Care of continent ileal reservoir (Koch pouch)

   a. Postop—catheter inserted and attached to drainage bag, q3h instill 10–20 mL NS into pouch, drain by gravity, kept in place 2 weeks

   b. To drain—lubricate catheter, insert 5 cm (2 inches), drain into toilet, wash and dry stoma

   c. If resistance, inject 20 mL air or water using syringe through catheter

D. Evaluation

   1. Has client accepted alteration in body image?

   2. Is client able to care for colostomy at home?

▶ CIRRHOSIS

A. Assessment

   1. Digestive disturbances

      a. Indigestion, dyspepsia

      b. Flatulence, constipation, diarrhea

      c. Anorexia, weight loss

      d. Nausea and vomiting

   2. Circulatory

      a. Esophageal varices, hematemesis, hemorrhage

      b. Ascites

      c. Hemorrhoids

      d. Increased bleeding tendencies, anemia

      e. Edema in extremities

      f. Spider angiomas

   3. Biliary

      a. Jaundice, pruritus

      b. Dark urine, clay-colored stools

      c. Increased abdominal girth

   4. Compensated

      a. Vascular spiders

      b. Ankle edema

      c. Indigestion

      d. Flatulence

      e. Abdominal pain

      f. Enlarged liver

   5. Decompensated

      a. Ascites

      b. Jaundice

      c. Weight loss

      d. Purpura

      e. Epistaxis

B. Diagnose

   1. Replacement of normal liver tissue with widespread fibrosis and nodule formation

      a. Alcoholic cirrhosis—due to alcoholism and poor nutrition

      b. Biliary cirrhosis—result of chronic biliary obstruction and infection

      c. Postnecrotic cirrhosis—result of previous viral hepatitis

   2. Complications

      a. Portal hypertension with esophageal varices due to elevated pressure throughout entire portal venous system

         1) Dilated tortuous veins usually found in the submucosa of the lower esophagus

             2) Hemorrhage from rupture leading cause of death in clients with cirrhosis

     b. Peripheral edema and ascites

             1) Ascites—accumulation of serous fluid in peritoneal and abdominal cavity

             2) Associated with dehydration and hypokalemia

     c. Hepatic encephalopathy (coma)

             1) Occurs with liver disease

             2) Results from accumulation of ammonia and other toxic metabolites in the blood

             3) Change in level of consciousness

             4) Symptoms of impending coma—disorientation to time, place, person, asterixis (flapping tremor of hand when arm extended and hand help upward [dorsiflexed])

             5) Jaundice

     d. Hepatorenal syndrome

             1) Functional renal failure

             2) Azotemia, ascites

C. Plan/Implementation

   1. Shunts to relieve portal hypertension

   2. Provide appropriate nutrition

     a. Early stages—high-protein, high-carbohydrate diet, supplemented with vitamin B complex

     b. Advanced stages—fiber, protein, fat, and sodium restrictions, high-calorie diet, protein foods of high biologic value

     c. Small, frequent feedings

     d. Fluid restriction

     e. Avoid alcohol

   3. Monitor for bleeding, administer blood products

   4. Observe vital signs for shock

   5. Monitor abdominal girth, daily weights

   6. Maintain skin integrity

     a. Avoid strong soaps

     b. Alleviate dry, itching skin

     c. Frequent position changes

   7. Assess degree of jaundice

   8. Promote rest

   9. Promote adequate respiratory function

  10. Reduce exposure to infection

  11. Promote safety

     a. Electric razor

     b. Soft-bristle toothbrush

     c. Pressure to site after venipuncture

12. Reduce ascites

    a. Sodium, fluid restrictions

    b. Diuretics

13. Treatment of bleeding esophageal varices

    a. Balloon tamponade—Sengstaken-Blakemore tube (see Figure 6), Minnesota tube

        1) Gastric inflation balloon—inflated with 100–200 mL air

        2) Gastric aspiration—connect to suction

        3) Esophageal inflation balloon—pressure on esophageal and gastric balloons 25–40 mm Hg, measured by manometer q 2–4 h

        4) Esophageal aspiration

        5) Tubing irrigated hourly

        6) Deflate balloons sequentially, esophageal balloon first

        7) Complications—necrosis of nose, stomach mucosa, or esophagus; asphyxiation

    b. Endoscopic sclerotherapy—injection of sclerosing agent into the esophagus, causes varices to become fibrotic

    c. Administration of vasopressin or propranolol IV or interarterial temporarily lowers portal pressure by constriction of splenic artery, IV octreotide

    d. Room-temperature saline lavage

    e. Esophageal banding therapy—modified endoscope with rubber band passed into esophagus, varices are banded

    f. Transjugular intrahepatic postsystemic shunting (TIPS)

    g. Surgical bypass

14. Treatment of hepatic encephalopathy

    a. Administer medications: lactulose, Neomycin

    b. Bedrest

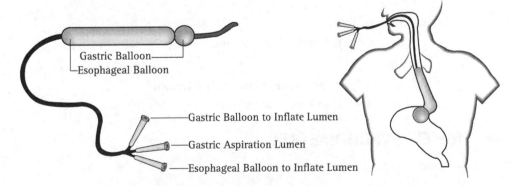

Gastric Balloon

Esophageal Balloon

Gastric Balloon to Inflate Lumen

Gastric Aspiration Lumen

Esophageal Balloon to Inflate Lumen

Figure 6. Sengstaken-Blakemore Tube

D. Evaluation

  1. Are client's vital signs stable?

  2. Has ascites been reduced?

▶ JAUNDICE

A. Assessment

1. Yellowish or greenish-yellow discoloration of skin and sclerae due to elevated bilirubin concentration in the blood

2. Dark-colored urine, clay-colored stools

3. Pruritus

B. Diagnose

1. Hemolytic—caused by destruction of great number of blood cells, leads to a high concentration of bilirubin that exceeds the liver's ability to excrete it

   a. Hemolytic transfusion reactions

   b. Hemolytic anemia

   c. Sickle-cell crisis

2. Intrahepatic—due to obstructed flow of bile through liver or biliary duct system

   a. Cirrhosis

   b. Hepatitis

3. Extrahepatic—due to obstructed flow of bile through liver or biliary duct system

   a. Cholelithiasis

   b. Tumors

   c. Adverse effect of medications—(e.g., phenothiazine, antithyroids, sulfonamides, tricyclic antidepressants, androgens, estrogens)

C. Plan/Implementation

1. Treat underlying cause

2. Relief of pruritus

   a. Medications: antihistamines

   b. Baking soda or alpha Keri baths

   c. Keep nails trimmed and clean; teach to rub with knuckles rather than nails

   d. Soft, old linen

   e. Moderate temperature (not too hot or cold)

D. Evaluation

1. Has cause of jaundice been identified and treated?

2. Has client's comfort been maintained?

▶ REYE'S SYNDROME (RS)

A. Assessment

1. Fever

2. Increased ICP

3. Decreased level of consciousness, coma

4. Decreased hepatic function

5. Diagnosed by liver biopsy

B. Diagnose
1. Acute metabolic encephalopathy of childhood that causes hepatic dysfunction
2. Causes
   a. Link between use of aspirin with viral illness
   b. Associated with viruses, especially URI, gastroenteritis
C. Plan/Implementation
1. Neurological checks
2. Maintain hydration and electrolytes with IV
3. Endotracheal tube and respirator may be needed
4. Monitor CVP or Swan-Ganz catheter
5. Promote family support
D. Evaluation
1. Has child recovered from Reye's syndrome with minimal or no neuropsychological deficit?
2. Have needs of family been met during acute phase of client's hospitalization?

▶ CHOLECYSTITIS, CHOLELITHIASIS

A. Assessment
1. Intolerance to fatty foods
2. Indigestion
3. Nausea, vomiting, flatulence, eructation
4. Severe pain in upper right quadrant of abdomen radiating to back and right shoulder (biliary colic)
5. Elevated temperature
6. Leukocytosis
7. Diaphoresis
8. Dark urine, clay-colored stools
B. Diagnose
1. Cholecystitis—inflammation of gallbladder
2. Cholelithiasis—presence of stones in gallbladder
3. Risk factors
   a. Obesity
   b. Sedentary lifestyle
   c. Women, especially multiparous
   d. Highest incidence 40+ years
   e. Pregnancy
   f. Familial tendency
   g. Hypothyroidism
   h. Increased serum cholesterol

C. Plan/Implementation

1. Rest

2. IV fluids

3. NG suction

4. Analgesics

5. Antibiotics

6. Low-fat liquids—powdered supplements high in protein, carbohydrates stirred into skim milk

7. Avoid fried foods, pork, cheese, alcohol

8. Laparoscopic laser cholecystectomy—removal of gallbladder by a laser through a laparoscope; laparoscope is attached to video camera and procedure is viewed through monitor; four small puncture holes made in abdomen

   a. Preoperative care

      1) NPO on day prior to outpatient (ambulatory) procedure

   b. Postoperative care

      1) Monitor for bleeding

      2) Resume normal activity in 1 week

      3) May need to be on low-fat diet for several weeks

9. Traditional cholecystectomy—removal of gallbladder through a high abdominal incision

   a. Preoperative care

      1) Nutritional supplements of glucose and protein hydrolysates to aid in would healing and prevent liver damage, if needed

      2) NG tube insertion before surgery

   b. Postoperative care

      1) Medicate for pain

      2) Monitor T-tube, if present—inserted to ensure drainage of bile from common bile duct until edema in area diminishes; keep T-tube drainage bag below level of gallbladder

      3) Maintain in semi-Fowler's position

      4) Observe for jaundice—yellow sclerae, stool that does not slowly progress from light to dark color after removal of T-tube

      5) Low-fat, high-carbohydrate, high-protein diet

D. Evaluation

1. Have postoperative complications been avoided?

2. Has client comfort been maintained?

▶ PANCREATITIS

A. Assessment

1. Abdominal pain, nausea, vomiting 24–48 hours after heavy meal or alcohol ingestion; pain relief with position change

2. Hypotension

3. Acute renal failure

4. Grey-blue discoloration in flank and around umbilicus

B. Diagnose

1. Acute pancreatitis (acute inflammation of the pancreas) is brought about by digestion of the organ by the enzymes it produces, principally trypsin

2. Chronic pancreatitis—progressive chronic fibrosis and inflammation of the pancreas, with obstruction of its ducts and destruction of its secreting cells

3. History

   a. Alcoholism

   b. Bacterial or viral infection

   c. Trauma

   d. Complication of mumps

4. Medications—thiazide diuretics, corticosteroids, oral contraceptives

C. Plan/Implementation

1. NPO, gastric decompression

2. Medications—antibiotics, opiods (meperidine avoided because of toxicity), histamine-blockers, proton pump inhibitors

3. Maintain fluid/electrolyte imbalance

4. Respiratory care—ABG, humidified oxygen, intubation, and ventilation

5. Cough and deep breathe q2h

6. Semi-Fowler's position or other position of comfort

7. Monitor for shock and hyperglycemia

8. PN

9. Long-term treatment includes avoidance of alcohol and caffeine; low-fat, bland diet; small, frequent meals

D. Evaluation

1. Is client knowledgeable about dietary restrictions?

2. Has client comfort been maintained?

▶ SYSTEMIC LUPUS ERYTHEMATOSUS (SLE)

A. Assessment

1. Musculoskeletal problems

   a. Polyarthralgia, arthritis, joint swelling

   b. Polymyositis—inflammation of skeletal muscle

2. Dermatological problems

   a. Butterfly rash across bridge of nose and cheeks—characteristic facial sign

   b. Papular rash; erythematous, purpuric lesions

   c. Oral ulcers

   d. Alopecia

3. Cardiopulmonary problems

   a. Pericarditis

   b. Pleural effusion

4. Renal problems
   a. Hematuria
   b. Proteinuria
   c. May end in renal failure
5. CNS problems
   a. Changes in behavior
   b. Psychosis
6. Vascular and lymphatic problems
   a. Papular, erythematous and purpuric lesions on fingertips, toes, forearms and hands
   b. Lymphadenopathy
   c. Raynaud's phenomenon–pain and color changes of extremities during exposure to cold

B. Diagnose

1. Chronic, systemic inflammatory disease of connective tissue that involves skin, joints, serous membranes, kidneys, hematologic system, CNS
2. Exaggerated production of autoantibodies
3. Diagnostic tests–rheumatoid factor (RF), antinuclear antibody (ANA), decreased C3 and C4 complement levels, increased immunoglobulin levels, increased anti-DNA levels, increased C-reactive protein levels
4. Potential nursing diagnosis
   a. Disturbed skin/tissue integrity
   b. Disturbed body image
   c. Fatigue

C. Plan/Implementation

1. Monitor for exacerbations–fever
2. Relieve pain and discomfort, NSAID therapy, acetaminophen
3. Antimalarial (e.g., hydroxychloroquine)
4. Protect skin from ultraviolet rays and sunlight because of photosensitivity, scaly and itchy rash
5. Corticosteroids for exacerbations
6. Immunosuppressive medications (cyclophosphamide, azathioprine)
7. Gamma globulins
8. Plasmapheresis
9. Education and support

D. Evaluation

1. Have complications been avoided?
2. Has client adjusted to living with a chronic disease?

► DERMATOLOGICAL DISORDERS

A. Assessment (see Table 10)

Table 10 SELECTED SKIN DISORDERS		
DISORDER	**ASSESSMENT**	**NURSING CONSIDERATIONS**
Impetigo	Reddish macule becomes honey-colored crusted vesicle, then crust; pruritus Caused by *Staphylococcus, Streptococcus*	Skin isolation: careful handwashing; cover draining lesions; discourage touching lesions Antibiotics—may be topical ointment and/or PO Loosen scabs with Burow's solution compresses; remove gently Restraints if necessary; mitts for infants to prevent secondary infection Monitor for acute glomerulonephritis (complication of untreated impetigo)
Herpes simplex type I	Pruritic vesicular groupings on nose, lips, and oral mucous membranes Chronically recurrent	Spread by direct contact, handwashing; bland, soft foods; mouth rinses with tetracycline- based preparations; avoid direct contact; administer antivirals (acyclovir, famciclovir and valacyclovir)
Herpes zoster	Vesicular eruption along nerve distribution Pain, tenderness, and pruritus over affected region Primarily seen on face, thorax, trunk	Caused by reactivation of chickenpox virus (varicella) Analgesics; compresses, antivirals Systemic corticosteroids to diminish severity Prevent spread—contagious to anyone who has not had chickenpox or who is immunosuppressed Antivirals: Famciclovir, valacyclovir
Scabies	Minute, reddened, itchy lesions Linear burrowing of a mite at finger webs, wrists, elbows, ankles, penis	Reduce itching—topical antipruritic (calamine lotion/topical steroids), permethrin 5% cream or crotamiton 10% Institute skin precautions to prevent spread Scabicide—lindane or crotamiton lotion; apply lotion (not on face) to cool, dry skin (not after hot shower because of potential for increased absorption); leave lindane on for 8-12 hours, then shower off; crotamiton may be applied at bedtime for 2 or more consecutive nights; treat all family members (infants upon recommendation of health care provider) Repeat in 10 days for eggs Launder all clothing and linen after above treatment The rash and itching may last for 2-3 weeks even though the mite has been destroyed; treat with antipruritic
Pediculosis (lice)	Scalp: white eggs (nits) on hair shafts, with itchy scalp Body: macules and papules Pubis: red macules	OTC pyrethrin, permethrin 1%, lindane Kills both lice and nits with one application May suggest to repeat in 7 d—depends on severity
Tinea	Pedis (athlete's foot)—vesicular eruptions in interdigital webs Capitis (ringworm)—breakage and loss of hair; scaly circumscribed red patches on scalp that spread in circular pattern; fluoresces green with Wood's lamp Corporis (ringworm of body)—rings of red scaly areas that spread with central clearing	Antifungal—topical ointment, creams, lotions; PO griseofulvin for resistant cases or if fingernails/toenails are involved; other topical antifungals include butenafine, ciclopirox, econazole, ketoconazole, miconazole, terbinafine Keep areas dry and clean Frequent shampoos

Table 10 SELECTED SKIN DISORDERS *(CONTINUED)*		
DISORDER	**ASSESSMENT**	**NURSING CONSIDERATIONS**
Psoriasis	Chronic recurrent thick, itchy, erythematous papules/plaques covered with silvery white scales with symmetrical distribution Commonly on the scalp, knees, sacrum, elbows, and behind ears Elevated sedimentation rate with negative rheumatoid factor	Topical administration of coal-tar preparations—protect from direct sunlight for 24 h Steroids followed by warm, moist dressings with occlusive outer wrapping (enhances penetration) Tar preparations—may stain skin Antimetabolites (e.g., methotrexate)—check liver function studies Ultraviolet light (wear goggles to protect eyes) Anthralin preparations—apply only to affected areas using tongue blade or gloves Counseling to support/enhance self-image/self-esteem Important for nurse to touch client to demonstrate acceptance
Acne vulgaris	Comedones (blackheads/whiteheads), papules, pustules, cysts occurring most often on the face, neck, shoulders, and back	Good hygiene and nutrition PO tetracycline (advise sunscreen with SPF of 15; avoid sun exposure) Antibacterial medications—azelaic acid, clindamycin, erythromycin Isotretinoin—risk of elevated LFTs, dry skin and fetal damage Drying preparations—Benoxyl/vitamin A may cause redness and peeling early in treatment and photosensitivity Ultraviolet light and surgery Monitor for secondary infection Emotional support Isotretinoin (contraindicated with pregnancy)
Eczema (Atropic dermatitis)	Children: rough, dry, erythematous skin lesions that progress to weeping and crusting; distributed on the cheeks, scalp, and extensor surfaces in infants and on flexor surfaces in children Adults: hard, dry, flaking, scaling on face, upper chest, and antecubital and popliteal fossa	Onset usually in infancy around 2–3 mo; often outgrown by 2–3 y May be precursor of adult asthma or hay fever Elimination from diet of common offenders, especially milk, eggs, wheat, citrus fruits, and tomatoes Eliminate clothing that is irritating (rough/wool) or that promotes sweating; cotton clothing is best Avoid soap and prolonged or hot baths/showers, which tend to be drying; may use warm colloid baths Lotions to affected areas Keep fingernails short and clean; arm restraints/mittens may be necessary Topical steroids Antihistamines

   B. Diagnose—potential nursing diagnoses

     1. Impaired tissue integrity

     2. Acute or chronic pain

     3. Risk for infection

     4. Impaired social interaction

   C. Plan/Implementation (see Table 10)

   D. Evaluation

     1. Has client comfort been maintained?

     2. Has spread of infection been prevented?

▶ PREOPERATIVE CARE

A. Assessment

    1. Stress—vasovagal responses

B. Diagnose

    1. Fears (see Table 1)

Table 1 FEARS OF SURGERY AT DIFFERENT DEVELOPMENTAL STAGES		
AGE GROUP	**SPECIFIC FEARS**	**NURSING CONSIDERATIONS**
Toddler	Separation	Teach parents to expect regression, e.g., in toilet training and difficult separations
Preschooler	Mutilation	Allow child to play with models of equipment Encourage expression of feelings, e.g., anger
School-ager	Loss of control	Explain procedures in simple terms Allow choices when possible
Adolescent	Loss of independence, being different from peers, e.g., alterations in body image	Involve adolescent in procedures and therapies Expect resistance Express understanding of concerns Point out strengths

C. Plan/Implementation

    1. Teaching (see Tables 2 and 3)

        a. Age-appropriate

            1) Toddler—simple directions

            2) Preschool and school-aged—allow to play with equipment

            3) Adolescent—expect resistance

        b. Family-oriented—have parents reinforce teaching

    2. Promote safe environment for hospitalized child

        a. Prevent or minimize the effects of separation on the child

            1) Encourage parental involvement in child's care, especially through rooming-in facilities

            2) Assign the same nurse to care for the child

            3) Provide objects that recreate familiar surroundings (e.g., toys from home)

Table 2 AGE-APPROPRIATE PREPARATION FOR HEALTH-CARE PROCEDURES		
AGE	SPECIAL NEEDS	TYPICAL FEARS
Newborn	Include parents Mummy restraint	Loud noises Sudden movements
6–12 month	Model desired behavior	Strangers, heights
Toddler	Simple explanations Use distractions Allow choices	Separation from parents Animals, strangers Change in environments
Preschooler	Encourage understanding by playing with puppets, dolls Demonstrate equipment Talk at child's eye level	Separation from parents Ghosts Scary people
School-ager	Allow questions Explain why Allow to handle equipment	Dark, injury Being alone Death
Adolescent	Explain long-term benefit Accept regression Provide privacy	Social incompetence War, accidents Death

3. Preparation for surgery
    a. Preoperative checklist
        1) Informed consent
        2) Lab tests, chest x-ray, EKG
        3) Skin prep
        4) Bowel prep
        5) IVs
        6) NPO
        7) Preop meds, sedation, antibiotics
        8) Removal of dentures, jewelry, nail polish
        9) Nutrition—may need PN or tube feedings preoperatively
4. Complementary/Alternative Therapies
    a. Supplements should not be taken near the time of surgery, may interact with anesthesia, may affect coagulation parameters
        1) Echinacea
        2) Garlic
        3) Ginkgo
        4) Ginseng
        5) Kava
        6) St. John's wort
    b. Eliminate all dietary supplements (other than multivitamins) at least 2–3 weeks before surgery
    c. May resume the supplements if health care provider advises

d. What to expect postoperatively

    1) Discuss postoperative procedures—deep breathing, leg exercises, moving in bed, incentive spirometer (sustained maximal inspiration device), equipment to expect postoperatively

    2) Explain importance of reporting pain or discomfort after surgery

    3) Explain pain relieve interventions, e.g., changing position, medication

    4) Provide for growth and development needs of children

Table 3 PREOPERATIVE TEACHING GUIDE
FACTORS FOR NURSE TO ASSESS BEFORE TEACHING
History of illness
Rationale for surgery
Nature of surgery—curative or palliative, minor or major, extent of disfigurement, potential alterations, e.g., ostomies
Factors related to client's readiness for learning—age, mental status, pre-existing knowledge about condition, concerns about condition, family's reaction to need for surgery
CONTENT AREAS TO COVER DURING TEACHING
Elicit client's concerns, e.g., fears about anesthesia
Provide information to clear up misconceptions
Explain preoperative procedures, remove jewelry, nail polish
Lab tests
Skin preparation—cleansing, possibly shaving
Enemas if indicated, e.g., before intestinal surgery
Rationale for withholding food and fluids (NPO)
Preoperative medications, IV line
Teach postoperative procedures—deep breathing, leg exercises, moving in bed, incentive spirometer (sustained maximal inspiration device), equipment to expect postoperatively
Explain importance of reporting pain or discomfort after surgery
Explain what will be done to relieve pain, e.g., changing position, medication
Provide for growth and development needs of children

D. Evaluation

    1. Is the preoperative check list complete?

    2. Is the client able to demonstrate postoperative exercises?

▶ INTRAOPERATIVE CARE

A. Assessment (see Table 4)

B. Diagnose (see Table 4)

Table 4 ANESTHESIA		
MEDICATION	ADVERSE EFFECTS	NURSING CONSIDERATIONS
General anesthesia via inhalation (Halothane)	Respiratory depression, circulatory depression Delirium during induction and recovery Nausea and vomiting, aspiration during induction, myocardial depression, hepatic toxicity	Check history of sensitization Maintain airway Protect and orient client Monitor vital signs, labs Prevent aspiration postop by elevating head of bed, turning head to side (unless contraindicated)
Nitrous oxide	Hypotension, postop nausea and vomiting	Monitor vital signs Adequate oxygenation is essential, especially during emergence
IV thiopental sodium	Respiratory depression, low BP, laryngospasm Poor muscle relaxation, hypotension, irritating to skin and subcutaneous tissue	Monitor vital signs, especially airway, breathing Straps for operative table, proper positioning Protect IV site, check for placement periodically
Spinal anesthesia Saddle	Hypotension, headache	Monitor vital signs Encourage oral fluids
Conduction blocks Epidural Caudal	Hypotension, respiratory depression	Headache not experienced Monitor vital signs
Local anesthesia Lidocaine hydrochloride	Excitability, toxic reactions such as respiratory difficulties, vasoconstriction if substance contains epinephrine	Monitor client Do not use local anesthesia with epinephrine on fingers (circulation is less optimal)
Moderate sedation Midazolam Diazepam	Respiratory depression, apnea, hypotension, bradycardia	Never leave the client alone Constantly monitor airway, level of consciousness, pulse oximetry, ECG Vital signs every 15–30 minutes Assess client's ability to maintain patent airway and respond to verbal commands

C. Plan/Implementation

    1. Monitor effects of anesthesia postinduction

    2. Continuously monitor vital signs

    3. Aseptic technique

    4. Appropriate grounding devices

    5. Fluid balance

    6. Perform sponge/instrument count

D. Potential complications

    1. Nausea and vomiting

    2. Hypoxia

3. Hypothermia

4. Malignant hyperthermia—inherited muscle disorder chemically induced by anesthesia; stop surgery, treated with 100% oxygen, skeletal muscle relaxant, sodium bicarbonate

E. Evaluation

1. Are client's vital signs stable?

2. Has the client's fluid balance been maintained?

▶ POSTOPERATIVE CARE

A. Assessment

1. Anesthesia, immobility, and surgery can affect any system in the body

2. Full systems assessment required

B. Diagnose

1. Neuropsychosocial

   a. Stimulate client postanesthesia

   b. Monitor level of consciousness

2. Cardiovascular

   a. Monitor vital signs q 15 min × 4, q 30 min × 2, q 1 hour × 2, then as needed

   b. Monitor I and O

   c. Check potassium level

   d. Monitor CVP

3. Respiratory

   a. Check breath sounds

   b. Turn, cough, and deep breathe (unless contraindicated, e.g., brain, spinal, eye surgery)

   c. Assess pain level—use verbal or visual scale, offer pain medication

   d. Teach how to use incentive spirometer—hold mouthpiece in mouth, exhale normally, seal lips and inhale slowly and deeply, keep ballsor cylinder elevated 2–3 seconds, exhale and repeat

   e. Teach how to use client-controlled analgesia (PCA)

   f. Get out of bed as soon as possible

4. Gastrointestinal

   a. Check bowel sounds in 4 quadrants for 5 minutes (high-pitched tympany is abnormal)

   b. Keep NPO until bowel sounds are present

   c. Provide good mouth care while NPO

   d. Provide antiemetics for nausea and vomiting

   e. Check abdomen for distention

   f. Check for passage of flatus and stool

5. Genitourinary
    a. Monitor I and O
    b. Encourage to void
    c. Notify health care provider if unable to void within 8 hours
    d. Catheterize if needed
6. Extremities
    a. Check pulses
    b. Assess color, edema, temperature
    c. Inform client not to cross legs
    d. Keep knee gatch flat
    e. Prohibit use of pillows behind knee
    f. Apply antiembolic stockings (TED hose) before getting out of bed
    g. Pneumatic compression devices (Venodynes)
    h. Assess for pain, swelling, and warmth in the distal extremity
7. Wounds
    a. Dressing
        1) Document amount and character of drainage
        2) Health care provider changes first postop dressing
        3) Use aseptic technique
        4) Note presence of drains
    b. Incision
        1) Assess site (e.g,. edematous, inflamed, excoriated)
        2) Assess drainage (e.g., serous, serosanguineous, purulent)
        3) Note type of sutures
        4) Note if edges of wound are well approximated
        5) Anticipate infection 3–5 days postop
        6) Debride wound, if needed, to reduce inflammation
        7) Change dressing frequently to prevent skin breakdown around site and minimize bacterial growth
8. Drains—prevent fluids from accumulating in tissues
9. GI tubes—check placement
    a. Upper GI tubes—used for gastric decompression
    b. Lower GI tubes—used to decompress bowel
10. Potential complications (see Table 5)

Table 5 POTENTIAL COMPLICATIONS OF SURGERY		
COMPLICATION	ASSESSMENT	NURSING CONSIDERATIONS
Hemorrhage	Decreased BP, increased pulse Cold, clammy skin	Replace blood volume Monitor vital signs
Shock	Decreased BP, increased pulse Cold, clammy skin	Treat cause Oxygen IV fluids

Table 5 POTENTIAL COMPLICATIONS OF SURGERY (CONTINUED)		
COMPLICATION	ASSESSMENT	NURSING CONSIDERATIONS
Atelectasis and pneumonia	Dyspnea, cyanosis, cough Tachycardia Elevated temperature Pain on affected side	Experienced second day postop Suctioning Postural drainage Antibiotics Cough and turn
Embolism	Dyspnea, pain, hemoptysis Restlessness ABG—low O_2, high CO_2	Experienced second day postop Oxygen Anticoagulants (heparin) IV fluids
Venous Thromboembolism	Positive ultrasound	Experienced 6–14 days up to 1 year later Anticoagulant therapy
Paralytic ileus	Absent bowel sounds, no flatus or stool	Nasogastric suction IV fluids Decompression tubes
Infection of wound	Elevated WBC and temperature Positive cultures	Experienced 3–5 days postop Antibiotics, aseptic technique Good nutrition
Dehiscence	Disruption of surgical incision or wound	Experienced 5–6 days postop Low Fowler's position, no coughing NPO Notify health care provider
Evisceration	Protrusion of wound contents	Experienced 5–6 days postop Low Fowler's position, no coughing NPO Cover viscera with sterile saline dressing or wax paper (if at home) Notify health care provider
Urinary retention	Unable to void after surgery Bladder distension	Experienced 8–12 hours postop Catheterize as needed
Urinary infection	Foul-smelling urine Elevated WBC	Experienced 5–8 days postop Antibiotics Force fluids
Psychosis	Inappropriate affect	Therapeutic communication Medication

▶ **BLOOD TESTS**

Table 1 LABORATORY TESTS			
TEST	PURPOSE/PREPARATION	CONVENTIONAL VALUES	SI;(INTERNATIONAL SYSTEM OF UNITS)
Red blood cell count (RBC), erythrocytes	Determines actual number of cells in relation to volume	Adult man—4.6–6.2 million/mm^3 Adult woman—4.2–5.4 million/mm^3 Child—3.2–5.2 million/mm^3	Adult man 4.6–6.2 x10^{12}/L Adult woman 4.2–5.4 x 10^{12}/L Child 3.2–5.2 x 10^{12}/L
White blood cell count (WBC), leukocytes	Establishes amount and maturity of white blood cell elements	Adult—4,500–11,000/mm^3 Child—5,000–13,000/mm^3	
Hemoglobin	Determines the amount of hemoglobin/100 mL of blood	Man—13–18 g/dL Woman—12–16 g/dL Child (3–12 years)—11–12.5 g/dL	Man 130–180g/L Woman 120–160 g/L Child (3–12 years) 110–125 g/L
Hematocrit	Measures percentage of red blood cells per fluid volume of blood	Man—42–52% Woman—35–47% Child (3–12 years)—35–45%	Man 0.42–0.52 Woman 0.35–0.47 Child (3–12 yrs) 0.35–0.45
Bleeding time	Measures duration of bleeding after standardized skin incision Used for preoperative screening	1.5–9.5 minutes	
Partial thromboplastin time (PTT)	Monitors effectiveness of heparin therapy Detects coagulation disorders	Lower limit of normal: 20–25 sec Upper limit of normal: 32–39 sec	
Platelet count (thrombocyte count)	Used to diagnose hemorrhagic diseases, thrombocytopenia	150,000–450,000/mm^3	150–450 x 10^9/L
Prothrombin time (PT)	Monitors effectiveness of warfarin therapy Detects coagulation disorders	9.5–12.0 seconds	
International normalized ratio (INR)	Monitors effectiveness of anticoagulation therapy	1.0 2–3 for therapy in atrial fibrillation, deep venous thrombosis, and pulmonary embolism 2.5–3.5 for therapy in prosthetic heart valves	
Sedimentation rate (ESR)	Speed at which RBCs settle in well-mixed venous blood Indicates inflammation	Man less than 50 yrs: less than 15 mm/h Man greater than 50 yrs: less than 20 mm/h Woman less than 50 yrs: less than 25 mm/h Woman greater than 50 yrs: less than 30 mm/h	

Table 1 LABORATORY TESTS *(CONTINUED)*			
TEST	PURPOSE/PREPARATION	CONVENTIONAL VALUES	SI;(INTERNATIONAL SYSTEM OF UNITS)
Glucose tolerance test (GTT)	Measures ability of body to secrete insulin in response to hyperglycemia	Fasting–60-110 mg/dL 1 hour–190 mg/dL 2 hours–140 mg/dL 3 hours–125 mg/dL	Fasting 3.3–6.1 mmol/L 1 hour 10.5 mmol/L 2 hours 7.8 mmol/L 3 hours 6.9 mmol/L
Total cholesterol	Evaluates tendency for athlerosclerosis Overnight fast	150–200 mg/dL	3.9–5.2 mmol/L
Low-density lipoproteins (LDL)	Determines whether elevated cholesterol levels are caused by increased LDL or HDL Fast for 12–14 hours	Less than 160 mg/dL if no CAD and less than 2 risk factors Less than 130 mg/dL if no CAD and 2 or more risk factors Less than 100 mg/dL if CAD present	Less than 4.1 mmol/L Less than 3.3 mmol/L Less than 2.6 mmol/L
High-density lipoproteins (HDL)	Same as for LDLs, above	Men 35–70 mg/dL, Women 35–85 mg/dL	Men 0.91–1.8 mmol/L Women 0.91–2.2 mmol/L
Creatinine (CR)	Test of renal function NPO 8 hours List medications client is taking on lab slip	Adult–0.7–1.4 mg/dL Child–0.4–1.2 mg/dl Infant–0.3–0.6 mg/dL	Adult 62–124 µmol/L Child 35–106 µmol/L Infant 27–53 µmol/L
Alkaline phosphatase	Evaluates liver and bone function NPO 8–12 hours List medications client is taking on lab slip	Adult–50–120 units/L Infant and adolescent up to 104 FU/L	
Creatine kinase (CK)	Used to diagnose acute MI Detected in blood in 3–5 hours	MM bands present = skeletal muscle damage MB bands present = heart muscle damage	
Serum albumin	Used to detect protein malnutrition	3.5–5.5 g/dL	35–55 g/L
BUN	Evaluate renal function	Values affected by protein intake, tissue breakdown, fluid volume changes 10–20 mg/dL	3.6–7.1 mmol/L
Triglycerides	Detect risk for atherosclerosis	100–200 mg/dL	1.13–2.26 mmol/L
Alanine aminotransferase (ALT)	Increase liver disease, hepatitis	10–40 units (males)	
Aspartate aminotransferase	Increase liver disease, hepatitis	10–40 units (males)	

▶ **ARTERIAL TESTS**

Table 2 ARTERIAL DIAGNOSTIC TESTS			
TEST	PURPOSE	PREPARATION/TESTING	POST–TEST NURSING CARE
Oscillometry	Abnormal findings help to pinpoint the level of arterial occlusion	Alterations in pulse volume are measured by placing a pneumatic cuff around the extremity at different levels, attached to a monitor	None
Skin temperature studies	Coldness of one or both extremities at normal room temperature implies poor circulation	Palpate and compare skin warmth or coolness in opposing limbs Use direct-reading skin temperature thermometer Immerse one extremity in warm water, and observe for rise in skin temperature in the other extremity, which should normally follow because of reflex vasodilation Place a hot water bottle on the client's abdomen and observe extremities for reflex rise in skin temperature	None
Angiography (arteriography)	Indicates abnormalities of blood flow due to arterial obstruction or narrowing	Contrast dye is injected into the arteries and x-ray films are taken of the vascular tree	Disadvantages include potential allergic reactions to radiopaque dye, potential irritation, or thrombosis of the injection site
Exercise tests for intermittent claudication	Claudication with exercise indicates inability of damaged arteries to increase the blood flow needed for increased tissue oxygenation	Client exercises until pain occurs; the length of time between start of exercise and the onset of pain is recorded	None
Lumbar sympathetic block	Decreased limb pain and increased temperature indicate sympathectomy could improve circulation to the extremities	Local anesthetic is injected into sympathetic ganglia, temporarily blocking the sympathetic vasomotor nerve fibers supplying an ischemic limb	Shock due to movement of blood from vital organs to peripheral vessels

▶ VENOUS TESTS

Table 3 VENOUS DIAGNOSTIC TESTS			
TEST	PURPOSE	PREPARATION/TESTING	POST-TEST NURSING CARE
Phlebography	Lack of filling of a vein is indicative of venous occlusion due to a thrombus	Thrombi are identified as radiolucent areas in opaque-filled veins	None
Venous pressure measurements	Significant only in early stages of thrombophlebitis before collateral veins develop	Venous occlusion in one leg causes venous pressure to be higher in other leg	None
Isotope studies	Helpful in diagnosing early formation of thrombi	Fibrinogen labeled with radioactive iodine molecules make up a clot along with naturally occurring fibrinogen Radioactivity counts are increased over thrombi	None
Ultrasonic flow detection—Doppler studies	Indicates obstruction in blood flow in extremities	Electronic stethoscope that detects sound of blood flow	None

▶ RESPIRATORY/CARDIAC TESTS

Table 4 RESPIRATORY/CARDIAC TESTS			
TEST	PURPOSE	PREPARATION/TESTING	POST-TEST NURSING CARE
Pulmonary function	Detects impaired pulmonary function Follows the course of pulmonary disease and evaluates treatment responses	Explain purpose No smoking 4 hours before test May withhold bronchodilator medications Asked to breathe into machine	Observe for dyspnea
Arterial blood gases (ABGs)	Measurements of tissue oxygenation, carbon dioxide removal, and acid-base balance pO_2—partial pressure oxygen pCO_2—partial pressure carbon dioxide Evaluates clients being mechanically ventilated or with cardiovascular disease	Perform Allen test—checks collateral circulation Arterial blood is obtained in heparinized syringe Unclotted blood is necessary Air bubbles cannot be present in specimen Results (see Table 5)	Apply pressure to site for 5 minutes to prevent hematoma (15 minutes if client is receiving anticoagulants) Send specimen on ice and occlude needle to avoid air in syringe Note on lab slip if client was breathing room air or oxygen (document liters) Check arm for swelling, discoloration, pain, numbness, tingling
Lung scan (VQ scan)	Evaluates pulmonary perfusion when pulmonary infarction or space-occupying disorders are suspected	Perfusion scan—intravenous injection of iodinated radioactive dye Significance—high level of radioactivity in areas of good perfusion; low levels of radioactivity in obstructed areas Ventilation scan—radioactive gas inhaled, should be equal distribution of gas	None

Table 4 RESPIRATORY/CARDIAC TESTS *(CONTINUED)*			
TEST	**PURPOSE**	**PREPARATION/TESTING**	**POST–TEST NURSING CARE**
Sputum analysis	Identify cause of pulmonary infection Identify abnormal lung cells	Encourage fluid intake night before test Instruct client to rinse mouth with water Do not brush teeth, eat, or use mouthwash before test Use sterile container Ultrasonic/heated nebulizer treatment 10-15 minutes prior aids in collection Teach client how to expectorate Collect early in the AM if possible	None
Bronchoscopy	Allows visualization of larynx, trachea, and mainstem bronchi Possible to obtain tissue biopsy, apply medication, aspirate secretions for laboratory examination, aspirate a mucus plug causing airway obstruction, or remove aspirated foreign objects	Explain procedure Maintain NPO for 6 hours before test Inspect mouth for infection Administer premedication—diazepam, midazolam, meperidine, atropine Remove dentures Prepare client for sore throat after procedure	Sit or lie on side, remain NPO until gag reflex returns Observe for respiratory difficulties
Thoracentesis	Aspiration of fluid or air from pleural space To obtain specimen for analysis, relieve lung compression, obtain lung tissue for biopsy, or instill medications into pleural space	Explain procedure Take vital signs Shave area around needle insertion site Position client sitting with arms on pillows on over-bed table or lying on side in bed Expect stinging sensation with injection of local anesthetic and feeling of pressure when needle inserted No more than 1,000 mL fluid removed at one time	Auscultate breath sounds frequently Monitor vital signs frequently Check for leakage of fluid, location of puncture site, client tolerance Sterile dressing after procedure
Chest x-ray	To identify abnormalities such as foreign bodies, fluid, infiltrates, tumors	Explain procedure Remove all jewelry from neck and chest Female clients of childbearing age wear a lead apron	None
Lung biopsy	Removal of lung tissue for culture or cytology	Explain procedure Administer premedication—sedatives or analgesics Have client hold breath in midexpiration Performed with fluoroscopic monitoring Position client as for thoracentesis	Monitor vital signs and breath sounds every 4 hours for 24 hours Report signs of respiratory distress Chest x-ray taken after procedure to check for complication of pneumothorax Sterile dressing applied after procedure
Computed tomography (CT)	Provides three-dimensional assessment of the lungs and thorax	Noninvasive	If dye, assess reaction

Table 4 RESPIRATORY/CARDIAC TESTS *(CONTINUED)*			
TEST	**PURPOSE**	**PREPARATION/TESTING**	**POST-TEST NURSING CARE**
Magnetic resonance imaging (MRI)	Provides detailed pictures of body structures	Explain procedure Assess the client for claustrophobia Remove all metal jewelry and metal objects Ask if client has metal implanted in body (pacemaker, clips)	None
Angiography	Evaluates specific areas of the arterial system	Explain procedure Remove all jewelry Client may experience nausea, flushing, warmth, salty taste with injection of dye	Assess for hematoma Assess distal pulses Compare skin temperature, color, sensation in both extremities Check vital signs frequently Notify health care provider if bleeding or change in vital signs occurs
Pulse oximetry	Measures oxygen saturation through the skin	Clean site using cotton ball with soap and water, then alcohol Dry skin	Rotate site every 4 hours to prevent skin irritation
Stress test	Assess cardiovascular response to increased workload	Client walks on treadmill, pedals stationary bicycle, or climbs set of stairs EKG monitored before, during, and after exercise testing	None
Ultrasound echocar-diogram	Noninvasive sound waves used to determine cardiac structures	None	None
Cardiac catheterization	Usually used with angiography Introduction of catheter into chambers of heart to evaluate ventricular function and obtain chamber pressures	NPO 8–12 hours Signed permit Empty bladder Check pulse Explain that client may experience feeling of heat, palpitations, desire to cough when dye injected	Monitor vital signs q 15 min for 2 hours, then q 30 min for 1 hour, then q 1 hour for 3 hours Check pulses, sensation, bleeding at insertion site q 30 min for 3 hours, then q 1 hour for 3 hours Bedrest 6–8 hours with insertion site extremity straight

Table 5 ARTERIAL BLOOD GASES (ABG)			
VALUE	**NORMAL**	**ACIDOSIS**	**ALKALOSIS**
pH	7.35–7.45	Below 7.35	Above 7.45
PaO_2	85–95 mm Hg		
SaO_2	95–99%		
$PaCO_2$	35–45 mm Hg	Respiratory greater than 45 mm Hg	Respiratory less than 35mm Hg
HCO_3	22–26 mEq/L	Metabolic less than 22 mEq/L	Metabolic greater than 26 mEq/L

▶ **NEUROLOGICAL TESTS**

Table 6 NEUROLOGICAL TESTS			
TEST	PURPOSE	PREPARATION/TESTING	POST-TEST NURSING CARE
Cerebral angiography	Indentifies aneurysms, vascular malformations, narrowed vessels	Informed consent Explain procedure: Lie flat; dye injection into femoral artery by needle/ catheter; fluoroscopy and radiologic films taken after injection Well hydrated Preprocedure sedation Skin prep, chosen site shaved Mark peripheral pulses May experience feeling of warmth and metallic taste when dye injected	Neurological assessment every 15–30 minutes until vital signs are stable Keep flat in bed 12–14 hours Check puncture site every hour Immobilize site for 6–8 hours Assess distal pulses, color, and temperature Observe symptons of complications, allergic response to dye, puncture site hematoma Force fluids, accurate intake and output
Lumbar puncture (LP)	Insertion of needle into subarachnoid space to obtain specimen, relieve pressure, inject dye or medications	Explain procedure Informed consent Procedure done at bedside or in treatment room Positioned in lateral recumbent fetal position at edge of bed	Neurological assessment every 15–30 minutes until stable Position flat for several hours Encourage PO fluid to 3,000 mL Oral analgesics for headache Observe sterile dressing at insertion site for bleeding or drainage
Electroencephalogram (EEG)	Records electrical activity of brain	Explain procedure Procedure done by technician in a quiet room Painless Tranquilizer and stimulant medications withheld for 24–48 hours pre-EEG Stimulants such as caffeine, cola, and tea, cigarettes withheld for 24 hours pre-EEG May be asked to hyperventilate 3–4 minutes and watch bright, flashing light Meals not withheld Kept awake night before test	Help client remove paste from hair Administer prescribed medication withheld before EEG Observe for seizure activity in seizure-prone clients
Echoencephalography	Evaluates brain structure through sound waves	Explain procedure–hand-held transducer used to record sound waves	None
CT (computed tomography)	Detects hemorrhage, infarction, abscesses, tumors	Informed consent Explain procedure Painless Immobile during exam If contrast dye used, may experience flushed, warm face, and metallic taste during injection	Assess for allergic responses to contrast dye (e.g., rash, pruritus, urticaria) Encourage PO fluids

Table 6 NEUROLOGICAL TESTS *(CONTINUED)*			
TEST	**PURPOSE**	**PREPARATION/TESTING**	**POST–TEST NURSING CARE**
Myelogram	Visualizes spinal column and subarachnoid space	Informed consent Explain procedure NPO for 4–6 hours before test Obtain allergy history Phenothiazines, CNS depressants, and stimulants withheld for 48 h prior to test Table will be moved to various positions during test	Neurologic assessment every 2–4 hours When metrizamide water-soluble dye used, head should be raised 30-45° for 3 hours Oral analgesics for headache Encourage PO fluids Assess for distended bladder Inspect injection site Assess for allergic responses to contrast dye (e.g., rash, pruritus, urticaria)
PET (positron emission tomography)	Used to assess metabolic and physio-logical function of brain; diagnose stroke, brain tumor, epilepsy, Parkinson's disease, head injury	Client inhales or is injected with radioactive substance, then is scanned Tell client may experience dizziness, headache Teach relaxation exercises	None

▶ LIVER FUNCTION TESTS

Table 7 LIVER FUNCTION TESTS			
TEST	**PURPOSE**	**PREPARATION/TESTING**	**POST–TEST NURSING CARE**
Pigment studies	Parameters of hepatic ability to conjugate and excrete bilirubin Abnormal in liver and gall bladder disorders, e.g., with jaundice Direct bilirubin increases in obstruction	Fast 4 h Normal Serum bilirubin, direct 0.1–0.4 mg/dL (1.7–3.1 mcmol/L) Serum bilirubin, total 0.3–1 mg/dL (5–17 mcmol/L) Urine bilirubin, total 0	Over 70% of the parenchyma of the liver may be damaged before liver function tests become abnormal
Protein studies Serum albumin	Proteins are produced by the liver Levels may diminish in hepatic disease Severely decreased serum albumin results in generalized edema	Normal 3.5–5.5 g/dL (35–55 g/L)	None
Coagulation studies Prothrombin time (PT) Partial thrombo-plastin time (PTT)	May be prolonged in hepatic disease In liver disease, PTT prolonged due to lack of vitamin K	Normal PT 9.5–12.0 seconds PTT Lower limit of normal 20–25 seconds; upper limit of normal 32–39 seconds	Put specimen in ice Apply pressure to site for 5 min (15 min if on anticoagulants)
Liver enzymes	With damaged liver cells, enzymes are released into bloodstream	Normal AST 10–40 units (males) ALT 10–40 units (males) LDH 90–176 units/L	None

Table 7	LIVER FUNCTION TESTS *(CONTINUED)*		
TEST	**PURPOSE**	**PREPARATION/TESTING**	**POST-TEST NURSING CARE**
Blood ammonia (arterial)	Liver converts ammonia to urea With liver disease, ammonia levels rise	Normal 15–45 mcg/dL (11–32 mcmol/L)	None
Abdominal X-ray	To determine gross liver size	None	None
Liver scan	To demonstrate size, shape of liver, visualize scar tissue, cysts, or tumors; use radiopaque dye	None	Question client about seafood (iodine) allergy before radiopaque dye administration; anaphylaxis common, aqueous-based dye available for hypersensitive individuals Resume diet
Cholecystogram and cholangiography	For gallbladder and bile duct visualization; radiopaque material injected directly into biliary tree	Fat-free dinner evening before exam Ingestion of dye in tablet form (Telepaque tablets—check history of allergies to iodine) evening before NPO after dye ingestion X-rays followed by ingestion of high-fat meal followed by further x-rays	Question client about seafood (iodine) allergy
Celiac axis arteriography	For liver and pancreas visualization; uses contrast media of organic iodine	None	Question client about seafood (iodine) allergy prior to radiopaque dye administration; anaphylaxis common
Splenoportogram (splenic portal venography)	To determine adequacy of portal blood flow; uses contrast media of organic iodine	None	Question client about seafood (iodine) allergy prior to radiopaque dye administration; anaphylaxis common
Liver biopsy	Sampling of tissue by needle aspiration	Administer vitamin K IM to decrease chance of hemorrhage NPO morning of exam (6 h) Sedative administration just before exam Teach client that he will be asked to hold his breath for 5–10 seconds Performed at bedside, supine position, lateral with upper arms elevated	Position on right side for 2–3 h with pillow under costal margin Frequent vital signs to detect hemorrhage and shock; check clotting time, platelets, hematocrit Expect mild local pain and mild pain radiating to right shoulder Client reports of severe abdominal pain immediately—may be indication of perforation of bile duct and peritonitis Avoid heavy lifting for 1 week
Bilirubin	Detect presence of bilirubin due to hemolytic or liver disease	Total bilirubin 0.3–1.0 mg/dL (5–17 mcmol/L) Direct (conjugated) bilirubin 0.1–0.4 mg/dL (1.7–3.7 mcmol/L) Indirect (unconjugated) bilirubin 0.2–0.6 mg/dL (3.4–11.2 mcmol/L)	None

▶ GASTROINTESTINAL TESTS

Table 8 GASTROINTESTINAL DIAGNOSTIC TESTS			
TEST	PURPOSE	PREPARATION/TESTING	POST–TEST NURSING CARE
Stomach/esophagus endoscopy	Visualization of esophagus and/or stomach by means of a lighted, flexible fiberoptic tube introduced through the mouth to the stomach to determine presence of ulcerations, tumors, or to obtain tissue or fluid samples	Verify that informed consent from client has been obtained Maintain NPO before procedure (at least 8 h) Teach client about numbness in throat due to local anesthetic applied to posterior pharynx by spray or gargle	Maintain NPO until gag reflex returns Observe for vomiting of blood, respiratory distress Inform client to expect sore throat for 3 to 4 days after procedure
Sigmoidoscopy/ Proctoscopy	Direct visualization of the sigmoid colon, rectum, and anal canal	Laxative night before exam and enema or suppository morning of procedure NPO at midnight	Allow client to rest Observe for hemorrhage, perforation Encourage fluids
Colonoscopy	Direct visualization of the colon; used as a diagnostic aid; removes foreign bodies, polyps, or tissue for biopsy	Clear liquid diet 24–72 h before exam (per health care provider order) Cathartic in evening for 2 days prior to exam Enema on morning of exam polyethelene glycol solution to cleanse bowel; clear liquid diet noon day before test	Allow to rest Observe for passage of blood and abdominal pain, signs of perforation, hemorrhage, or respiratory distress Follow-up x-rays Resume diet
Ammonia	Detect liver disorders	Normal 15–45 mcg/dL (11–32 mcmol/L) Avoid smoking before test	None
Amylase	Diagnose pancreatitis and acute cholecystitis	Normal 6–160 Somogyi U/dL Restrict food 1–2 hours before test Avoid opiates 2 hours before test	None
Lipase	Diagnose acute and chronic pancreatitis, biliary obstruction, hepatitis, cirrhosis	Normal less than 200 U/mL NPO 8–12 hrs before test Avoid opiates 24 hrs prior to test	None
Gastric aspirate	Aspiration of gastric contents to evaluate for presence of abnormal constituents such as blood, abnormal bacteria, abnormal pH, or malignant cells	NPO before test NG tube passed, stomach contents aspirated and sent for evaluation Histamine is sometimes used to stimulate hydrochloric acid secretion pH—measures acid/alkaline range; (4.5–7.5); normal gastric pH less than 4; generally overly acidic environment can lead to ulcerative activity Guaiac—tests for presence of blood; normally, blood absent	Encourage fluids
Upper GI series Barium swallow	Ingestion of barium sulfate to determine patency and size of esophagus, size and condition of gastric walls, patency of pyloric valve, and rate of passage to small bowel	Maintain NPO after midnight Inform client that stool will be light-colored after proccdure	Encourage fluids Laxatives to prevent consti-pation Stool will be white from barium

Table 8 GASTROINTESTINAL DIAGNOSTIC TESTS *(CONTINUED)*			
TEST	**PURPOSE**	**PREPARATION/TESTING**	**POST–TEST NURSING CARE**
Lower GI series Barium enema	Instillation of barium (radiopaque substance) into colon via rectum for fluoroscopy x-rays to view tumors, polyps, strictures, ulcerations, inflammation, or obstructions of colon	Low-residue diet for 1–2 days Clear liquid diet and laxative evening before test; cleansing enemas until clear morning of test	Cleansing enemas after exam to remove barium and prevent impaction X-rays may be repeated after all barium is expelled
Paracentesis	Needle aspiration of fluid in abdominal cavity used for diagnostic examination of ascitic fluid and treatment of massive ascites resistant to other therapies	Done at bedside—client in semi-Fowler's position or sitting upright on edge of bed Empty bladder prior to procedure to avoid accidental perforation	Check vital signs frequently for shock and/or infection Report elevated temperature and/or abdominal pain to health care provider Observe for sign of hypovolemic shock

▶ REPRODUCTIVE TESTS

Table 9 REPRODUCTIVE TESTS AND PROCEDURES			
TEST	**PURPOSE**	**PREPARATION/TESTING**	**POST–TEST NURSING CARE**
Culdoscopy	Visualization of ovaries, fallopian tubes, uterus via lighted tube inserted into vagina and through cul-de-sac	Local anesthetic and/or light sedation Knee-chest position during procedure	Position on abdomen after procedure Observe for vaginal bleeding Avoid douching and intercourse for 2 weeks
Colposcopy	Similar to pelvic exam	Performed between menstrual periods Takes 20 minutes Lithotomy position Cervix is washed with dilute acetic acid	None
Laparoscopy	Visualization of pelvic cavity through an incision beneath the umbilicus to view structures	Carbon dioxide introduced to enhance visualization General anesthesia Foley catheter inserted for bladder decompression	Out of bed after procedure Regular diet
Cultures and smears	Samples of tissues are taken to identify infectious processes or identify abnormal cells	No anesthetic needed Chlamydia smear needs media preparation by laboratory	None
Cervical biopsy	Sample tissue taken to identify unusual cells	No anesthesia used May have cramping sensation	Provide written instructions Restrictions on intercourse, douching, and swimming for 3 days

▶ **URINARY SYSTEM TESTS**

Table 10 URINARY SYSTEM DIAGNOSTIC TESTS			
TEST	**PURPOSE**	**PREPARATION/TESTING**	**POST–TEST NURSING CARE**
Urinalysis	Detect kidney abnormalities	Advise client to save first am specimen Overnight specimen is more concentrated pH 4.5–8 Specific gravity 1.010–1.030	None
Urine culture and sensitivity	Identify bacteria in urine	Cleanse external meatus with povidone-iodine or soap and water before test Obtain midstream specimen Normal—less than 100,000 colonies/mL	None
Cystometrogram	Test of muscle tone	Prepare client for Foley catheter Instillation of saline may cause feeling of pressure in bladder during test	Advise client to report any post-test symptoms
Creatinine clearance	Evaluate renal function	24-hour urine collection Blood drawn for creatinine level at end of urine collection Normal—1.42–2.08 mL/min (males)	None
BUN	Evaluate renal function	Values affected by protein intake, tissue breakdown, fluid volume changes 10–20 mg/dL (3.6–7.1 mmol/L)	None
Cystoscopy	Direct visualization by cystoscope of bladder and urethra	Bowel preparation Teach client to deep-breathe to decrease discomfort NPO if general anesthesia used	Monitor character and volume of urine Check for abdominal distention, urinary frequency, fever Urine usually pink-tinged Abdominal or pelvic pain indicates trauma Provide antimicrobial prophylaxis
Cystourethrogram	X-ray study of bladder and urethra	Explain procedure to client: catheter inserted into urethra, radiopaque dye injected, client voids, x-rays taken during voiding	Advise client to report any symptoms
Intravenous pyelogram	Provides x-ray visualization of kidneys, ureters, and bladder	Bowel preparation NPO after midnight Check allergies to shellfish or iodine, chocolate, eggs, milk Burning or reports of salty taste may occur during injection of radiopaque dye into vein X-rays are taken at intervals after dye injection	Post procedure x-rays usually done Client should be alert to signs of dye reaction: edema, itching, wheezing, dyspnea
Renal scan	Evaluation of kidneys	Radioactive isotope injected IV Radioactivity measured by radioactivity counter Fluids forced before procedure	None

Table 10 URINARY SYSTEM DIAGNOSTIC TESTS *(CONTINUED)*			
TEST	PURPOSE	PREPARATION/TESTING	POST-TEST NURSING CARE
Ultrasound	Images of renal structures obtained by sound waves	Noninvasive procedure No preparation required Full bladder required	None
Kidney biopsy	Kidney tissue obtained by needle aspiration for pathological evaluation	NPO 6–8 hours X-ray taken prior to procedure Skin is marked to indicate lower pole of kidney (fewer blood vessels) Position: prone Client instructed to hold breath during needle insertion	Pressure applied to site for 20 minutes Keep on affected side for 30-60 minutes Pressure dressing applied Check vital signs q 15–15 min for 1 h Client kept flat in bed Bedrest for 6–8 hours Intake 3,000/day Observe for hematuria and site bleeding
Schilling test	Diagnoses vitamin B_{12} deficiency (pernicious anemia)	Radioactive vitamin B_{12} is administered to the client Low value excreted in urine indicates pernicious anemia, (normal is greater than 10% of dose excreted in 24 hours)	Vitamin B_{12} (cyancobalamin injection for life)

THERAPEUTIC PROCEDURES *Unit 5*

▶ CHEST PHYSIOTHERAPY

A. Breathing exercises
   1. Diaphragmatic or abdominal breathing
      a. Client positioned on back with knees bent
      b. Place hands on abdomen
   2. Pursed lip breathing
      a. Breathe in through nose
      b. Purse lips and breathe out through mouth
      c. Exhalation should be twice as long as inspiration

B. Coughing techniques
   1. Instruct client to lean slightly forward and take three slow, deep breaths though the nose, exhaling slowly through slightly parted or pursed lips
   2. Client should then take another deep breath and cough several times during expiration
   3. Client must be encouraged to cough from deep within the chest and avoid nonproductive coughing that wastes energy

C. Postural drainage—uses gravity to facilitate removal of bronchial secretions
   1. Client is placed in a variety of positions to facilitate drainage into larger airways
   2. Five positions used—head down, prone, right and left lateral, upright
   3. Stay in each position 10–15 minutes
   4. Breathe in slowly through nose; breathe out through pursed lips
   5. Performed 2–4 times daily before meals and at hs
   6. Secretions may be removed by coughing or suctioning

D. Percussion and vibration—usually performed during postural drainage to augment the effect of gravity drainage
   1. Percussion—rhythmic striking of chest wall with cupped hands over areas where secretions are retained
   2. Vibration—hand and arm muscles of person doing vibration are tensed, and a vibrating pressure is applied to the chest as the client exhales
   3. Place towel over area
   4. Percussion alternated with vibration, 5 min in each position

E. Incentive spirometer—used to maximize respiration and mobilize secretions
   1. Client must inhale deeply and hold breath for 3–5 seconds to achieve effective lung expansion
   2. Client must form seal around mouthpiece with lips
   3. Sitting in semi-Fowler's position
   4. Do 10 breaths/h while awake

▶ SUCTIONING

A. Procedure

1. Wear protective eyewear

2. Hyperoxygenate before, during, and after suctioning—100% oxygen for 3 minutes or 3 deep breaths

3. Explain procedure to client (potentially frightening procedure)

4. Semi-Fowler's position

5. Lubricate catheter with sterile saline and insert without applying suction

6. Advance catheter as far as possible or until client coughs; do not apply suction

7. Withdraw catheter 1–2 cm, apply suction and withdraw catheter with a rotating motion for no more than 10 seconds; wall suction set between 80–120 mm Hg

8. Repeat procedure after client has rested

9. Hyperoxygenate for 1–5 minutes after suctioning endotracheal tube or tracheostomy tube suctioned, then mouth is suctioned; provide mouth care

B. Complications

1. Hypoxia

2. Bronchospasm

3. Vagal stimulation

4. Tissue trauma

5. Cardiac dysrhythmias

6. Infection

▶ TRACHEOSTOMY CARE

A. Procedure

1. Perform every 8 hours and as needed

2. Explain procedure

3. Hyperoxygenate or deep breathe

4. Suction tracheostomy tube

5. Remove old dressings

6. Open sterile tracheostomy care kit

7. Put on sterile gloves

8. Remove inner cannula (permanent or disposable)

9. Clean with hydrogen peroxide if permanent inner cannula

10. Rinse with sterile water, dry

11. Reinsert into outer cannula

12. Clean stoma site with hydrogen peroxide and sterile water, then dry

13. Change ties or velcro tracheostomy tube holders as needed; old ties must remain in place until new ties are secured; tie on side of neck, allowing 2 fingers to be inserted under tie

14. Apply new sterile dressing; do not cut gauze pads

15. Document site of tracheostomy, type/quantity of secretions, client tolerance of procedure

16. Purpose of cuff—prevents aspiration of fluids; inflated during continuous mechanical ventilation, during and after eating, during and 1 hour after a tube feeding, when client is unable to handle oral secretions, when client may aspirate; check cuff pressure q 8 hours, maintain at less than 25 cm/H_2O

B. Complications

1. Airway obstruction

2. Trachial necrosis

3. Infection

▶ OXYGEN THERAPY

Table 1 OXYGEN ADMINISTRATION		
METHOD	OXYGEN DELIVERED	NURSING CONSIDERATIONS
Nasal cannula or prongs	23–42% at 1–6 L/min	Assess patency of nostril Apply water-soluble jelly to nostrils every 3–4 hours Perform good mouth care
Face mask	40–60% at 6–8 L/min (oxygen flow minimum 5 L)	Remove mask every 1–2 hours Wash, dry, apply lotion to skin Emotional support to decrease feeling of claustrophobia
Partial rebreather mask	50–75% at 8–11 L/min	Adjust oxygen flow to keep reservoir bag two-thirds full during inspiration
Nonrebreather mask	80–100% at 12 L/min	Adjust oxygen flow to keep bag two-thirds full
Venturi mask	24–40% at 4–8 L/min	Provides high humidity and fixed concentrations Keep tubing free of kinks
Tracheostomy collar or T-piece	30–100% at 8–10 L/min	Assess for fine mist Empty condensation from tubing Keep water container full
Oxygen hood	30–100% at 8–10 L/min	Used for infants and young children Provides cooled humid air Check O_2 concentration with O_2 analyzer every 4 hours Refill humidity jar with sterile distilled water Clean humidity jar daily Cover client with light blanket and towel or cap for head Change linen frequently Monitor client's temperature frequently

Table 2 HAZARDS OF OXYGEN ADMINISTRATION	
COMPLICATION	NURSING CONSIDERATIONS
Infection	Change masks, tubing, mouthpieces daily
Drying and irritation of mucosa	Administer humidified oxygen
Respiratory depression (CO_2 narcosis)	Monitor respiratory rates frequently Alternate between breathing room air and O_2 at prescribed intervals Administer mixed O_2 (air and O_2) rather than pure O_2 Administer minimal concentrations necessary Periodically inflate the lungs fully
Oxygen toxicity	Premature infants exposed to excessive amounts of O_2 for prolonged periods may develop retinopathy of prematurity (ROP); may result in irreversible blindness from vasoconstriction of the retinal blood vessels Lungs of clients on respirators (children and adults) are most susceptible to pulmonary damage Pulmonary damage includes atelectasis, exudation of protein fluid into alveoli, damage to and proliferation of pulmonary capillaries, and interstitial hemorrhage Early symptoms include cough, nasal congestion, sore throat, reduced vital capacity, and substernal discomfort
Combustion	Be sure electrical plugs and equipment are properly grounded Enforce no-smoking rules Do not use oils on the client or on O_2 equipment

▶ CHEST TUBES

A. Intrapleural drainage system with one or more chest catheters held in pleural space by suture to chest wall, attached to drainage system

B. Nursing care (see Figures 1 and 2)

1. Fill water-seal chamber with sterile water to the level specified by manufacturer

2. If suction is to be used, fill the suction control chamber with sterile water to the 20-cm level, or as ordered by the health care provider

3. Encourage the client to change position and cough and deep breathe frequently

4. The drainage system must be maintained below the level of insertion, without kinks in tubing

5. Chest tubes are clamped *only momentarily* to check for air leaks and to change the drainage apparatus

6. Observe for fluctuations of fluid in water-seal chamber; stops fluctuating when:

   a. Lung re-expands

   b. Tubing is obstructed

   c. Loop hangs below rest of tubing

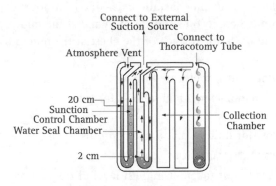
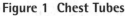

Figure 1 Chest Tubes

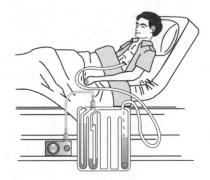

Figure 2 Pleur-evac

C. Removal of the chest tube
   1. Instruct the client to do the Valsalva maneuver (forcibly bear down while holding breath)
   2. Chest tube is clamped and quickly removed by the health care provider
   3. Occlusive dressing is applied to the site

D. Complications
   1. Observe for constant bubbling in the water-seal chamber; this indicates air leak in the drainage system; report to health care provider
   2. If the chest tube becomes dislodged, apply pressure over the insertion site with a dressing that is tented on one side to allow for the escape of air; immediately report to health care provider
   3. If the tube becomes disconnected from the drainage system, cut the contaminated tip off of the tubing, insert a sterile connector, and reattach to the drainage system; otherwise immerse the end of the chest tube in 2 cm of sterile water until the system can be re-established; report to health care provider.

▶ CENTRAL VENOUS PRESSURE (CVP)

A. Purpose
   1. Measurement of effective blood volume and efficiency of cardiac pumping
   2. Indicates ability of right side of heart to manage a fluid load
   3. Guide to fluid replacement

B. Equipment
   1. Central line threaded into right atrium
   2. Water manometer with three-way stopcock
   3. IV fluids

C. Procedure (see Figure 3)
   1. Client has catheter in jugular, subclavian, or antecubital vein
   2. Attach manometer to a three-way stopcock that also connects IV to central catheter

3. Zero on manometer placed at the phlebostatic axis—line from fourth intercostal space at point where it joins the sternum and a line midway between the anterior and posterior surface of the chest at the outermost point of the sternum

4. Measured with client flat in bed or elevated up to 45°

5. Stopcock opened to the manometer, which allows for filling with IV fluid to level of 18–20 cm

6. Stopcock turned to allow for fluid in manometer to flow to client

7. Level of fluid fluctuates with respirations

8. When level stabilizes, reading is taken at highest level of fluctuation

9. Return stopcock to proper position and adjust IV flow rate

10. Normal reading: 4-12 mm Hg

   a. Elevated: greater than 12 mm hypervolemia or poor cardiac contractility

   b. Lowered: less than 4 mm hypovolemia

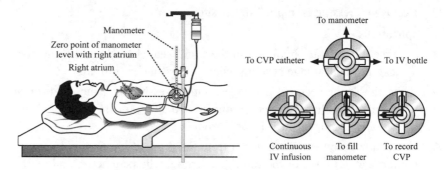

Figure 3 Central Venous Pressure

D. Potential complications

1. Pneumothorax from catheter insertion

2. Air embolism

3. Infection at insertion site

E. Nursing care

1. Dry, sterile dressing

2. Change dressing, IV fluid bag, manometer, and tubing every 24 hours

3. Instruct client to hold breath (Valsalva maneuver) when inserted and withdrawn or when tubing is changed to prevent air embolism

4. Check and secure all connections

▶ EAR PROCEDURES

A. Ear irrigations

1. Tilt head toward side of affected ear, gently direct stream of fluid against sides of canal

2. After procedure, instruct client to lie on affected side to facilitate drainage

3. Contraindicated if there is evidence of swelling or tenderness

B. Ear drops

1. Position the affected ear uppermost

2. Pull outer ear upward and backward for adult

3. Pull outer ear downward and backward for child

4. Place drops so they run down the wall of ear canal

5. Have client lie on unaffected ear to encourage absorption

▶ EYE PROCEDURES

A. Eye irrigation

1. Tilt head back and toward the side of affected area

2. Allow irrigating fluid to flow from the inner to the outer canthus

3. Use a small bulb syringe or eye dropper to dispense fluid

4. Place small basin close to head to collect excess fluid and drainage

B. Eyedrop instillation

1. Equipment must be sterile

   a. Wash hands, before instillation

   b. Do not allow dropper to touch eye

   c. Do not allow drops from eye to flow across nose into opposite eye

2. Tilt head back and look up; pull lid down

3. Place drops into center of lower conjunctival sac

   a. Instruct client not to squeeze eye

   b. Teach client to blink between drops

4. To prevent systemic absorption, press the inner canthus near the bridge of the nose for 1–2 minutes

▶ NASOGASTRIC TUBES

A. Types

1. Levin—single-lumen stomach tube used to remove stomach contents or provide tube feeding

2. Salem sump—double-lumen stomach tube; most frequently used tube for decompression with suction

3. Sengstaken-Blakemore—triple-lumen gastric tube with inflatable esophagus balloon, stomach ballon, gastric suction lumen used for treatment of bleeding esophageal varices

4. Keofeed/Dobhoff—soft silicone rubber, medium-length tube used for long-term feedings; placement verified by x-ray; takes 24 hours to pass from stomach into intestines; lay on right side to facilitate passage

5. Cantor—single-lumen tube with mercury-filled balloon and suction port

6. Miller-Abbott—double-lumen tube with mercury-filled balloon and suction

7. Harris—single-lumen tube with mercury-filled balloon and suction port

B. Insertion of Levin/Salem sump

1. Measure distance from tip of nose to earlobe plus distance from earlobe to bottom of xiphoid process

2. Mark distance on tube with tape and lubricate end of tube with water-soluble jelly

3. Insert tube through the nose to the stomach

4. Offer sips of water and advance the tube gently; bend the head forward (closes the epiglottis, closing the trachea)

5. Observe for respiratory distress, an indication that tube is misplaced in the lungs; if in correctly, secure tube with hypoallergenic tape

C. Verify placement of tube initially and before administering feeding

1. X-ray is only sure way to verify placement

2. Aspirate gastric contents

3. Observe color—gastric aspirate usually cloudy and green but may also be off-white, tan, bloody, or brown

4. Measure pH of aspirate

    a. Gastric—usually less than or equal to 4

    b. Intestinal—usually greater than 4

    c. Respiratory—usually greater than 5.5

D. Nursing care of Levin/Salem pump

1. Check residual before intermittent feeding and q 4 hours with continuous feeding; hold feeding if more than 100 mL

2. Instill 15–30 mL saline or water according to agency policy

    a. Before and after each dose of medications and each tube feeding

    b. After checking residuals and pH

    c. Every 46 hours with continuous feedings

    d. When feeding is discontinued

3. Control rate of feeding—use enteral pump or count drops in gravity administration

4. Administer fluid at room temperature

5. Change bag every 24–72 hours

6. Elevate head of bed 30° while feeding is running and for 30 min after feeding

7. Check patency every 4 h; document drainage

8. Measure I and O

9. Good mouth care, lubricate tube around nares with water-soluble jelly

10. Hang the amount of fluid that will be infused in 4 hours

E. Irrigation of Levin/Salem sump

1. Verify placement of tube

2. Insert 30–50 mL syringe filled with normal saline into tube, inject slowly

3. If resistance felt, check to see if tube is kinked, have client change position

4. Pull back on plunger or bulb to withdraw solution; if irrigating solution not removed, record as input

5. Repeat if needed

F. Removal of Levin/Salem sump

   1. Clamp tube, remove tape

   2. Instruct client to exhale and remove tube with smooth, continuous pull

G. Insertion of intestinal tubes (Cantor, Miller-Abbott, Harris)

   1. Mechanical passage into stomach; same as NG tube

   2. Passage of tube along intestines is aided by gravity, weight of mercury, and peristalsis

   3. After tube is in stomach, have client lie on right side, then on back (in Fowler's position), and then on left side to use gravity to position tube

   4. Position of tube is ascertained by x-ray—do not tape tube to face, but coil loosely on bed

   5. Position of tube and absence of telescoping of bowel from weight of tube is ascertained daily by x-ray

H. Nursing care of intestinal tubes

   1. Measure drainage every shift

   2. General care of client with NG tube

   3. Report signs of return of peristalsis, e.g., bowel sounds, flatus

I. Removal of intestinal tubes

   1. Clamp tube, remove tape

   2. Deflate balloon or aspirate contents of intestine tube balloon

   3. Instruct client to exhale

   4. Remove 6 inches every 10 minutes until it reaches stomach, then remove completely with smooth continuous pull

▶ SURGICAL DRAINS

Table 3 SURGICAL DRAINS		
TYPE	DESCRIPTION	NURSING CONSIDERATIONS
Penrose	Simple latex drain	Note location Usually not sutured in place, but layered in gauze dressing Expect drainage on dressing
T tube	Used after gallbladder surgery Placed in common bile duct to allow passage of bile	Monitor drainage Fasten tubing to dressings Keep below waist May clamp for 1 hour before and after each meal May be discharged with T tube in place Remove 7–14 days Teach client about care

Table 3 SURGICAL DRAINS *(CONTINUED)*		
TYPE	DESCRIPTION	NURSING CONSIDERATIONS
Jackson-Pratt	Portable wound self-suction device with reservoir	Monitor amount and character of drainage Notify health care provider if it suddenly increases or becomes bright red
Hemovac	Larger portable wound self-suction device with reservoir Used after mastectomy	Monitor and record amount and character of drainage Notify health care provider if it suddenly increases or becomes bright red Empty when full or every 8 h Remove plug (maintain sterility), empty contents, place on flat surface, cleanse opening and plug with alcohol sponge, compress evacuator completely to remove air, replace plug, check system for operation

▶ ENEMAS

A. Types

   1. Oil retention—softens feces

   2. Soapsuds—irritates colon, causing reflux evacuation

   3. Tap water—softens feces, stimulating evacuation, volume expander

B. Procedure—instillation of solution into rectum and sigmoid colon; promote defecation by stimulating peristalsis

   1. Explain procedure to client

   2. Position in Sims' position with right knee flexed

   3. Use tepid solution

   4. Hold irrigation set at 12–18 inches for high enema, 3 inches for low enema

   5. Insert tube no more than 3–4 inches for adult, 2–3 inches for child, 1–1.5 inches for infant

   6. Ask client to retain solution for 5–10 minutes

   7. Do not administer in presence of abdominal pain, nausea, vomiting, or suspected appendicitis

▶ URINARY CATHETERS

A. Types of catheters (see Table 4)

B. Procedure for catheterization

   1. Female

     a. Explain procedure to client

     b. Assemble equipment

     c. Client should be placed in dorsal recumbent position or in Sims' position

    d. Drape client with sterile drapes using sterile technique

    e. Apply sterile gloves

    f. Lubricate catheter tip and place in sterile catheter tray

    g. Separate labia with thumb and forefinger and wipe from the meatus toward the rectum with sterile povidone-iodine swab and discard swab

    h. Insert catheter 2 to 3 inches into the urethra

    i. Insert catheter an additional inch after urine begins to flow to ensure balloon portion of catheter is in the bladder

    j. Inflate balloon

    k. Gently apply traction to the catheter

    l. Tape drainage tubing to client's thigh

  2. Male

    a. If uncircumcised, retract the foreskin to expose urinary meatus

    b. Cleanse glans and meatus with sterile povidone-iodine swabs in circular motion

    c. Hold penis perpendicular to the body; insert catheter into urethra 6–7 inches

    d. Replace the foreskin

Table 4 URINARY CATHETERS		
TYPE	**CHARACTERISTICS**	**COMMENTS**
Whistle-tip	Straight	For blood clot removal
Coude	Curved	For BPH to avoid prostate trauma
Robinson	Hollow—2 openings	For intermittent catheterizations
Filiform	Stiff	For urethral strictures
Foley	Double lumen with inflatable balloon toward tip	Indwelling for urinary drainage
Pezzer	Mushroom tip, otherwise like a Foley	Indwelling for urinary drainage
Malecot	Wing-shaped tip	Used as nephrostomy tube—anchored in renal pelvis through flank incision
Suprapubic	Placed in bladder via abdominal incision Dressing over site	Used in conjunction with urethral drainage

    e. Inflate balloon

    f. Gently apply traction to the catheter until resistance is felt, indicating the catheter is at the base of the bladder

    g. Tape drainage tubing to client's thigh

C. Principles of drainage system care

  1. Catheter should not be disconnected from drainage system, except to perform ordered irrigations

2. Urine samples should be obtained from drainage port with a small-bore needle using sterile technique; clamp tubing below port

3. Drainage bags should not be elevated above level of cavity being drained (to prevent reflux)

4. Avoid kinks in tubing

5. Avoid removing more than 1000 mL at one time; if more urine in bladder clamp after 1000 mL, wait 15–30 min, then continue or follow facility policy.

6. Coil excess tubing on bed

D. Catheter irrigation

1. Purpose—prevent obstruction of flow and catheter or remove buildup of sediment in long-term use

2. Procedure—urethral catheter irrigation

   a. Closed urethral catheter irrigation

      1) Draw solution into syringe using sterile technique

      2) Clamp catheter below injection port

      3) Cleanse port with antiseptic swab

      4) Insert needle into injection port at 30° angle

      5) Slowly inject fluid

      6) Withdraw needle

      7) Remove clamp

      8) Solution drains into the bag

   b. Open urethral catheter irrigation

      1) Use sterile technique

      2) Cleanse around catheter; disconnect tubing

      3) Gently instill 30 mL of solution

      4) Allow fluid to drain by gravity into sterile basin

      5) If solution is easily instilled but does not return, have client turn to side; if still doesn't return, depress the syringe bulb to provide gentle suction

      6) Disinfect ends of catheter tubing and reconnect

E. Nursing care

1. Use aseptic technique on insertion

2. Do not disturb integrity of closed drainage system

3. Check for kinks

4. Perineal care with soap and water 2–3 times daily, then apply antimicrobial ointment to insertion site

5. Keep urine collection bag below the level of the urinary bladder

6. Secure to leg to prevent traction

7. Monitor I and O; minimum urinary drainage catheter output should be 30 mL/h

8. Monitor for signs and symptoms of infection (foul-smelling urine with pus, blood, or mucus streaks)

9. Adhere to special precautions for type of catheter used

   a. Ureterostomy tube—never irrigate

   b. Straight catheter—do not remove more than 1,000 mL at one time

   c. Nephrostomy tube—never clamp

10. Clamp indwelling catheters intermittently prior to removal

F. Intermittent self-catheterization

1. Used to treat neurogenic bladder caused by spinal cord injury, multiple sclerosis (MS), brain injury

   a. Caused by neurologic conditions: spinal cord injury, multiple sclerosis (MS), brain injury

2. Preparation

   a. Gather equipment

      1) Straight or curved-tip 12 or 14 Fr Tiemann catheter (most common for male clients)

      2) Clean container or plastic bag

      3) Water-soluble lubricant

      4) Washcloth with soap and water

      5) Container for urine

   b. Wash hands

   c. Wash catheter with warm water and soap, rinse, and dry completely

3. Insertion

   a. Clear perineum with soap and water

   b. Lubricate catheter with water-soluble lubricant

   c. Locate catheter insertion point

      1) Female: combination visualization and palpation

      2) Male: visualize penile meatus

   d. Insert catheter slowly until urine returns, then advance 1/2–1 inch

   e. Press down with abdominal muscles to promote complete emptying

   f. Once bladder is drained, remove gently

   g. Immediately rinse catheter with cool tap water to remove residue, dry thoroughly

   h. Wash hands

4. Client teaching

   a. Should be done every 4–6 hours

   b. Should be performed at consistent times daily

   c. Uses clean technique, not sterile technique

   d. Removes 350–400 ml each time

   e. Performed in a comfortable postition, sitting or standing

   f. Use catheter for 2–4 weeks and then discard

   g. Store catheter in sandwich-sized bag or clean container

   h. Never store catheter wet or in antiseptic solution

   i. Should drink 250 ml at 2-hour intervels or up to 2 L at regular intervals

Chapter 5

PHYSIOLOGICAL INTEGRITY: PHYSIOLOGICAL ADAPTATION

Units

1. **Medical Emergencies**

2. **Fluid and Electrolyte Imbalances**

3. **Alterations in Body Systems**

4. **Cancer**

▶ **UPPER AIRWAY OBSTRUCTION**

A. Assessment

   1. Inability to breathe or speak

   2. Cyanosis

   3. Collapse

   4. Death can occur within 4–5 minutes

B. Diagnose—potential nursing diagnosis

   1. Airway clearance, ineffective

C. Planning/Implementation

   1. If conscious

      a. Give 5 back blows between shoulder blade with heel of hand

      b. Give 5 abdominal thrusts (Heimlich maneuver)

      c. Alternate between 5 back blows and 5 thrusts until the blockage is dislodged

   2. If unconscious

      a. Begin CPR

      b. Remove object if it becomes visible

   3. Intubation (see Table 1 and Figure 1)

Table 1 AIRWAY INTUBATION	
METHOD	**NURSING CONSIDERATIONS**
Endotracheal tube—tube passed through the nose or mouth into the trachea	Assess for bilateral breath sounds and bilateral chest excursion Mark tube at level it touches mouth or nose Secure with tape to stabilize Encourage fluids to facilitate removal of secretions

Tracheostomy—surgical incision made into trachea via the throat; tube inserted through incision into the trachea	Cuff is used to prevent aspiration and to facilitate mechanical ventilation
	Maintain cuff pressure at 14–20 mm Hg
	Encourage fluids to facilitate removal of secretions
	Sterile suctioning if necessary
	Frequent oral hygiene
	Indications for suctioning tracheostomy
	  • Noisy respirations
	  • Restlessness
	  • Increased pulse
	  • Increased respirations
	  • Presence of mucus in airway

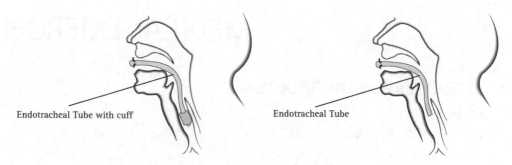

Figure 1   Endotracheal Tube

4. Tracheostomy (see Table 1 and Figure 2)

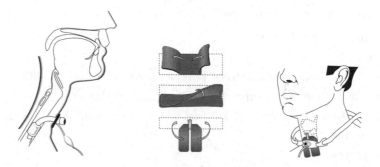

Figure 2   Tracheostomy Tube

5. Suctioning

6. Mechanical ventilation

   a. Prepare client psychologically for use of ventilator

   b. Monitor client's response to the ventilator

      1) Assess vital signs at least q 4 hours

      2) Listen to breath sounds (crackles, wheezes, equal breath sounds, decreased or absent breath sounds)

      3) Assess need for suctioning

      4) Respiratory monitoring

      5) Evaluate ABGs, continuous pulse oximetry monitoring

      6) Check for hypoxia (restlessness, cyanosis, anxiety, tachycardia, increased respiratory rate)

      7) Check neurologic status

      8) Check chest for bilateral expansion

   c. Provide good oral hygiene at least twice each shift

   d. Assess need for tracheal/oral/nasal suctioning q 2 hours and perform as necessary

   e. Move endotracheal tube to opposite side of mouth q 24 hours to prevent ulcers

   f. Monitor intake and output

   g. Create alternative methods of communication with client (letter board, pencil and paper); provide access to call light

h. Perform and document ventilator and equipment checks—care for client first, ventilator second

    1) Check ventilator settings as ordered by health care provider— tidal volume (TV), respiratory rate, pO_2 (fraction of inspired oxygen), mode of ventilation, sigh button/cycle (usually 1–3/h) (may cause lung damage from excessive pressure)

    2) Check that alarms are set (low pressure and low exhaled volume)

    3) Check temperature and level of water in humidification system

    4) Check PEEP (positive end-expiratory pressure) maintained at end of expiration to open collapsed alveoli and improve oxygenation

    5) Drain condensation from tubing away from client

    6) Verify that tracheostomy or endotracheal cuff is inflated to ensure tidal volume

i. Observe for gastrointestinal distress (diarrhea, constipation, tarry stools)

j. Document observations/procedures in medical record

7. Oxygen administration

D. Evaluation

1. Does respiratory rate return to normal?

2. Is client able to speak?

► CARDIOPULMONARY ARREST

A. Assessment

1. Breathless

2. Pulseless

3. Unconscious

B. Diagnose

1. Failure to institute ventilation within 4–6 minutes will result in cerebral anoxia and brain damage

2. Purpose—to re-establish CO_2/O_2 exchange and adequate circulation

C. Plan/Implementation

1. Basic Life Support

a. Recognition

    1) All ages: unresponsive

    2) Adults: no breathing or no normal breathing (i.e., only gasping)

    3) Children and infants: no breathing or only gasping

    4) No pulse palpated within 10 seconds (HCP only)

b. Activate EMS system

c. CPR sequence: C-A-B

d. Compression rate: at least 100/minute

      e. Compression depth

         1) Adults: at least 2 inches (5 cm)

         2) Children: at least ½ anterior posterior diameter or about 2 inches (5 cm)

         3) Infants: at least ¼ anterior posterior diameter or about 1 ½ inches (4 cm)

      f. Chest wall recoil

         1) Allow complete recoil between compressions

         2) HCPs rotate compressors every 2 minutes

      g. Compression interruptions

         1) Minimize interruptions in chest compressions

         2) Attempt to limit interruptions to less than 10 seconds

      h. Airway

         1) Head tilt-chin lift

         2) HCP suspected trauma; jaw thrust

      i. Compression-to-ventilation ratio (until advance airway placed)

         1) Adult: 30:2; 1 or 2 rescuers

         2) Children and infants: 30:2 single rescuer; 15:2 2 HCP rescuers

      j. Ventilations when rescuer untrained or trained and not proficient: compressions only

      k. Ventilations with advanced airway (HCP)

         1) 1 breath every 6–8 seconds (8–10 breaths/minute)

         2) Asynchronous with chest compressions

         3) About 1 second per breath

         4) Visible chest rise

      l. Defibrillation

         1) Attach and use AED as soon as possible

         2) Minimize compressions before and after shock

         3) Resume CPR beginning with compressions immediately after each shock

   2. Continue CPR until one of the following occurs

      a. Victim responds

      b. Another qualified person takes over

      c. Victim is transferred to an emergency room

      d. Rescuer is physically unable to continue

D. Evaluation

   1. Has cardiac function been re-established?

   2. Has cerebral anoxia been prevented?

▶ CROUP SYNDROMES: ACUTE EPIGLOTTITIS, ACUTE LARYNGOTRACHEOBRONCHITIS

A. Assessment

1. Barklike cough, use of accessory muscles
2. Dyspnea, inspiratory stridor, cyanosis
3. Decrease in noisy respirations may indicate decompensation

B. Diagnose

1. Viral—infection in the area of the larynx
2. Medical emergency due to narrowed airway in children
3. Potential nursing diagnoses
   a. Risk for suffocation
   b. Anxiety

C. Plan/Implementation

1. Care at home
   a. Steamy shower
   b. Sudden exposure to cold air
   c. Sleep with cool humidified air
2. Hospitalization required
   a. Increasing respiratory distress
   b. Hypoxia or depressed sensorium
   c. High temperature (102°F)
3. Nursing care if hospitalized
   a. Maintain airway (keep tracheostomy set at bedside)
   b. Oxygen hood
   c. Monitor heart rate and respiration for early sign of hypoxia
   d. Oxygen with humidification
   e. IV fluids
   f. Medications—antipyretics, bronchodilators, nebulized epinephrine, steroids
   g. Position in infant seat or prop with pillow

D. Evaluation

1. Does the child have adequate respirations and airway clearance?
2. Is there a reduction in the child's anxiety?

▶ MYOCARDIAL INFARCTION (MI)

A. Assessment

1. Symptoms vary depending on whether pain, shock, or pulmonary edema dominates clinical picture
2. Chest pain—severe, crushing, prolonged; unrelieved by rest or nitroglycerin; often radiating to one or both arms, jaw, neck, and back (see Figure 3); women may present with atypical symptoms (fatigue, shortness of breath)

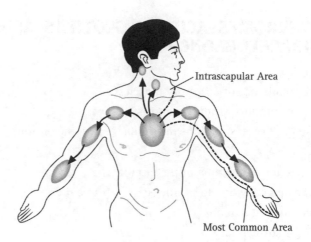

Figure 3 Ischemic Pain Patterns

3. Dyspnea

4. Nausea, vomiting, gastric discomfort, indigestion

5. Apprehension, restless, fear of death

6. Acute pulmonary edema, sense of suffocating

7. Cardiac arrest

8. Shock—systolic blood pressure below 80 mm Hg, gray facial color, lethargy, cold diaphoresis, peripheral cyanosis, tachycardia or bradycardia, weak pulse

9. Oliguria—urine output of less than 20 ml/hour

10. Low-grade fever—temperature rises to 100°–103°F (38°–39° C) within 24 hours and lasts 3 to 7 days

11. Dysrhythmias, heart block, asystole

12. WBC—leukocytosis within 2 days, disappears in 1 week

13. Erythrocyte sedimentation rate (ESR)—elevated

14. CK–MB—first enzyme tube to be elevated after MI; appears 3–6 hours; peaks 18–24 hours

15. LDH—appears 12–24 hours; peaks 48–72 hours; lasts 6–12 days

16. Troponin—peaks in 4–12 hours; remains elevated for up to 2–3 weeks

17. Myoglobin—begins to rise within 1 hour; peaks in 4–6 hours; returns to normal in less than 24 hours

18. Electrocardiogram—ST segment elevation, T wave inversion, Q wave formation

B. Diagnose

1. Formation of localized necrotic areas within the myocardium, usually following the sudden occlusion of a coronary artery and the abrupt decrease of blood and oxygen to the heart muscle

2. Causes

   a. Complete or near complete occlusion of a coronary vessel (most common)

   b. Decreased blood and oxygen supply to the heart muscle; vasospasm

      c. Hypertrophy of the heart muscle from CHF or hypertension

      d. Embolism to a coronary artery

  3. Potential nursing diagnoses

      a. Risk for decreased cardiac output

      b. Anxiety/fear

      c. Deficient knowledge

C. Plan/Implementation

  1. Provide thrombolytic therapy—streptokinase or tissue-type plasminogen activator (t-PA) to dissolve thrombus in coronary artery within 6 hours of onset

  2. Relieve client's and family's anxiety

  3. Bedrest to decrease stress on heart, allow to use bedside commode for bowel movement; semifowler's position

  4. Monitor vital signs, pain status, lung sounds, level of consciousness, ECG, oxygen saturation

  5. Monitor intake and output

      a. Intake—fluid intake 2,000 ml daily; too much may precipitate CHF, and too little may result in dehydration

      b. Output—Foley catheter, if necessary; oliguria indicates inadequate renal perfusion, concentrated urine indicates dehydration

  6. Carefully monitor IV infusion—vein should be kept open in case emergency IV drugs are necessary

  7. Administer medications: beta blockers (e.g., propranolol), morphine sulfate for pain (reduces preload, afterload pressures, and decreases anxiety), antidysrhythmics (e.g., lidocaine, verapamil, solalol, propafenone), anticoagulant medications (e.g., heparin, warfarin)

  8. Administer oxygen

  9. Prevent complications

      a. Dysrhythmias

      b. Shock

      c. Congestive heart failure

      d. Rupture of heart muscle

      e. Pulmonary embolism

      f. Recurrent MI

  10. Teaching

      a. Healing not complete for 6–8 weeks

      b. Modify lifestyle

         1) Stop smoking

         2) Reduce stress

         3) Decrease caffeine

         4) Modify intake of calories, sodium, and fat

      c. Maintain regular physical activity

      d. Medication schedule and adverse effects

D. Evaluation

1. Does client experience relief of pain and reduction in anxiety?
2. Does client institute lifestyle changes to decrease stress?
3. Does client comply with medication, diet, and activity recommendations?

▶ RHYTHM DISTURBANCES (DYSRHYTHMIAS)

A. Assessment

1. Dizziness, syncope
2. Chest pain, palpitations, abnormal heart sounds
3. Nausea, vomiting
4. Dyspnea
5. Abnormal pulse rate—increased, decreased, or irregular

B. Diagnose

1. Caused by interruption in normal conduction process
2. Can occur at any point in the normal conduction pathway
3. Types of dysrhythmias

    a. <u>Sinus dysrhythmias</u>—dysrhythmias originate in the sinoatrial node and are conducted along the normal conductive pathways

        1) *Tachycardia*—sympathetic nervous system increases the automaticity of the SA node

            a) Heart rate is increased above 100 beats per minute

            b) Causes—pain, exercise, hypoxia, pulmonary embolism, hemorrhage, hyperthyroidism, or fever

            c) Symptoms—dizziness, dyspnea, hypotension, palpitations

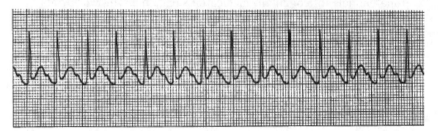

Rules for Sinus Tachycardia

            d) Treatment—treat underlying problem, beta blockers (metoprolol), calcium channel blockers (diltiazem), or cardio version

        2) *Bradycardia*—parasympathetic nervous system (vagal stimulation) causes automaticity of the SA node to be depressed

            a) Heart rate decreased to below 60 beats per minute

            b) Causes—myocardial infarction, the Valsalva maneuver, or vomiting, arteriosclerosis in the carotid sinus area, ischemia of SA node, hypothermia, hyperkalemia, or drugs such as digitalis and propranolol

c) Symptoms—Pale, cool, hypotension, syncope, dyspnea, weakness

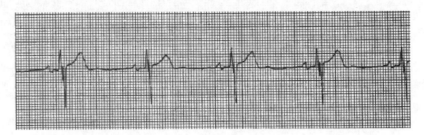

Rules for Sinus Bradycardia

d) Treatment—Atropine or possible pacemaker

b. <u>Atrial dysrhythmias</u>—abnormal electrical activity that results in stimulation outside the SA node but within the atria

1) *Premature atrial contractions (PAC)*

a) Ectopic focus within one of the atria fires prematurely

b) Causes—Normal phenomenon in some individuals, but may be caused by emotional disturbances, fatigue, tobacco, or caffeine

c) Symptoms—"sense of skipped beat"

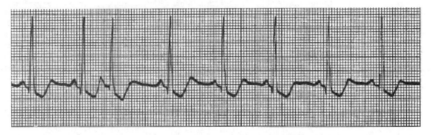

Rules for Premature Atrial Contraction

d) Treatment—treat the underlying cause

2) *Atrial flutter*

a) Arises from an ectopic focus in the atrial wall causing the atrium to contract 250–400 times per minute (AV node blocks most of the impulses, thereby protecting the ventricles from receiving every impulse)

b) Causes—stress, hypoxia, drugs, or disorders such as chronic heart disease, hypertension

c) Symptoms—chest discomfort, dyspnea, hypotension

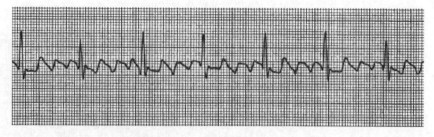

Rules for Atrial Flutter

      d) Treatment—Vagal maneuvers, adenosine, cardioversion or ablation

   3) *Atrial fibrillation*

      a) Uncoordinated atrial electrical activation that causes a rapid, disorganized uncoordinated twitching of the atrial muscle. (Most common atrial dysrhythmia) (presents with a grossly irregular pulse rate)

      b) Causes—chronic lung disease, heart failure, and rheumatic heart disease, chronic hypertension

      c) Symptoms—stroke symptoms, hypotension, syncope, dyspnea

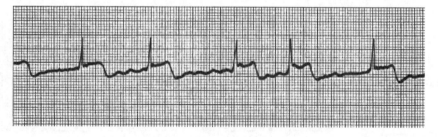

Rules for Fibrillation

      d) Treatment—address underlying cause, calcium channel blockers (diltiazem), beta blockers (metoprolol), digoxin, cardioversion, warfarin

  c. <u>Ventricular dysrhythmias</u>—occur when one or more ectopic foci arise within the ventricles

   1) *Premature ventricular contractions (PVCs)*

      a) One or more ectopic foci stimulate a premature ventricular response

      b) Causes—ischemia due to a myocardial infarction, infection, mechanical damage due to pump failure, deviations in concentrations of electrolytes (e.g., potassium, calcium), nicotine, coffee, tea, alcohol, drugs such as digitalis and reserpine, psychogenic factors (stress, anxiety, fatigue), and acute or chronic lung disease

      c) Symptoms—Angina, shortness of breath, "heart flip" feeling

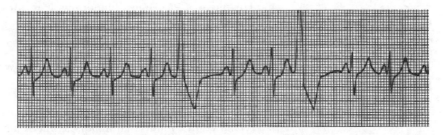

Rules for Premature Ventricular Contractions

    d) Treatment—amiodarone, beta blockers (metoprolol), procainamide

2) *Ventricular tachycardia*

    a) Three or more PVCs occurring in a row at a rate exceeding 100 bpm (severe myocardial irritability)

    b) Causes—large MI, low ejection fraction, same as for PVCs

    c) Symptoms—hypotension, pulmonary edema, confusion, cardiac arrest

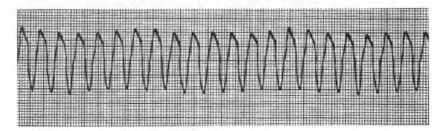

Rules for Ventricular Tachycardia

    d) Treatment—determine if monomorphic (procainamide, sotalol, amiodarone) or polymorphic (magnesium, isoproterenol), pulseless (CPR, defibrillation, epinephrine, amiodarone)

3) *Ventricular fibrillation*

    a) Several ectopic foci within the ventricles are discharged at a very rapid rate. Most serious of all dysrhythmias because of potential cardiac standstill

    b) Causes—acute myocardial infarction, hypertension, rheumatic or arteriosclerotic heart disturbances, or hypoxia

    c) Symptoms—unresponsive, pulseless, apneic

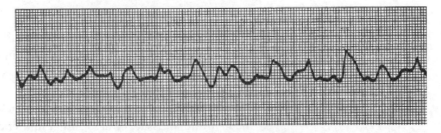

Rules for Ventricular Fibrillation

      d) Treatment—CPR; Unless blood flow is restored (by CPR) and the dysrhythmia is interrupted (by defibrillation), death will result within 90 seconds to 5 minutes

  d. <u>Heart block</u>—delay in the conduction of impulses within the atrioventricular system

    1) *First-degree block*

      a) AV junction conducts all impulses, but at a slower-than-normal rate

      b) Causes—digitalis, calcium channel blockers, beta blockers, MI, and/or increased vagal tone.

      c) Symptoms—asymptomatic

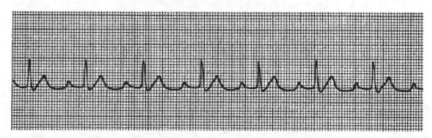

Rules for First-Degree Heart Block

      d) Treatment—Address underlying cause

    2) *Second-degree block (Type I and Type II)*

      a) AV junction conducts only some impulses arising in the atria

      b) Causes—infections, digitalis toxicity, coronary artery disease

      c) Symptoms—May note hypotension, dyspnea, syncope

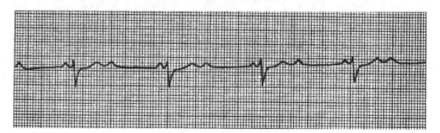

Rules for Classic Second-Degree Heart Block

      d) Treatment—Atropine, pacemaker

    3) *Third-degree heart block*

      a) AV junction blocks all impulses to the ventricles, causing the atria and ventricles to dissociate and beat independently (each with its own pacemaker establishing a rate, ventricular rate is low, 20 to 40 beats per minute)

      b) Causes—congenital defects, vascular insufficiency, fibrosis of the myocardial tissue, or myocardial infarction

      c) Symptoms—shock symptoms, syncope

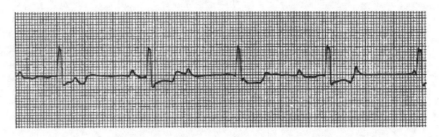

Rules for Third-Degree Heart Block

    d) Treatment—Pacemaker, atropine dopamine, epinephrine. If not treated immediately, may lead to death

4. Diagnostic tests

    a. EKG (see Figure 4)

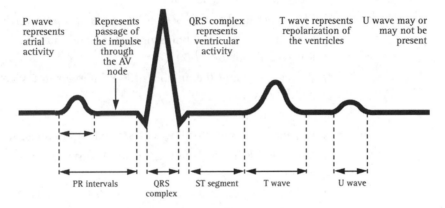

Figure 4. Components of an EKG

    b. ABGs

    c. Holter recorder

       1) 24-hour continuous EKG tracing

       2) Client keeps diary of activities

    d. Cardiac catheterization and coronary angiography (see Reduction of Risk Potential)

    e. Echocardiogram—noninvasive, sound waves used to examine cardiac structures

    f. Stress testing—client walks on treadmill, pedals stationary bicycle, or climbs set of stairs, EKG monitored before, during, and after exercise testing

C. Plan/Implementation

    1. Vital signs

    2. Frequent assessment of cardiac monitor

    3. Administer medication as needed/ordered

    4. Evaluateneed of oxygen

    5. Cardiac monitor identifies changes in rhythm and rate (see Figure 5)

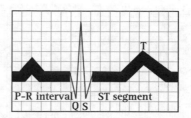

Figure 5. Components of an EKG

a. Determine rate

  1) Each small box = 0.04 seconds

  2) 1,500 small boxes = 1 minute

  3) Each large box = 0.2 seconds (5 small boxes)

  4) 15 large boxes = 3 seconds

  5) EKG paper marked at 3-second intervals at top by vertical line

  6) If regular, count the number of 0.04–second intervals between two R waves, divide by 1,500

  7) If irregular, count the number of R-R intervals in 6 seconds, multiply by 10

b. Determine rhythm

  1) Presence or absence of P wave—SA node originated impulse

  2) Measure P-R interval—normal: 0.12–0.20 seconds (each small box = 0.04 seconds)

  3) Measure QRS duration—normal: 0.04–0.12 seconds

  4) Check P wave, QRS complex, ST segment, and T wave

Table 2 DEFIBRILLATION VERSUS CARDIOVERSION		
	DEFIBRILLATION	CARDIOVERSION
Indication	Emergency treatment of ventricular fibrillation	Elective procedure for dysrhythmias such as atrial fibrillation
Action	Completely depolarizes all myocardial cells so SA node can re-establish as pacemaker	Same
Nursing considerations	Start CPR before defibrillation Plug in defibrillator and turn on Turn on monitor and attach leads to client Apply gel or paste to paddles (rub paddle surfaces together) Select electric charge as ordered Paddles placed over right sternal-border and over the apex of the heart Person with paddles calls "all clear" Push discharge button Check monitor between shocks for rhythm Don't stop to check pulse after shocks, continue CPR, intubate, start IV Epinephrine given 1 mg IV push every 3–5 minutes Sodium bicarbonate given to treat acidosis	Informed consent Diazepam IV Digoxin withheld for 48 hours prior to procedure Synchronizer turned on, check at the R wave Oxygen discontinued Assess airway patency Plug in defibrillator and turn on Turn on oscilloscope and attach leads to client Apply gel or paste (rub paddle surfaces together) Voltage 25–360 joules Paddles placed over right sternal border and over the apex of the heart Person with paddles calls "all clear" Push discharge button Check monitor between shocks for rhythm After procedure, assess vital signs every 15 minutes for 1 hour; every 30 minutes for 2 hours; then every 4 hours

    c. Medications

        1) Antiarrhythmics (e.g., lidocaine, quinidine, procanimide)

        2) Antilipid medications (e.g., lovastatin, cholestyramine)

6. Defibrillation (see Table 2)

7. Pacemakers—apparatus used to initiate heartbeat when the SA node is seriously damaged and unable to act as a pacemaker (see Table 3)

Table 3 PACEMAKERS			
TYPES	ACTION	COMPLICATIONS	NURSING CONSIDERATIONS
Demand (synchronous; noncompetitive)	Functions when heart rate goes below set rate	Dislodgement and migration of endocardial leads	Assess for infection, bleeding
Fixed rate (asynchronous; competitive)	Stimulates ventricle at preset constant rate	Wire breakage Cracking of insulation surrounding wires	Monitor heart rate and rhythm; for preset rate pacemakers, client's rate may vary 5 beats above or below set rate
Temporary	Used in emergency situations (after MI with heart block, cardiac arrest with bradycardia) Inserted through peripheral vein, tip of catheter is placed at apex of right ventricle	Infection of sites surrounding either pacing wires or pulse generator Interference with pacemaker function by exposure to electro-magnetic fields (old microwave ovens, MRI equipment, metal detectors at airports)	Provide emotional support Check pulse daily, report any sudden increase or decrease in rate Carry ID card or wear identification Request hand scanning at security check points at airports
Permanent	Lead is passed into right ventricle, or right atrium and right ventricle, and generator is implanted under skin below clavicle or in abdominal wall	Perforation of myocardium or right ventricle Abrupt loss of pacing	Avoid situations involving electromagnetic fields Periodically check generator Take frequent rest periods at home and at work Wear loose clothing over area of pacemaker All electrical equipment used in vicinity of client should be properly grounded Immobilize extremity if temporary electrode pacemaker is used to prevent dislodgement Document model of pacemaker, date and time of insertion, location of pulse generator, stimulation threshold, pacer rate Place cell phone on side opposite generator

D. Evaluation

   1. Is client free from dysrhythmias as evidenced by stable vital signs?

   2. Have complications been prevented?

▶ **HEAD INJURY**

A. Assessment

   1. Skull fracture—Battle's sign (ecchymosis over mastoid bone), raccoon eyes (bilateral periorbital ecchymosis), rhinnorrhea, otorrhea

   2. Concussion—transient mental confusion or loss of consciousness, headache, no residual neurological deficit, possible loss of memory surrounding event, long-term effects (lack of concentration, personality changes)

   3. Contusion—varies from slight depression of consciousness to coma, with decorticate posturing (flexion and internal rotation of forearms and hands) or decerebrate posturing (extension of arms and legs, pronation of

arms, plantar flexion, opisthotonos), indicates deeper dysfunction, generalized cerebral edema

4. Laceration—penetrating trauma with bleeding

5. Hematoma

   a. Epidural—short period of unconsciousness, followed by lucid interval with ipsilateral pupillary dilation, weakness of contralateral extremities

   b. Subdural—decreased level of consciousness, ipsilateral pupillary dilation, contralateral weakness, personality changes

B. Diagnose

1. Skull is a closed vault with a volume ratio of three components: brain tissue, blood, and CSF; sudden increase in any of these can cause brain dysfunction

2. Ingestion of drugs and alcohol may delay manifestations of symptoms of damage

3. Generalized brain swelling occurs in response to injury

4. Diagnosed by x-ray, CT scan, lumbar puncture (LP), EEG, MRI

5. May be two points of impact of brain with skull

   a. Coup (direct impact)

   b. Contrecoup (rebound to skull wall opposite direct impact)

6. May cause twisting of brain stem

C. Plan/Implementation

1. Evaluate level of consciousness; check vital signs, pupil size, shape, equality, and reaction to light; check nose and ears for CSF leakage

2. Neurological assessment

3. Monitor level of consciousness, careful I and O

4. Seizure precautions, prophylactic anticonvulsants

5. Elevate the head of bed 30° to decrease intracranial pressure; monitor neurologic status after position change

6. Regulate hydration according to I and O, avoid overhydration

7. Prevent infection of open wound, keep dressing dry and intact

8. Manage increased intracranial pressure (ICP) and cerebral edema, administer glucocorticoids (e.g., dexamethasone), mannitol, furosemide

9. Hypothermia—to decrease metabolic demands

10. Barbiturate therapy—to decrease cerebral metabolic rate

11. Minimal procedures (e.g., suctioning, turning, positioning)

12. Prevent complications of immobility

D. Evaluation

1. Have complications been prevented?

2. Is client alert and oriented?

▶ **CHEST TRAUMA**

A. Assessment

1. Flail chest—affected side goes down with inspiration and up during expiration

2. Open pneumothorax

   a. Sucking sound on both inspiration and expiration

   b. Pain

   c. Hyperresonance

   d. Decreased respiratory excursion

   e. Diminished/absent breath sounds on affected side

   f. Weak, rapid pulse

   g. Anxiety, diaphoresis

   h. Altered ABGs

3. Pneumothorax

   a. Dyspnea, pleuritic pain

   b. Absent or restricted movement on affected side

   c. Decreased or absent breath sounds, cyanosis

   d. Cough and fever

   e. Hypotension

B. Diagnose

1. Flail chest—fracture of multiple adjacent ribs causing the chest wall to become unstable and respond paradoxically

2. Open pneumothorax—penetrating chest wound causing the intrapleural space to be open to atmospheric pressure and resulting in collapse of lung

3. Pneumothorax—collapse of lung due to air in the pleural space caused by surgery, disease, or trauma (see Figure 6)

   a. Spontaneous—without a known cause

   b. Tension—pressure builds up; shifting of heart and great vessels

   c. Hemothorax—blood in pleural space

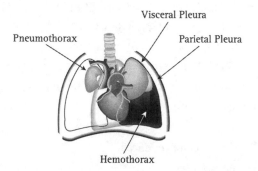

Figure 6. Pneumothorax and Hemothorax

    4. Potential nursing diagnoses

        a. Ineffective breathing pattern

        b. Impaired gas exchange

        c. Anxiety

        d. Acute pain

C. Plan/Implementation

    1. Flail chest

        a. Monitor for shock

        b. Humidified O_2

        c. Pain management

        d. Monitor ABGs

        e. Encourage turning, deep breathing, and coughing

    2. Open pneumothorax

        a. Thoracentesis

        b. Chest tubes (see Reduction of Risk Potential)

D. Evaluation

    1. Has the client's breathing pattern returned to normal?

    2. Has the client's oxygenation been maintained?

▶ ABDOMINAL INJURIES

A. Assessment

    1. Penetrating—symptoms of hemorrhage

    2. Blunt—abdominal pain, rigidity, distension; nausea and vomiting; shock; ecchymosis (around umbilicus—Cullen's-sign; in either flank—Turner's sign) indicative of retroperitoneal bleeding; bruits indicate renal artery injury; resonance over spleen with client on left side (Balance's sign) indicates rupture of spleen; resonance over liver indicates pathology

    3. Diagnosis—X-ray, CT scan; exploratory laparotomy

B. Diagnose

    1. Penetrating—open wound resulting in hemorrhage if major blood vessels/ liver/spleen/pancreas/kidney are involved; increased risk of infection (peritonitis) from rupture of bowel

    2. Blunt—usually injury to solid organs (spleen, liver, pancreas)

C. Plan/Implementation

    1. Penetrating—NPO, NG tube, monitor drainage, bowel sounds; indwelling catheter, monitor output carefully, assess for hematuria

    2. Blunt—IV with large-bore needle in upper extremities; monitor CVP; check hematological values, ABGs, serum electrolytes, liver and kidney function, and clotting studies; cardiac monitor; indwelling catheter

D. Evaluation

    1. Has shock been prevented?

    2. Are client's vital signs stable?

▶ SHOCK

A. Assessment

1. Cool, clammy skin, cyanosis, decreased capillary refill
2. Restlessness, decreased alertness, anxiety
3. Weakness
4. Tachycardia, weak or absent pulse, decreased blood pressure
5. Metabolic acidosis
6. Oliguria, increased urine specific gravity
7. Respirations shallow, rapid
8. Increased muscle weakness

B. Diagnose

1. Sudden reduction of oxygen and nutrients; decreased blood volume causes a reduction in venous return, decreased cardiac output, and a decrease in arterial pressure

2. Types of shock

   a. Hypovolemic shock—loss of fluid from circulation

      1) Hemorrhagic shock (external or internal)
      2) Cutaneous shock, e.g., burns resulting in external fluid loss
      3) Diabetic ketoacidosis
      4) Gastrointestinal obstruction, e.g., vomiting and diarrhea
      5) Diabetes insipidus
      6) Excessive use of diuretics
      7) Internal sequestration, e.g., fractures, hemothorax, ascites

   b. Cardiogenic shock—decreased cardiac output

      1) Myocardial infarction
      2) Dysrhythmias
      3) Pump failure

   c. Distributive shock—inadequate vascular tone

      1) Neural-induced loss of vascular tone
         a) Anesthesia
         b) Pain
         c) Insulin shock
         d) Spinal cord injury
      2) Chemical-induced loss of vascular tone
         a) Toxic shock
         b) Anaphylaxis
         c) Capillary leak—burns, decreased serum protein levels

C. Plan/Implementation

1. Maintain adequate oxygenation
2. Increase tissue perfusion
3. Maintain systolic BP greater than 90 mm Hg
4. Treat acidosis

5. Maintain patent airway
   a. If necessary, ensure ventilation by Ambu bag or ventilator assistance
   b. Provide supplemental oxygen to maintain adequate blood pO_2
6. Indwelling catheter, hourly outputs
7. Assess CVP
8. Assess ABGs
9. Treat acidosis
10. Keep warm (maintain body temperature)
11. Intravenous administration of blood or other appropriate fluids (plasma expanders, electrolyte solutions)
12. Large amounts of fluid may be pushed until systemic blood pressure, urine volume, and lactate levels return to a relatively normal level or central venous or pulmonary artery pressures, or both, become elevated
    a. Crystalloids—normal saline, Ringer's lactate (isotonic)
    b. Colloids—blood, packed red cells, plasma, plasma expanders e.g., hetastarch
13. Medications
    a. Antibiotics—when shock is due to an infection (septic shock), antibiotic therapy should be instituted immediately; blood, urine, sputum, and drainage of any kind should be sent for culture and sensitivity (C and S); usually use combination of ampicillin, polymyxin, and cephalothin
    b. Medications to vasoconstrict and improve myocardial contractility
    c. Medications to maintain adequate urine output, e.g., mannitol, furosemide
    d. Medications used to restore blood pressure, adrenergics/ sympathomimetics (e.g., dobutamin hydrochloride)
    e. Low-dose corticosteroids for septic shock
14. Infuse and assess large volumes of fluids

D. Evaluation
   1. Is client's systolic blood pressure maintained over 90 mm Hg?
   2. Has the client's normal circulation been restored?
   3. Is client's urinary output greater than 30 ml/hour?

▶ INCREASED INTRACRANIAL PRESSURE

A. Assessment
   1. Altered LOC—often earliest sign
   2. Glasgow coma scale (see Table 4)
      a. Level of consciousness
      b. Score of 3–8 indicates severe head trauma; score of 15 indicates client is alert and oriented

Table 4 GLASGOW COMA SCALE																					
Eyes Open	Spontaneously	4																			
	To speech	3																			
	To pain	2																			
	None	1																			
Best Verbal Response	Oriented	5																			
	Confused	4																			
	Inappropriate words	3																			
	Incomprehensible sounds	2																			
	None	1																			
Best Motor Response	Obeys commands	6																			
	Localizes pain	5																			
	Flexes to pain	4																			
	Flexor posture	3																			
	Extensor posture	2																			
	No response	1																			

3. Confusion, restlessness (early signs)

4. Pupillary changes (early signs)

5. Vital signs changes—increased BP, decreased pulse (late changes)

B. Analysis

1. Diagnostic tests

   a. Neurological tests (e.g., lumbar puncture, EEG, myelogram)

2. Causes

   a. Cerebral edema

   b. Hemorrhage

   c. Space-occupying lesions

3. Complications

   a. Cerebral hypoxia

   b. Decreased cerebral perfusion

   c. Herniation—pupil constriction

C. Plan/Implementation

1. Monitor vital signs hourly—be alert for increased systolic pressure, widening pulse pressure, and bradycardia (Cushing's triad—very late sign)

2. Monitor pupillary reactions

3. Monitor muscle strength

4. Monitor verbal response and change in level of consciousness

5. Monitor Glasgow coma scale

6. Maintain respiratory function

7. Elevate head 30–45° to promote venous drainage from brain

8. Avoid neck flexion, head rotation, coughing, sneezing, and bending forward—support in cervical collar or neck rolls

9. Reduce environmental stimuli

10. Prevent the Valsalva maneuver, teach client to exhale while turning or moving in bed

11. Administer stool softeners (e.g., docusate)

12. Restrict fluids to 1,200–1,500 ml/day

13. Administer medications

    a. Osmotic diuretics—to reduce fluid volume (e.g., mannitol)

    b. Corticosteroid therapy—to reduce cerebral edema (e.g., dexamethazone)

    c. Antiseizure medications–(e.g., diazepam, phenytoin, phenobarbital)

D. Evaluation

1. Have complications of increased intracranial pressure been prevented?

2. Is the client alert and oriented?

▶ SEIZURES

A. Assessment (see Table 5)

1. Episodes of abnormal motor, sensory, autonomic, or psychic activity due to abnormal discharge from brain cells

B. Analysis

1. Causes

    a. Epilepsy

    b. Fever in child

    c. Head injury

    d. Hypertension

    e. CNS infection

    f. Brain tumor or metastasis

    g. Drug withdrawal

    h. Stroke

C. Plan/Implementation

1. During seizure

    a. Protect from injury

    b. Raise side rails or ease client to floor and protect client from injury

    c. Use padded side rails according to agency policy

    d. Loosen restrictive clothing

    e. Do not restrain

    f. Do not try to insert a bite block, padded tongue blade, or oral airway

    g. Protect nurse—client may be flailing arms

    h. Place client on side with head extended

    i. Monitor onset, duration, pattern of seizure

    j. Administer medications for status epilepticus

Table 5 SEIZURES		
TYPE	AGE GROUP	ASSESSMENT
Generalized seizures Tonic-clonic	All	Aura Usually starts with tonic or stiffening phase, followed by clonic or jerking phase May have bowel/bladder incontinence; in postictal phase, sleeps, hard to arouse
Absence	Usually children	Staring spell, or staring spell with lip smacking, chewing
Myoclonic	Onset in children	Brief muscular contraction involving one or more limbs, trunk
Infantile spasms	Infants and children	Gross flexion, extension of limbs Treated with ACTH
Atonic seizures	Infants and children	Sudden loss of muscle tone and posture control, causing child to drop to floor
Tonic seizures	Infants and children	Stiffening of limbs
Partial seizures Seizures beginning locally	All	Jacksonian, or focal seizure, starting at one location, may spread
Sensory	All	Tingling, numbness of a body part; visual, olfactory, taste symptoms
Affective	All	Inappropriate fear, laughter, dreamy states, depersonalization
Complex partial seizures Temporal lobe/ psychomotor seizures	All	Aura complex Most commonly involves automatism—lip-smacking, picking at clothing, dreamy states, feelings of déja vu, hallucinations; may have antisocial, violent behavior, somatosensory reports, bizarre behavior
Partial seizures with secondary generalization	All	May spread from an original discharge site to other parts of the brain and become generalized

2. After seizure
   a. Position on side to prevent aspiration, reduce environmental stimuli
   b. Provide oxygen and suction equipment, if needed
   c. Reorient as needed
   d. Provide description of seizure in record
      1) Circumstances surrounding seizure
      2) How seizure started (location of first tremors or stiffness)
      3) Type of body movements
      4) Areas of body involved

      5) Presence of automations (involuntary motor activities, e.g., lip smacking)

      6) Incontinence

      7) Duration of each phase

      8) Unconsciousness during seizure or paralysis after seizure

      9) Actions after seizures (e.g., confusion, sleep, speech)

  3. To prevent seizures

    a. Administer anticonvulsant medications (e.g., phenytoin,phenobarbital)

      1) Don't discontinue abruptly

      2) Avoid alcohol

      3) Good oral hygiene

      4) Carry medical identification

    b. Avoid seizure triggers

      1) Alcoholic beverages

      2) Stress

      3) Caffeine

      4) Fever

      5) Hyperventilation

    c. Complementary/Alternative therapies

      1) Ketogenic diet to prevent seizures

        a) Diet high in fat and low in carbohydrates mimics effects of fasting and places the body in a constant state of ketosis

        b) Suppresses many types of seizures (tonic-clonic, absence, complex partial) and is effective when other methods of seizure control fail

D. Evaluation

  1. Is client compliant with medication regimen?

  2. Have injuries from seizure been prevented?

▶ STROKE

A. Assessment

  1. Confusion/disorientation

  2. Changes in vital signs and neurological signs

  3. Change in level of consciousness, seizures

  4. Aphasia

  5. Hemiplegia

  6. Bladder and/or bowel incontinence

  7. Headache, vomiting

  8. Hemianopsia—loss of half of visual field

  9. Dysphagia—difficulty swallowing

  10. Decreased sensation/neglect syndrome

  11. Emotional lability

B. Diagnose

1. Abrupt onset of neurological deficits resulting from interference with blood supply to the brain

2. Causes

   a. Thrombosis

   b. Embolism

   c. Hemorrhage

3. Risk factors

   a. Age

   b. Hypertension

   c. Transient ischemic attacks (TIAs)

   d. Diabetes mellitus

   e. Smoking

   f. Obesity

   g. Elevated blood lipids

   h. Oral contraceptives

   i. Atrial fibrillation

C. Plan/Implementation

1. Immediate care

   a. Maintain patent airway

   b. Minimize activity

   c. Keep head of bed elevated 15–30° to prevent increased intracranial pressure

   d. Maintain proper body alignment

   e. Keep side rails in upright position

   f. Administer thrombolytics within 3 hours of onset of symptoms

2. Intermediate care and rehabilitative needs

   a. Position for good body alignment and comfort

   b. Institute measures that facilitate swallowing

      1) Allow client to sit in upright position with head flexed slightly

      2) Instruct client to use tongue actively

      3) Administer liquids slowly, avoid milk-based products

      4) Place food on unaffected side of mouth

      5) Provide semisolid foods (easiest to swallow)

      6) Instruct to swallow while eating; maintain upright position for 30–45 minutes after eating

   c. Monitor elimination patterns

   d. Provide skin care

   e. Perform passive and/or active range-of-motion exercises

   f. Orient to person, time, and place

   g. Move affected extremities slowly and gently

   h. Teach use of supportive devices (e.g., commode, trapeze, cane)

     i. Address communication needs—face client and speak clearly and slowly; give the client time to respond; use verbal and nonverbal communication

     j. Do not approach from visually impaired side

     k. Encourage use of affected side

D. Evaluation

  1. Are client's vital signs stable?

  2. Has client regained mobility?

  3. Is client oriented?

▶ SPINAL CORD INJURY

A. Assessment

  1. Loss of motor and sensory function below level of injury (see Table 6)

  2. Spinal shock symptoms

     a. Flaccid paralysis of skeletal muscles

     b. Complete loss of all sensation

     c. Decreased pulses, bradycardia

     d. Suppression of somatic (pain, touch, temperature) and visceral reflexes

  3. Postural hypotension

  4. Circulatory problems—edema

  5. Alteration in normal thermoregulation

B. Diagnose

  1. Types of spinal cord injuries

     a. Concussion without direct trauma

     b. Penetrating wound or fracture dislocation

     c. Hemorrhage

     d. Laceration—damage related to level of cord affected

     e. Compression—often dural/epidural hematoma; if pressure on the cord is not relieved early, will cause ischemia, cord necrosis, and permanent damage

  2. Categories of neurological deficit

     a. Complete—no voluntary motor activity or sensation below level of injury

     b. Incomplete—some voluntary motor activity or sensation below level of injury

     c. Paraplegia—thoracic vertebral injury or lower; lower extremity involvement

     d. Tetraplegia (quadriplegia)—cervical/vertebral injury; all 4 extremities involved

  3. Causes

     a. Trauma due to accidents

       1) Car accidents, falls, sports, and industrial accidents

          2) Occurs predominantly in young white males (ages 15–30)

          3) May be related to substance abuse

      b. Neoplasms

    4. Diagnosis—neurological examination, x-rays, CT scan, MRI, myelography, digital rectal exam to determine extent of neurological deficit

C. Plan/Implementation

    1. Prevention

      a. Drive within the speed limit

      b. Use seat belts in car

      c. Wear helmets when riding motorcycles and bicycles

      d. Don't drink and drive

    2. Assessment (triage)

      a. Airway, breathing, circulation (ABC)

      b. Stabilization of vital signs

      c. Head-to-toe assessment

    3. Immobilize cervical spine

      a. Skeletal traction—Gardner-Wells, Crutchfield, Vinke tongs, halo traction

      b. Surgical stabilization—reduction and stabilization by fusion, wires, and plates

    4. Administer steroid therapy and antispasmodics

    5. Administer antispasmodics—baclofen, diazepam

    6. Hyperbaric oxygen therapy

    7. Move client by log-rolling technique; use turning frames

    8. Provide good skin care

    9. Provide emotional support

    10. Ensure adequate nutrition

    11. Reduce aggravating factors that cause spasticity

    12. Bladder and bowel training, catheterization

    13. Client and family education to cope with detailed care at home

    14. Prevent complication of autonomic hyperreflexia (dysreflexia)

      a. Usually caused by bladder or bowel distention; other causes: pain, tactile stimulation

      b. Occurs in clients with spinal cord lesions at or above T6 after spinal shock has subsided

      c. Symptoms—pounding headache, profuse sweating, especially of forehead, nasal congestion, piloerection (goose flesh), bradycardia, hypertension

      d. Place client in sitting position

      e. Catheterize or irrigate existing catheter to re-establish patency

      f. Check rectum for fecal mass

      g. Hydralazine may be given slowly IV

D. Evaluation

1. Is client able to regain optimal functioning?

2. Have complications been prevented?

Table 6 SPINAL CORD INJURY		
LEVEL OF INJURY	FUNCTIONAL ABILITY	SELF-CARE CAPABILITY
C3 and above	Inability to control muscles of breathing	Unable to care for self, life-sustaining ventilatory support essential
C4	Movement of trapezius and sternocleidomastoid muscles, no upper extremity muscle function, minimal ventilatory capacity	Unable to care for self, may self-feed with powered devices (depending on respiratory function)
C5	Neck movement, possible partial strength of shoulder and biceps	Can drive electric wheelchair, may be able to feed self with powered devices
C6	Muscle function in C5 level; partial strength in pectoralis major	May self-propel a lightweight wheelchair, may feed self with devices, can write and care for self, can transfer from chair to bed
C7	Muscle function in C6 level, no finger muscle power	Can dress lower extremities, minimal assistance needed, independence in wheelchair, can drive car with hand controls
C8	Muscle function in C7 level, finger muscle power	Same as C7; in general, activities easier
T1–T4	Good upper extremity muscle strength	Some independence from wheelchair, long leg braces for standing exercises
T5–L2	Balance difficulties	Still requires wheelchair, limited ambulation with long-leg braces and crutches
L3–L5	Trunk-pelvis muscle function intact	May use crutches or canes for ambulation
L5–S3	Waddling gait	Ambulation

FLUID AND ELECTROLYTE IMBALANCES Unit 2

▶ FLUID VOLUME IMBALANCES

A. Assessment (see Table 1)

B. Diagnose (see Table 1)

C. Plan/Implementation (see Table 1)

Table 1 FLUID VOLUME IMBALANCES		
	VOLUME DEFICIT	**VOLUME OVERLOAD**
Assessment	Thirst (early sign)	No change in temperature
	Temperature increases	Pulse increases slightly and is bounding
	Rapid and weak pulse Respirations increase	Respirations increase, shortness of breath, dyspnea, rales (crackles)
	Poor skin turgor–skin cool, moist	Peripheral edema–bloated appearance, weight gain
	Hypotension	
	Emaciation, weight loss	Hypertension
	Dry eye sockets, mouth and mucous membranes	May have muffled heart sounds
		Jugular vein distention
	Anxiety, apprehension, exhaustion	Urine specific gravity less than 1.010
	Urine specific gravity greater than 1.030	Apprehension
	Decreased urine output	Increased venous pressure
	Increased hemoglobin, hematocrit, Na$^+$, serum osmolality	Decreased hematocrit BUN, hemoglobin, Na$^+$, serum osmolality
	Headache, lethargy, confusion, disorientation, weight loss	
Diagnose	Isotonic loss	Isotonic gain, increase in the interstitial compartment, intravascular compartment, or both
	Vomiting Diarrhea	
	GI suction	CHF
	Sweating	Renal failure
	Decreased intake	Cirrhosis of the liver
	Hemorrhage	Excessive ingestion of sodium
	Third space shift	Excessive or too rapid intravenous infusion
Plan/Implementation	Force fluids	Administer diuretics
	Provide isotonic IV fluids: lactated ringer's or 0.9% NaCl	Restrict fluids
		Sodium-restricted diet (average daily diet–6–15 mg Na$^+$)
	I and O, hourly outputs	
	Daily weights (1 liter fluid = 1 kg or 2.2 lb)	Daily weight
	Monitor vital signs	Assess breath sounds
	Check skin turgor	Check feet/ankle/sacral region for edema
	Assess urine specific gravity	Semi-Fowler's position if dyspneic

D. Evaluation

1. Has client's fluid and electrolyte balance been re-established?

2. Have complications been prevented?

▶ **ADH DISORDERS**

   A. Assessment (see Table 2)

   B. Analysis (see Table 2)

   C. Plan/Implementation (see Table 2)

   D. Evaluation

      1. Has the client's fluid and electrolyte balance been maintained?

      2. Is client knowledgeable about medications?

Table 2 ADH DISORDERS		
	DIABETES INSIPIDUS (DECREASED ADH)	**SIADH—SYNDROME OF INAPPROPRIATE ANTIDIURETIC HORMONE SECRETION (INCREASED ADH)**
Assessment	Excessive urine output Chronic, severe dehydration Excessive thirst Anorexia, weight loss Weakness Constipation	Anorexia, nausea, vomiting Lethargy Headaches Change in level of consciousness Decreased deep tendon reflexes Tachycardia Increased circulating blood volume Decreased urinary output

Diagnose	Head trauma
	Brain tumor
	Meningitis
	Encephalitis
	Deficiency of ADH
	Diagnosis tests:
	   Low urine specific gravity
	   Urinary osmolality below plasma level
	High serum sodium
		Small cell carcinoma of lung
		Pneumonia
		Positive-pressure ventilation
		Brain tumors
		Head trauma
		Stroke
		Meningitis
		Encephalitis
		Feedback mechanism that regulates ADH does not function properly; ADH is released even when plasma hypo-osmolality is present
		Diagnostic tests:
		   Serum sodium decreased, plasma osmolality decreased
		Increased urine specific gravity

Nursing considerations	Record intake and output Monitor urine specific gravity, skin condition, weight, blood pressure, pulse, temperature Administer vasopressin	Restrict water intake (500-600 ml/24 h) Administer diuretics to promote excretion of water Hypertonic saline (3% NaCl) IV Administer demeclocycline Weigh daily I and O Monitor serum Na^+ levels Assess LOC

▶ POTASSIUM IMBALANCES

A. Assessment (see Table 3)

B. Diagnose (see Table 3)

C. Plan/Implementation (see Table 3)

Table 3 POTASSIUM IMBALANCES		
	HYPOKALEMIA	HYPERKALEMIA
Assessment	less than 3.5 mEq/L (3.5 mmol/L) Anorexia, nausea, and vomiting Muscle weakness, paresthesias Dysrhythmias, increased sensitivity to digitalis	greater than 5.0 mEq/L (5 mmol/L) EKG changes, dysrhythmias, cardiac arrest Muscle weakness Paralysis Nausea Diarrhea
Diagnose	Potassium—main intracellular ion; involved in cardiac rhythm, nerve transmission Normal level—3.5–5.0 mEq/L (3.5-5 mmol/L) Causes—vomiting, gastric suction, diarrhea, diuretics and steroids, inadequate intake	Causes—renal failure, use of potassium supplements, burns, crushing injuries

Plan/Implementation	Administration of oral potassium supplements—dilute in juice to avoid gastric irritation
	
	Increase dietary intake—raisins, bananas, apricots, oranges, beans, potatoes, carrots, celery
	
	IV supplements—40 mEq/L usual concentration; cannot give concentration greater than 40 mEq/L into peripheral IV or without cardiac monitor
	
	Increases risk of digoxin toxicity
	
	    Protect from injury
	
	    Assess renal function prior to administration
		Restrict dietary potassium and potassium-containing medications
		
		Sodium polystyrene sulfonate—cation exchange resin (causes diarrhea)
		
		Orally—dilute to make more palatable
		
		Rectally—give in conjunction with sorbitol to avoid fecal impaction
		
		In emergency situation, calcium gluconate given IV, sodium bicarbonate given IV, regular insulin and dextrose
		
		IV administration of regular insulin and dextrose shifts potassium into the cells
		
		Peritoneal or hemodialysis
		
		Diuretics

D. Evaluation

    1. Has client's fluid and electrolyte balance been re-established?

    2. Have complications been prevented?

▶ SODIUM IMBALANCES

A. Assessment (see Table 4)

B. Diagnose (see Table 4)

C. Plan/Implementation (see Table 4)

Table 4 SODIUM IMBALANCES		
	HYPONATREMIA	HYPERNATREMIA
Assessment	Less than 135 mEq/L (135 mmol/L) Nausea Muscle cramps Increased intracranial pressure, confusion, muscular twitching, convulsions	greater than 145 mEq/L (145 mmol/L) Elevated temperature Weakness Disorientation Delusion and hallucinations Thirst, dry swollen tongue, sticky mucous membranes Postural hypotension with decreased ECF Hypertension with normal or increased ECF Tachycardia
Diagnose	Sodium—main extracellular ion; responsible for water balance Normal—135–145 mEq/L (135–145 mmol/L) Causes—vomiting, diuretics, excessive administration of dextrose and water IVs, prolonged low-sodium diet, excessive water intake	Causes—hypertonic tube feedings without water supplements, diarrhea, hyperventilation, diabetes insipidus, ingestion of OTC drugs such as Alka-Seltzer, inhaling large amounts of salt water (near-drowning), inadequate water ingestion
Plan/Implementation	Oral administration of sodium-rich foods—beef broth, tomato juice IV lactated Ringer's or 0.9% NaCl Water restriction (safer method) I and O Daily weight	IV administration of hypotonic solution—0.3% NaCl or 0.45% NaCl; 5% dextrose in water Offer fluids at regular intervals Decrease sodium in diet Daily weight

D. Evaluation

    1. Has client's fluid and electrolyte balance been re-established?

    2. Have complications been prevented?

▶ CALCIUM IMBALANCES

A. Assessment (see Table 5)

B. Diagnose (see Table 5)

C. Plan/Implementation (see Table 5)

D. Evaluation

    1. Has client's fluid and electrolyte balance been re-established?

    2. Have complications been prevented?

Table 5 CALCIUM IMBALANCES		
	HYPOCALCEMIA	**HYPERCALCEMIA**

Assessment	Ionized serum calcium less than 4.5 mg/dL or total serum calcium less than 8.6 mg/dL (2.2 mmol/L) (total serum calcium levels used)
	
	Nervous system becomes increasingly excitable
	
	Tetany
	  Trousseau's sign—inflate BP cuff on upper arm to 20 mm Hg above systolic pressure; carpal spasms within 2–5 minutes indicate tetany
	  Chvostek's sign—tap facial nerve 2 cm anterior to the earlobe just below the zygomatic arch; twitching of facial muscles indicates tetany
	
	Seizures
	
	Confusion
	
	Paresthesia
	
	Irritability
		Ionized serum calcium greater than 5.1 mg/L or total serum calcium greater than 10.2 mg/dL (2.5 mmol/L)(total serum calcium levels used)
		
		Sedative effect on central and peripheral nervous system
		
		Muscle weakness, lack of coordination, constipation, abdominal pain, and distension
		
		Confusion
		
		Depressed or absent tendon reflexes
		
		Dysrhythmias

Diagnose	Calcium—needed for blood clotting, skeletal muscle contraction Ionized serum calcium less than 4.5 mg/dL or total serum calcium less than 8.6 mg/dL (2.2 mmol/L) Regulated by parathyroid hormone and vitamin D, which facilitates reabsorption of calcium from bone and enhances absorption from the GI tract Causes—hypoparathyroidism, pancreatitis, renal failure, steroids and loop diuretics, inadequate intake, post-thyroid surgery	Causes—malignant neoplastic diseases, hyperparathyroidism, excessive intake, immobility, excessive intake of calcium carbonate antacids
Plan/ Implementation	Orally—calcium gluconate (less concentrated) or calcium chloride; administer with orange juice to maximize absorption Parenterally—calcium gluconate Effect is transitory and additional doses may be necessary Use caution with digitalized clients because both are cardiac depressants Calcium may cause vessel irritation and should be administered through a long, stable intravenous line Avoid infiltration since tissue can become necrotic and slough Administer at a slow rate to avoid high serum concentrations and cardiac depression Seizure precautions Maintain airway because laryngeal stridor can occur Maintain safety needs since confusion is often present Increase dietary intake of calcium, calcium supplements Regular exercise Administer phosphate-binding antacids, calcitriol, vitamin D	IV administration of 0.45% NaCl or 0.9% NaCl Encourage fluids furosemide Calcitonin—decreases calcium level Mobilize the client Restrict dietary calcium Prevent development of renal calculi Increase fluid intake Maintain acidic urine Prevent UTI Surgical intervention may be indicated in hyperparathyroidism Injury prevention Limit intake of calcium carbonate antacids

▶ MAGNESIUM IMBALANCES

A. Assessment (see Table 6)

B. Analysis (see Table 6)

C. Plan/Implementation (see Table 6)

D. Evaluation

1. Has client's fluid and electrolyte balance been re-established?

2. Have complications been prevented?

Table 6 MAGNESIUM IMBALANCES		
	HYPOMAGNESEMIA	HYPERMAGNESEMIA
Assessment	less than 1.3 mEq/L (0.53 mmol/L)	greater than 2.3 mEq/L (0.95 mmol/L)
	Magnesium acts as a depressant	Depresses the CNS
	Increased neuromuscular irritability	Depresses cardiac impulse transmission
	Tremors, tetany, seizures	Hypotension
	Dysrhythmias	Facial flushing, muscle weakness
	Depression, confusion	Absent deep tendon reflexes, paralysis
	Dysphagia	Shallow respirations
Diagnose	Normal–1.3–2.3 mEq/L (0.53-0.95 mmol/L)	Causes–renal failure, excessive magnesium administration (antacids, cathartics)
	Causes–alcoholism, GI suction, diarrhea, intestinal fistulas, abuse of diuretics or laxatives	
	Usually seen with other electrolyte deficits	
Plan/Implementation	Increased intake of dietary Mg–green vegetables, nuts, bananas, oranges, peanut butter, chocolate	Discontinue oral and IV Mg
		Emergency
	Parenteral administration of supplements–magnesium sulfate	Support ventilation
		IV calcium gluconate
	Monitor cardiac rhythm and reflexes to detect depressive effects of magnesium	Hemodialysis
		Monitor reflexes
	Keep self-inflating breathing bag, Monitor respiratory status airway and oxygen at bedside, in case of respiratory emergency	Teach about OTC drugs containing Mg
		Monitor cardiac rhythm; have calcium preparations available to antagonize cardiac depression
	Calcium preparations may be given to counteract the potential danger of myocardial dysfunction that may result from magnesium intoxication secondary to rapid infusions	
	Oral–long-term maintenance with oral magnesium	
	IV administration–assess renal function	
	Monitor for digitalis toxicity	
	Maintain seizure precautions	
	Provide safety measures because confusion is often present	
	Test ability to swallow before PO fluids/ food because of dysphagia	

▶ BURNS

A. Assessment

1. "Rule of Nines" (see Figure 1)

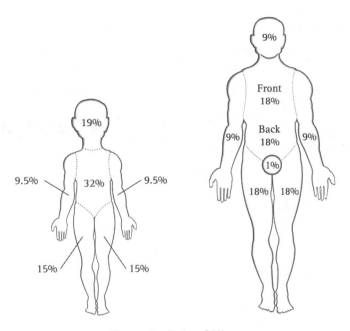

Figure 1   Rule of Nines

2. Determination of intensity (see Table 7)

Table 7 CLASSIFICATION OF BURNS				
SUPERFICIAL	**SUPERFICIAL PARTIAL–THICKNESS**	**DEEP PARTIAL–THICKNESS**	**FULL–THICKNESS**	**DEEP FULL–THICKNESS**
Similar to first-degree	Similar to second-degree	Similar to second-degree	Similar to third-degree	Similar to third-degree
Skin pink to red Painful	Skin pink to red Painful	Skin red to white Painful	Skin red, white, brown, black Pain possible	Skin black No pain
Epidermis Sunburn	Epidermis and dermis Scalds, flames	Epidermis and dermis Scalds, flames, tar, grease	All skin layers Prolonged contact with hot objects	All skin layers, possibly muscles and tendon Flames, electricity
Heals in 3 to 5 days	Heals in 2 weeks	Heals in 1 month Possible grafting	Heals in weeks to months	Heals in weeks to months Escharotomy Grafting

B. Analysis (see Table 8)

1. At risk

   a. Young children

   b. Elderly

2. Prevention

    a. Keep all matches and lighters away from children

    b. Do not leave children alone around fires

    c. Install and maintain smoke detectors

    d. Set water-heater temperature no higher than 120°F (48.9°C)

    e. Do not smoke in bed or fall asleep while smoking

    f. Use caution when cooking

    g. Keep a working fire extinguisher in the home

3. Thermal—contact with hot substance (solids/liquids/gases)

Table 8 NURSING CARE FOR BURN CLIENT	
GOAL	**NURSING CONSIDERATIONS**

Correct fluid and electrolyte imbalance	First 24–48 h (emergent/resuscitative phase):
	
	    IV fluids balanced salt solution (Lactated Ringers), plasma
	
	    Rapid for first 8 h, more slowly over remaining 16 h
	
	2–5 d after burn (intermediate phase):
	
	    Packed RBCs
	
	    Indwelling catheter to monitor hourly output; should be at least 30 ml/h
	
	    Careful administration of IV fluids; check for signs of fluid overload versus dehydration
	
	    Monitor blood pressure, TPR, wt, serum electrolytes

Promote healing	Cap, gown, mask, and gloves worn by nurse Wound care at least once a day Debridement (removal of nonviable tissue)—hydrotherapy is used to loosen dead tissue, 30 min maximum Escharotomy (incising of leathery covering of dead tissue conducive to bacterial growth)—used to alleviate constriction, minimize infection Dressing: careful sterile technique, avoid breaking blisters, wound may be covered or left exposed Application of topical antibacterial medications: silver sulfadiazine—closed method; monitor for hypersensitivity, rash, itching, burning sensation in areas other than burn, decreased WBC; mafenide—open method; monitor acid/base balance and renal function; remove previously applied cream; Silver nitrate—keep dressings wet with solution to avoid over concentrations; handle carefully; can leave a gray/black stain Grafting: biological (human amniotic membrane, cadaver, allograft); autografting when granulation bed is clean and well vascularized Tetanus prophylaxis Avoid hypothermia and add humidity
Support nutrition	High-caloric, high-carbohydrate, high-protein diet; may require PN or tube feeding; oral nutrient supplements; vitamins B, C, and iron; H2 histamine blockers and antacids to prevent stress ulcer (Curling's ulcer) NG tube to prevent gastric distention, early acute gastric dilation, and paralytic ileus associated with burn shock; monitor bowel sounds
Control pain	Pain medication (morphine)—given IV at first due to impaired circulation and poor absorption Monitor VS frequently; analgesic 30 min before wound care

Table 8 NURSING CARE FOR BURN CLIENT *(CONTINUED)*	
GOAL	**NURSING CONSIDERATIONS**
Prevent complications of immobility	Prevent contractures—maintain joints in neutral position of extension; shoes to prevent foot drop; splints; active and passive ROM exercises at each dressing change; turn side to side frequently; skin care to prevent breakdown
	Stryker frame or Circ-O-Lectric bed may facilitate change of position
	Facial exercises and position that hyperextends neck for burns of face and neck
	Consult with physical therapist
Support client	Counsel client regarding change in body image
	Encourage expression of feelings and demonstrate acceptance of client
	Evaluate client's readiness to see scarred areas, especially facial area
	Assist client's family to adjust to changed appearance
	Consider recommending client for ongoing counseling
	Support developmental needs of children, e.g., sick children need limits on behavior
	Assist client in coping with immobilization, pain, and isolation
	Prepare client for discharge—anticipate readmission for release of contractures/cosmetic surgery; proper use of any correctional orthopedic appliances, pressure garments (used to decrease scarring); how to change dressings

4. Chemical—contact with strong acids or strong bases; prolonged contact with most chemicals

5. Electrical—contact with live current; internal damage may be more severe than expected from external injury

6. Radiation—exposure to high doses of radioactive material

C. Plan/Implementation

1. Emergency care—on the scene

   a. Stop the burning process

   b. Thermal—smother; stop, drop, and roll

   c. Chemical—remove clothing and flush/irrigate skin/eyes

   d. Electrical—shut off electrical current or separate person from source with a nonconducting implement

   e. Ensure airway, breathing, and circulation

   f. Immediate wound care—keep person warm and dry; wrap in clean, dry sheet/blanket

2. Nursing care (see Table 8)

3. Stages following severe burns (see Table 9)

Table 9 PHASES FOLLOWING SEVERE BURNS	
EMERGENT/RESUSCITATIVE	INTERMEDIATE/ACUTE
First 24–48 hours	Begins 36–48 hours after burn
Fluid loss through open wound or extrava-sation into deeper tissues	Decrease in peripheral edema
Hypovolemia	Blood volume restored
Renal complications possible	Diuresis if renal system unimpaired
K^+ (hyperkalemia)	K^+ (hypokalemia)
↓ BP, ↑ Pulse	↑ BP

D. Evaluation

    1. Have client's physical needs been met?

    2. Have complications from the burn been prevented?

▶ ADRENAL DISORDERS

A. Assessment (see Table 10)

B. Analysis (see Table 10)

    1. Adrenal cortex

        a. Glucocorticoids

        b. Mineralocorticoids

        c. Androgen and estrogen

    2. Adrenal medulla

        a. Norepinephrine

        b. Epinephrine

C. Plan/Implementation

    1. Addison's disease

        a. High-protein, high-carbohydrate, high-sodium, low-potassium diet

        b. Wear Medic-Alert bracelet

        c. Protect from infection

        d. Monitor for hypoglycemia, hyponatremia

        e. Assist with 24-hour urine collection for 17-hydroxycorticosteroids (refrigerate urine during collection)

        f. Administer hormonal replacement—may be lifelong

        g. Avoid factors that precipitate Addisonian crisis

            1) Physical stress

            2) Psychological stress

            3) Inadequate steroid replacement

Table 10 ADRENAL DISORDERS		
	ADDISON'S DISEASE	**CUSHING'S SYNDROME**
Assessment	Fatigue, weakness, dehydration, ↓ BP, hyperpigmentation, ↓ resistance to stress, alopecia Weight loss, pathological fractures Depression, lethargy, emotional lability	Fatigue, weakness, osteoporosis, muscle wasting, cramps, edema, ↑ BP, purple skin striations, hirsutism, emaciation, depression, decreased resistance to infection, moon face, buffalo hump, obesity (trunk), mood swings, masculinization in females, blood sugar imbalance

Diagnose	Hyposecretion of adrenal hormones (mineralocorticoids, glucocorticoids, androgens)
	
	Pathophysiology:
	   ↓ Na^+ dehydration
	   ↓ Blood volume + shock
	   ↑ K^+ metabolic acidosis + arrhythmias
	   ↓ Blood sugar + insulin shock
	Diagnostic tests:
	   CT and MRI
	   Hyperkalemia and hyponatremia
	   ↓ Plasma cortisol
	   ↓ Urinary 17-hydroxycorticosteroids and 17-ketosteroids
	ACTH stimulation test
	Treatment: hormone replacement
		Hypersecretion of adrenal hormones (mineralocorticoids, glucocorticoids, androgens)
		
		Pathophysiology:
		   ↑ Na^+ ↑ blood volume + ↑ BP
		   ↓ K^+ metabolic alkalosis + shock
		   ↑ Blood sugar + ketoacidosis
		Diagnostic tests:
		   Skull films
		   Blood sugar analysis
		   Hypokalemia and hypernatremia
		   Plasma cortisol level
		Urinary 17-hydroxycorticosteroids and 17-ketosteroids
		Treatment: hypophysectomy, adrenalectomy

h. Observe for clinical manifestations of Addisonian crisis (precipitated by physical or emotional stress, sudden withdrawal of hormones)

   1) Nausea and vomiting

   2) Abdominal pain

   3) Fever

   4) Extreme weakness

   5) Severe hypoglycemia, hyperkalemia, and dehydration develop rapidly

   6) Blood pressure falls, leading to shock and coma; death results if not promptly treated

      i. Treatment of Addisonian crisis

        1) Administer and assess hydrocortisone therapy

        2) Carefully monitor IV infusion of 0.9% NaCl or D_5W/NaCl

        3) Administer IV glucose, glucagon

        4) Administer insulin with dextrose in normal saline; administer potassium-binding and excreting resin (e.g., sodium polystyrene sulfonate)

        5) Monitor vital signs

  2. Cushing's syndrome

    a. Assure the client that most physical changes are reversible with treatment

    b. High-protein, low-carbohydrate, high-potassium, low-sodium, low-calorie diet; fluid restriction

    c. Use careful technique to prevent infection

    d. Eliminate environmental hazards for pathological fractures

    e. Observe for hyperactivity, GI bleeding, fluid volume overload

    f. Administer aminoglutethimide or metyrapone to decrease cortisolproduction

    g. Provide postadrenalectomy care

      1) Flank incision—painful to breathe, so encourage coughing and deep breathing

      2) Ensure client safety to decrease risk of fractures

      3) Monitor for shock

      4) Monitor for hypertension

      5) Administer cortisone and mineralocorticoids as ordered

    h. Anticipate slow recovery from anesthesia in obese client

    i. Anticipate slow wound healing

    j. Monitor glucose level, monitor urine output

D. Evaluation

  1. Has the client's fluid and electrolyte balance been maintained?

▶ PHEOCHROMOCYTOMA

A. Assessment

  1. Intermittent hypertension

  2. Increased heart rate, palpitations during hypertensive episodes

  3. Nausea and vomiting, weight loss

  4. Hyperglycemia, glucosuria, polyuria

  5. Diaphoresis, pallor, tremor, nervousness during hypertensive episodes

  6. Pounding headache, weakness, visual disturbances during hypertensive episodes

  7. Pain

8. Urinary vanillylmandelic acid (VMA) test
   a. 24-hour urine for VMA—breakdown product of catecholamine metabolism
   b. Normal results: 1–5 mg, positive for tumor if significantly higher
   c. Foods affecting VMA excretion excluded 3 days before test
      1) Coffee
      2) Tea
      3) Bananas
      4) Vanilla
      5) Chocolate
   d. All drugs discontinued during test
   e. Urine collected on ice or refrigerated with preservative
9. Clonidine suppression test—conidine levels not decreased

B. Diagnose
   1. Definition—hypersecretion of catecholamines (epinephrine and norepinephrine) activate fight-or-flight response due to secreting tumors of the adrenal medulla; tumor can also occur anywhere, from neck to pelvis, along course of sympathetic nerve chain
   2. Potential nursing diagnoses
      a. Deficient knowledge
      b. Decreased cardiac output/ineffective tissue perfusion

C. Plan/Implementation
   1. Avoid physical and emotional stress
   2. Monitor blood pressure in lying and sitting positions
   3. Frequent bathing, but avoid chilling
   4. Administer analgesics for pain, sedatives and tranquilizers for rest and relaxation
   5. Increase caloric, vitamin, and mineral intake due to increased metabolic demand
   6. Avoid coffee, tea, cola, and foods containing tyramine
   7. Limit activity
   8. Administer adrenergic-blocking medications
   9. Administer apresoline for hypertensive crisis
   10. Allow time to verbalize concerns to decrease nervousness and tremors
   11. Provide postsurgical care—adrenalectomy or medullectomy

D. Evaluation
   1. Has the client's fluid and electrolyte balance been maintained?
   2. Have complications been prevented?

ALTERATIONS IN BODY SYSTEMS

▶ CHRONIC OBSTRUCTIVE PULMONARY DISEASE (COPD)

A. Assessment

1. Change in skin color—cyanosis or reddish color
2. Weakness, weight loss
3. Risk factors
   a. Smoking tobacco
   b. Passive tobacco smoke
   c. Occupational exposure
   d. Air pollution, coal, gas, asbestos exposure
   e. Genetic abnormalities—alpha 1antitrypsin deficiency
4. Use of accessory muscles of breathing, dyspnea
5. Changes in posture—day and hs
6. Cough, changes in color, consistency of sputum
7. Abnormal ABGs—PaO_2, and $PaCO_2$
8. Adventitious breath sounds
9. Changes in sensorium, memory impairment

B. Diagnose

1. Most common cause of lung disease in United States
2. Group of conditions associated with obstruction of air flow entering or leaving the lungs; genetic and environmental causes—smoking and air pollution
   a. Asthma—chronic disease with episodic attacks of breathlessness
   b. Emphysema—overinflation of alveoli resulting in destruction of alveolar walls; predisposing factors: smoking, chronic infections,and environmental pollution
   c. Chronic bronchitis—inflammation of bronchi with productive cough
   d. Cystic fibrosis—hereditary dysfunction of exocrine glands causing obstruction because of flow of thick mucus
      1) Causes—sweat gland dysfunction, respiratory dysfunction, GI dysfunction
      2) Diagnostic tests
         a) Sweat chloride analysis test—elevated levels of sodium and chloride
         b) GI enzyme evaluation—pancreatic enzyme deficiency
3. Potential nursing diagnoses
   a. Ineffective airway clearance
   b. Imbalanced nutrition: less than body requirements
   c. Anxiety
   d. Compromised family coping
   e. Activity intolerance

      f. Deficient knowledge

      g. Social interaction, impaired

      h. Risk for infection

      i. Impaired gas exchange

C. Plan/Implementation

  1. Assess airway clearance

  2. Listen to breath sounds

  3. Administer low-flow oxygen to prevent CO_2 narcosis for emphysema

  4. Encourage fluids (6–8 glasses, 3000 ml/24 hours), provide small, frequent feedings

  5. Administer medications: bronchodilators, mucolytics, corticosteroids, anticholinergics, leukotriene inhibitors, influenza and pneumococcal vaccines

  6. Metered dose inhalers (MDI)

      a. May be used with or without spacers

      b. Delivers medication directly to lungs

      c. Medications used with inhalers

        1) Beta-2 adrenergic drugs: albuterol, metaproterenol, terbutaline, salmeterol

        2) Corticosteriods: fluticasone, prednisone

        3) Cromolyn sodium and nedocromil

        4) Anticholinergics: ipratropium, tiotropium

      d. Medications should be administered so that bronchodilators are given first to open the airways, and then other medications are given

      e. Spacers attach to the MDI to hold medication in the chamber long enough for the client to inhale medication directly to the airways

      f. Teach proper use of MDI and spacers

      g. Caution against overuse

      h. Teach client to report decreasing effectiveness of medication and adverse effects

      i. Teach client to clean equipment thoroughly

      j. Teach client to rinse mouth thoroughly with water after steriod treatment to minimize risk of infection from oral candidiasis

  7. Client teaching

      a. Breathing exercises

      b. Stop smoking

      c. Avoid hot/cold air or allergens

      d. Instructions regarding medications

      e. Avoid close contact with persons who have respiratory infections or "flu"

      f. Avoid crowds during times of the year when respiratory infections most commonly occur

      g. Maintain a high resistance with adequate rest, nourishing diet, avoidance of stress, and avoidance of exposure to temperature extremes, dampness, and drafts

      h. Practice frequent, thorough oral hygiene and handwashing

      i. Advise about prophylactic influenza vaccines

      j. Instruct to observe sputum for indications of infection

D. Evaluation

   1. Are client's ABGs stable?

   2. Has client stopped smoking?

   3. Has airway clearance been maintained?

   4. Does client perform self-care?

   5. Are breathing patterns improved?

   6. Does client cope with chronic disease?

▶ PNEUMONIA

A. Assessment

   1. Fever, chills

   2. Cough productive of rust-colored, green, whitish-yellow sputum (depending on organism)

   3. Dyspnea, pleuritic pain, accessory muscle use, upright position

   4. Tachycardia, crackles, sonorous wheezes, bronchial breath sounds

   5. Elevated WBC count, sputum culture and sensitivity, blood culture and sensitivity

B. Diagnose

   1. Causes include bacteria, fungus, virus, parasite, chemical

   2. Inflammatory process that results in edema of lung tissues and extravasion of fluid into alveoli, causing hypoxia

   3. Risk factors

      a. Community-acquired pneumonia

         1) Older adult

         2) Has not received pneumococcal vaccination

         3) Has not received yearly flu vaccine

         4) Chronic illness

         5) Exposed to viral infection or flu

         6) Smokes or drinks alcohol

      b. Hospital-acquired pneumonia

         1) Older adult

         2) Chronic lung disease

         3) Aspiration

         4) Presence of endotracheal, tracheostomy, or nasogastric tube

         5) Mechanical ventilation

         6) Decreased levels of consciousness

         7) Immunosuppression (disease or pharmacologic etiology)

    4. Potential nursing diagnoses

        a. Ineffective airway clearance

        b. Activity intolerance

        c. Deficient knowledge

        d. Deficient fluid volume

C. Plan/Implementation

    1. Assess vital signs every 4 hours

    2. Cough and breathe deeply every 2 hours

    3. Assess breath sounds, and oxygen saturation

    4. Incentive spirometer—5–10 breaths per hour while awake

    5. Chest physiotherapy

    6. Encourage fluids to 3,000 ml/24 h

    7. Suction as needed

    8. Oxygen therapy

    9. Semi-Fowler's position/bedrest

    10. Teach about fluid intake and smoking cessation

    11. Medications

        a. Mucolytics

        b. Expectorants

        c. Bronchodilators (e.g., beta-2 agonists)—nebulizer or MDI

        d. Antibiotics

D. Evaluation

    1. Is there improved airway clearance?

    2. Is there a reduction in symptoms?

    3. Are the client's vital signs stable?

▶ CONGENITAL HEART ANOMALIES

A. Assessment (see Table 1)

B. Diagnose

    1. History-predisposing factors

        a. Maternal rubella during pregnancy

        b. Maternal alcoholism

        c. Maternal age over 40 years

        d. Maternal insulin-dependent diabetes (IDDM)

        e. Sibling(s) with heart disease

        f. Parent with congenital heart disease

        g. Other congenital anomalies

Table 1 CONGENITAL HEART ANOMALIES	
ACYANOTIC TYPE	**CYANOTIC TYPE**
Normal color	Cyanosis usually from birth; clubbing of fingers
Normal CNS function	May have seizures due to hypoxia; fainting; confusion
Possible exercise intolerance	Marked exercise intolerance; may have hypoxic spells following exercise; squats to decrease respiratory distress
Possible weight loss or gain (with fluid retention)	Difficulty eating because of inability to breathe at the same time, with subsequent weight loss
Small stature; failure to thrive	Small stature; failure to thrive
Characteristic murmur; increased frequency of respiratory infections	Characteristic murmur; frequent and severe respiratory infections

2. General effects of heart malformation
   a. Increased workload—overloading of chambers results in hypertrophy and tachycardia
   b. Pulmonary hypertension (increased vascular resistance) results in dyspnea, tachypnea, and recurrent respiratory infections
   c. Inadequate systemic cardiac output results in exercise intolerance and growth failure
   d. Arterial desaturation from shunting of deoxygenated blood directly into the systemic circulation results in polycythemia, cyanosis, cerebral changes, clubbing, squatting
   e. Murmurs due to abnormal shunting of blood between two heart chambers or between vessels
3. Types of defects (see Figure 1)
   a. Increased pulmonary blood flow (acyanotic)
      1) Ventricular septal defect (VSD)—abnormal opening between right and left ventricles; may vary in size from pinhole to absence of septum
         a) Characterized by loud, harsh murmur
         b) May close spontaneously by age 3—surgery may be indicated (purse-string closure of defect or pulmonary artery banding)

2) Atrial septal defect (ASD)—abnormal opening between the two atria; severity depends on the size and location

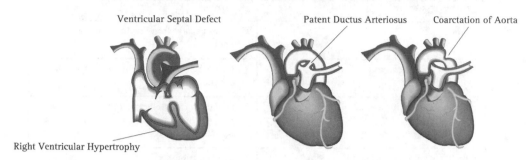

Figure 1. Congenital Heart Defects

a) Small defects high on the septum may not cause clinical symptoms

b) Murmur audible and distinct for defect

c) Unless defect is severe, prophylactic closure is done in later childhood

3) Patent ductus arteriosus (PDA)—failure of that fetal structure to close after birth (in fetus, ductus arteriosis connects the pulmonary artery to the aorta to shunt oxygenated blood from placenta directly into systemic circulation, bypassing the lungs)

a) PDA allows blood to be shunted from aorta (high pressure) to pulmonary artery (low pressure), causing additional blood to be reoxygenated in the lungs; result is increased pulmonary vascular congestion and right ventricular hypertrophy

b) Characteristic murmur, widened pulse pressure, bounding pulse, and tachycardia

c) Treatment is surgical intervention to divide or ligate the patent vessel

b. Obstruction to blood flow from ventricles (acyanotic)

1) Coarctation of the aorta—narrowing of the aorta

a) High blood pressure and bounding pulses in areas receiving blood from vessels proximal to the defect; weak or absent pulses distal to the defect, cool extremities, and muscle cramps

b) Murmur may or may not be present

c) Surgical treatment involves resection of the coarcted portion and end-to-end anastomosis or replacement of the constricted section using a graft

d) High incidence of complications if left untreated

2) Pulmonic stenosis—narrowing at the entrance to the pulmonary artery

a) Resistance to blood flow causes right ventricular hypertrophy

b) Commonly seen with PDA

c) Severity depends on degree of defect

d) Surgery recommended for severe defect (pulmonary valvotomy)

3) Aortic stenosis—narrowing of aortic valve causes decreased cardiac output

 a) Murmur usually heard

 b) Surgery recommended

c. Decreased pulmonary blood flow (cyanotic)

 1) Tetralogy of Fallot—four defects: ventricular septal defect, pulmonic stenosis, overriding aorta, right ventricular hypertrophy (first three are congenital, fourth is acquired due to increased pressure within the right ventricle)

 a) Cyanosis, clubbing of fingers, delayed physical growth and development

 b) Child often squats or assumes knee-chest position

 c) Treatment is surgical correction

d. Mixed blood flow (cyanotic)

 1) Transposition of the great vessels—pulmonary artery leaves from the left ventricle and the aorta leaves from the right ventricle

 a) Unless there is an associated defect to compensate, this condition is incompatible with life

 b) Depending on severity of condition—severe cyanosis to mild HF

 c) Treatment is surgical correction

 2) Truncus arteriosus—failure of normal septation and embryonic division of pulmonary artery and aorta, resulting in a single vessel that overrides both ventricles, giving rise directly to the pulmonary and systemic circulations

 a) Blood from both ventricles enters the common artery and flows either to the lungs or the aortic arch and body

 b) Cyanosis, left ventricular hypertrophy, dyspnea, marked activity intolerance, and growth retardation

 c) Harsh murmur audible; congestive heart failure usually develops

 d) Palliative treatment—banding both pulmonary arteries to decrease the amount of blood going to lungs

 e) Corrective treatment—closing ventricular septal defect so truncus originates from left ventricle, and creating pathway from right ventricle

 3) Total anomalous venous return—absence of direct communication between pulmonary veins and left atrium; pulmonary veins attach directly to the right atrium or to various veins draining toward the right atrium

 a) Cyanosis, pulmonary congestion, and heart failure

 b) Audible murmur

 c) Surgical correction involves restoring the normal pulmonary venous circulation

4. Compensatory mechanisms observed in cyanotic heart disease
   a. Tachycardia
   b. Polycythemia
   c. Posturing—squatting, knee-chest position
5. Potential nursing diagnoses
   a. Decreased cardiac output
   b. Excess fluid volume
   c. Risk for impaired gas exchange
   d. Activity intolerance
   e. Deficient knowledge
   f. Disabled family coping

C. Plan/Implementation
1. Prevent congenital heart disease
   a. Optimal maternal nutrition, prenatal care, and avoidance of drugs and alcohol
   b. Immunization against rubella in females
2. Recognize early symptoms—cyanosis, poor weight gain, poor feeding habits, exercise intolerance, unusual posturing; carefully evaluate heart murmurs
3. Monitor vital signs and heart rhythm
4. Provide support for client as well as restful environment
5. Prepare client for invasive procedures
6. Monitor intake and output
7. Provide calm environment and promote rest
8. Medications
   a. Digoxin
   b. Iron preparations
   c. Diuretics
   d. Potassium
9. Change feeding pattern for infant
   a. Small amounts every 2 hours
   b. Enlarged nipple hole
   c. Diet—low sodium, high potassium

D. Evaluation
1. Does child demonstrate good growth and development patterns?
2. Do family and child cope with alterations caused by congenital defect?

▶ **HEART FAILURE (HF)**

A. Assessment (see Table 2)
B. Diagnose
1. Failure of the cardiac muscle to pump sufficient blood to meet the body's metabolic needs
2. Ventricles cannot empty completely, which causes backup of circulation
3. Causes of heart failure (see Table 3)

Table 2 HEART FAILURE	
LEFT-SIDED FAILURE	**RIGHT-SIDED FAILURE**
Dyspnea, paroxysmal nocturnal dyspnea	Dependent edema (ankle, lower extremities)
Orthopnea	Liver enlargement and abdominal pain
Pleural effusion	Anorexia, nausea, bloating
Cheyne-Stokes respirations	Coolness of extremities secondary to venous congestion in major organs
Pulmonary edema, rales (crackles)	Anxiety, fear, depression
Cough with frothy, blood-tinged sputum	Weight gain
Decreased renal function—elevated BUN, albuminuria	
Edema, weight gain	
Changes in mental status (cerebral anoxia)	
Fatigue, muscle weakness	
S3 gallop	

4. Potential nursing diagnoses

   a. Decreased cardiac output

   b. Activity intolerance

   c. Anxiety

   d. Deficient knowledge

   e. Impaired gas exchange

   f. Ineffective tissue perfusion (cerebral)

C. Plan/Implementation

1. Administer cardiac glycosides

   a. Digoxin—fundamental drug in the treatment of heart failure, especially when associated with low cardiac output

   b. Two categories of dosages

      1) Rapid digitalization —aimed at administering the drug rapidly to achieve detectable effect

      2) Gradual digitalization—client placed on smaller amounts, designed to replace the digoxin lost by excretion while maintaining "optimal" cardiac functioning

2. Administer angiotensin-converting enzyme (ACE) inhibitors or angiotensin-receptor blockers (ARBs)—decrease afterload and improve myocardial contractility

3. Administer diuretics—thiazide diuretics, carbonic anhydrase inhibitors, aldosterone antagonists, loop diuretics

4. Administer vasodilators—decrease afterload and improve contractility

5. Administer morphine—decrease afterload

6. Administer inotropic medications—improve cardiac contractility

7. Administer Human B–type natriuretic peptides—vasodilates

8. Administer beta-adrenergic blockers—decrease myocardial oxygen demand

9. Diet
   a. Restricted sodium diet
      1) Normal intake: 6–15 g/day
      2) No table salt: 1.6–2.8 g/day
      3) No salt: 1.2–1.4 g/day
      4) Strict low-sodium diet: 0.2–1 g/day
   b. Low calorie, supplemented with vitamins—promotes weight loss, thereby reducing the workload of the heart
   c. Bland, low residue—avoids discomfort from gastric distention and heartburn
   d. Small, frequent feedings to avoid gastric distention, flatulence, and heartburn

Table 3 CAUSES OF HEART FAILURE		
DISEASE	PATHOLOGY	RESULT
Hypertensive disease	Vessels become narrowed; peripheral resistance increases	Cardiac muscle enlarges beyond its oxygen supply
Arteriosclerosis	Degenerative changes in arterial walls cause permanent narrowing of coronary arteries	Cardiac muscle enlarges beyond its oxygen supply
Valvular heart disease	Stenosed valves do not open freely; scarring and retraction of valve leaflets result in incomplete closure	Workload increases until heart fails
Rheumatic heart disease	Infection causes damage to heart valves, making them incompetent or narrowed	Incompetent valves cause blood to regurgitate backward; workload increases until heart fails
Ischemic heart disease	Coronary arteries are sclerosed or thrombosed	Blood supply is insufficient to nourish heart
Constrictive pericarditis	Inflamed pericardial sac becomes scarred and constricted, causing obstruction in blood flow	Low cardiac output and increased venous pressure. Decreases filling of heart
Circulatory overload (IV fluid over-load; sodium retention; renal shutdown)	Excessive fluid in circulatory system	Overwhelms heart's ability to pump
Pulmonary disease	Damage to arterioles of lungs causes vascular constriction; this increases workload of heart	Right ventricular enlargement and failure
Tachydysrhythmias	Decreases ventricular filling time	Decreased cardiac output

10. Record I and O
11. Weigh daily
12. Oxygen therapy and continuous positive airway pressure (CPAP)
13. Teach about disease process, medications and energy management

D. Evaluation

1. Is client able to perform activities of daily living without difficulty?

2. Is client knowledgeable about dietary restrictions?

▶ ANGINA PECTORIS

A. Assessment

1. Pain—may radiate down left arm; arm pain associated with stress, exertion, or anxiety

2. Relieved with rest and nitroglycerin

B. Diagnose

1. Cause—coronary atherosclerosis

2. Risk factors for coronary artery disease

    a. Nonmodifiable (client has no control)

        1) Increasing age

        2) Family history of coronary heart disease

        3) Men more likely to develop heart disease than premenopausal women

        4) Race

    b. Modifiable risk factors (client can exercise control)

        1) Elevated serum cholesterol

        2) Cigarette smoking and/or secondhand exposure

        3) Hypertension

        4) Diabetes mellitus

        5) Physical inactivity

        6) Obesity

        7) Depression or chronic stress

        8) Oral contraceptive use or hormone replacement therapy

        9) Substance abuse-methamphetamines or cocaine

3. Significance—warning sign of ischemia

C. Plan/Implementation

1. Health promotion

    a. No smoking

    b. Follow balanced diet that limits intake of fat and sodium

    c. Check blood pressure and cholesterol regularly

    d. Engage in regular physical activity—goal is reduction of blood pressure and pulse rate upon exertion

2. Administer vasodilators, aspirin, glycoprotein, IIb/IIIa inhibitors, beta blockers, angiotensin receptor blockers, calcium channel blockers

3. Exercise program—goal is reduction of blood pressure and pulse rate upon exertion

4. Percutaneous transluminal coronary angioplasty (PTCA) and stent placement

    a. Balloon-tipped catheter inserted under fluoroscopy to the occluded coronary artery

      b. Plaque is compressed against wall to open lumen of vessel

      c. IV heparin by continuous infusion is used to prevent thrombus formation

      d. IV or intracoronary nitroglycerin or sublingual nifedipine is given to prevent coronary vasospasm

      e. Monitor for complications (closure of vessel, bleeding, reaction to the dye, hypotension, hypokalemia, dysrhythmias)

      f. Health care provider will prescribe long-term nitrate, calcium channel blocker, and aspirin therapy

  5. Coronary artery bypass graft surgery (CABG)

      a. Indications—to increase blood flow to heart muscle in clients with severe angina

      b. Saphenous vein or internal mammary artery used for graft; as many as five arteries may be bypassed

      c. Preoperative

         1) Educational and psychological preparation

         2) Medications discontinued—digitalis 12 hours preop, diuretics 2–3 days preop, aspirin and anitcoagulants 1 week preop

         3) Medications administered—potassium chloride to maintain normal potassium level, beta blockers, calcium-channel blockers, antiarrhythmics, antihypertensives, prophylactic antibiotics 20–30 minutes before surgery

      d. Postoperative

         1) Receives mechanical ventilation for 6–24 hours

         2) Connect chest tubes to water-seal drainage system

         3) Ground epicardial pacer wire and tape to client

         4) Assess pulmonary artery and arterial pressures and heart rate and rhythm

         5) Pain relief

         6) Monitor for complications—fluid and electrolyte imbalance, hypotension or hypertension, hypothermia, bleeding, cardiac tamponade, altered cerebral perfusion

         7) Be alert to psychological state, disorientation, or depression

         8) Provide activity as tolerated with progress as ordered, from feet dangling over side of bed, to sitting in chair, to walking in room by third day

      e. Provide guidance concerning long-term care and follow-up

D. Evaluation

  1. Does client experience relief of pain and reduction of anxiety?

  2. Does client institute lifestyle changes to decrease stress?

  3. Does client comply with medication, diet, and activity recommendations?

▶ PERIPHERAL VASCULAR DISEASE

A. Assessment (see Table 4)

B. Diagnose

  1. Predisposing factors (see Table 4)

C. Plan/Implementation (see Table 4)

D. Evaluation

  1. Has adequate tissue perfusion been re-established?

  2. Does the client have stable vital signs, good color, and adequate peripheral pulses?

  3. Is client free from infection?

  4. Is client free from pain?

  5. Do client and significant others understand and comply with activity restrictions?

Table 4 PERIPHERAL VASCULAR DISEASE			
TYPE	ASSESSMENT	PREDISPOSING FACTORS	TREATMENT/NURSING CONSIDERATIONS
Arterial (Arteriosclerosis, Raynaud's disease, Buerger's disease)	Dependent rubor Cool, shiny skin Cyanosis Ulcers, gangrene Impaired sensation Intermittent claudication Decreased peripheral pulses Pallor with extremity elevation Rest pain	Smoking Exposure to cold Emotional stress Diabetes mellitus High-fat diet Hypertension Obesity	Monitor peripheral pulses Good foot care Do not cross legs Regular exercise Stop smoking Transluminal angioplasty Arterial bypass Endarterectomy Amputation Vasodilators Anticoagulants Antiplatelet medications
Venous (Varicose veins, Thrombophlebitis)	Cool, brown skin Edema, ulcers, pain Normal or decreased pulses	Immobility Pregnancy Hereditary Obesity Surgery CHF Injury to vein wall Hypercoagulability	Monitor peripheral pulses Thrombectomy Avoid extremes of temperature Elastic stockings, TED hose, intermittent pneumatic compression devices (IPC) Anticoagulants Activity as ordered Encourage early ambulation Elevate legs Warm moist packs

▶ HYPERTENSION

A. Assessment

  1. May be no symptoms

  2. Headache, dizziness, facial flushing

  3. Anginal pain

4. Intermittent claudication

5. Retinal hemorrhages and exudates

6. Severe occipital headaches associated with nausea, vomiting, drowsiness, giddiness, anxiety, and mental impairment

7. Polyuria, nocturia, protein and RBCs in urine, diminished ability of kidneys to concentrate urine

8. Dyspnea upon exertion—left-sided heart failure

9. Edema of the extremities—right-sided heart failure

B. Diagnose

1. Persistent elevation of the systolic blood pressure above 140 mm Hg and diastolic blood pressure above 90 mm Hg

2. Causes

   a. Risk factors

      1) Family history of hypertension

      2) Excessive sodium intake

      3) Excessive intake of calories

      4) Physical inactivity

      5) Excessive alcohol intake

      6) Contributing factors—history of renal and/or cardiovascular disease

      7) Low potassium intake

      8) Stressful lifestyle

      9) Age

   b. Primary (essential or idiopathic)—constitutes 90% of all cases; may be benign (gradual onset and prolonged course) or malignant(abrupt onset and short dramatic course, which is rapidly fatal unless treated)

   c. Secondary—develops as a result of another primary disease of the cardiovascular system, renal system, adrenal glands, or neurological system, medications

3. Complications

   a. Renal failure

   b. Stroke

   c. Transient ischemic attacks (TIAs)

   d. Retinal hemorrhages

4. Potential nursing diagnoses

   a. Knowledge deficit

   b. Management of therapeutic regimen: individual, ineffective

   c. Noncompliance related to medications

C. Plan/Implementation

1. Administer antihypertensive medications—diuretics, calcium-channel blockers, ACE inhibitors, angiotensin receptor blocker, beta blockers, aldosterone blockers, central alpha antagonists

2. Teaching

   a. Medication adverse effects and compliance with medication

   b. Dietary restriction of sodium and fat

    c. Weight control

    d. Moderate alcohol intake

    e. Increase physical activity

    f. Stop smoking

    g. Health care follow-up

    h. Change positions slowly because of possible orthostatic hypotension

D. Evaluation

    1. Is client's blood pressure within normal limits?

    2. Is client compliant with therapeutic regime?

▶ ANEMIA

A. Assessment

    1. Mild

        a. Hemoglobin 13–18 g/dL male (130-180 g/L): usually asymptomatic

        b. Symptoms usually follow strenuous exertion: palpitations, dyspnea, diaphoresis

    2. Moderate

        a. Dyspnea, palpitations

        b. Diaphoresis

        c. Chronic fatigue

    3. Severe

        a. Pale, exhausted all the time

        b. Severe palpitations

        c. Sensitivity to cold

        d. Loss of appetite

        e. Profound weakness

        f. Dizziness, syncope

        g. Headache

        h. Cardiac complications—CHF, angina pectoris

B. Diagnose

    1. A decrease in the number of erythrocytes or a reduction in hemoglobin

C. Plan/Implementation

    1. Identify cause

    2. Frequent rest periods

    3. Frequent turning and positioning

    4. Diet high in protein, iron, vitamins

    5. Small, easily digestible meals

    6. Good oral hygiene

    7. Monitor blood transfusions

    8. Protect from sources of infection

D. Evaluation

    1. Does client maintain normal hemoglobin and erythrocyte levels?

    2. Does client maintain adequate tissue perfusion and gas exchange?

▶ IRON DEFICIENCY ANEMIA

A. Assessment

1. Fatigue
2. Decreased serum albumin, gamma globulin, and transferrin
3. Glossitis (inflammation of tongue)
4. "Spoon" fingernails (koilonychia)
5. Impaired cognition

B. Diagnose

1. Most common type
2. Causes: decreased dietary intake; malabsorption after gastric resection; blood loss due to ulcers, gastritis, GI tumors, menorrhagia (excessive menstrual bleeding); poor absorption due to high-fiber diet

C. Plan/Implementation

1. Dietary addition of iron-rich foods
2. Iron supplements IM or IV iron dextran (IV route is preferred), IM route causes pain, skin staining, and higher incidence of anaphylaxis; take oral supplements with meals if experience GI upset, then resume between meals for maximum absorption, take with ascorbic acid; use straw if liquids are used
3. Iron Preparations

D. Evaluation

1. Serum values within normal limits.
2. Client experiences a reduction of symptoms.

▶ VITAMIN B$_{12}$ ANEMIA AND PERNICIOUS ANEMIA

A. Assessment

1. Pallor
2. Fatigue
3. Weight loss
4. Sore, red tongue
5. Balance and gait disturbances
6. Paresthesias in hands and feet

B. Diagnose

1. Pernicious anemia: gastric mucosa fails to secrete sufficient intrinsic factor required for absorption of vitamin B$_{12}$; diagnosed by Schilling test (fast for 12 hours; given small dose of radioactive B$_{12}$ in water to drink, followed by large, nonradioactive dose IM, 24-hour urine specimen collected, measured for radioactivity)
2. Inadequate dietary intake (can occur with vegans who eat no meat or meat products)
3. Bone marrow produces fewer, larger (macrocytic) red blood cells

C. Plan/Implementation

1. Initial IM administration of 25 to 100 micrograms of vitamin B_{12}, followed by 500 to 1,000 micrograms every 1 to 2 months or cyanocobalamin nasal spray

2. Vegetarians prevent or treat by taking vitamins or fortified soy milk

D. Evaluation

1. Serum values remain within normal limits

2. Client experiences a reduction of symptoms

▶ SICKLE CELL DISEASE

A. Assessment

1. Pain (may be severe)

2. Swelling of joints during crisis

3. Fever

4. Jaundice (especially of sclerae)

5. Tachycardia, cardiac murmurs

6. Hemoglobin 7–10 g/dL (70-100 g/L); sickled cells on peripheral blood smear

B. Diagnose

1. Severe hemolytic anemia resulting from defective hemoglobin, hemoglobin becomes sickle-shaped in presence of low oxygenation

2. Symptoms are caused by hemolysis and thrombosis

C. Plan/Implementation

1. Check joint areas for pain and swelling

2. Check for signs of infection (osteomyelitis and pneumonia common)

3. Promptly treat infection (to prevent crisis)

4. Avoid high altitudes and exposure to extreme temperature

5. Encourage fluid intake (dehydration promotes crisis)

6. Administer folic acid daily

7. During crisis provide analgesics (PCA with morphine sulfate or hydromorphone) and hydration (3–5 L of IV fluids/day for adults; 1600 ml/m2/day for child)

8. Administer hydroxyurea; risk of leukemia and bone marrow suppression

D. Evaluation

1. Has client comfort been maintained?

2. Are parents knowledgeable about ways to prevent sickle cell crisis?

▶ HEMOPHILIA

A. Assessment

1. Spontaneous easy bruising

2. Joint pain with bleeding

3. Prolonged internal or external bleeding from mild trauma, gingival bleeding, GI bleeding, hematuria

4. Pallor

B. Diagnose

1. Causes

a. Sex-linked, transmitted to male by female carrier, recessive trait

b. Factor VIII deficiency—hemophilia A—most common

2. Treatment

a. Plasma or factor VIII cryoprecipitate

b. Bedrest

c. Analgesics (aspirin contraindicated)

C. Plan/Implementation

1. Assess forinternal bleeding

2. Analgesics for joint pain—not aspirin

3. Avoid IM injections

4. Bedrest during bleeding episodes

5. Assist with coping with chronic disease and altered lifestyle

6. Teach to avoid contact sports; engage in activities such as golf, swimming

7. Teach about replacement of clotting factor

D. Evaluation

1. Is normal blood volume maintained?

2. Is client aware of restrictions on use of analgesics?

▶ PITUITARY DISORDERS

A. Assessment (see Table 5)

B. Diagnose (see Table 5)

1. Anterior hormones—Growth, TSH, ACTH, LH, FSH

2. Posterior hormones—oxytocin, vasopressin, ADH

C. Plan/Implementation (see Table 5)

Table 5 PITUITARY DISORDERS		
	DWARFISM (HYPOPITUITARISM)	ACROMEGALY
Assessment	Height below normal, body proportions normal, bone/tooth development retarded, sexual maturity delayed, skin fine, features delicate	Body size enlarged, coordination poor, flat bones enlarged, sexual abnormalities, deep voice, skin thick and soft, visual field changes
Diagnose	Hyposecretion of growth hormone; occurs before maturity Etiology unclear; predisposition—pituitary tumors, idiopathic hyperplasia Treatment: hormone replacement (human growth hormone, thyroid growth hormone, testosterone) Complication: diabetes	Hypersecretion of growth hormone occurs after maturity Etiology: unclear Diagnosis: growth hormone measured in blood plasma Treatment: external irradiation of tumor, atrium-90 implant transnasally, hypophysectomy (removal of pituitary or portion of it with hormone replacement)
Potential nursing diagnosis	Self-esteem disturbance Risk for sexual dysfunction	Body image disturbance Nutrition, altered Chronic pain Risk for sexual dysfunction

Plan/Implementation	Monitor growth and development
	Provide emotional support
	Assess body image
	Refer for psychological counseling as needed
	Monitor medications
	Hormone replacement therapy
	Thyroid hormone replacement
	Testosterone therapy
	Human chorionic gonadotropin (hCG) injections
		Monitor blood sugar level
		Provide emotional support
		Provide safety due to poor coordination and vision
		Administer dopamine agonists; somatostatin analogs; growth hormone receptor blockers
		Provide care during radiation therapy
		Provide posthypophysectomy care:
		  Elevate head
		  Check neurological status and nasal drainage
		  Monitor BP frequently
		  Observe for hormonal deficiencies (thyroid, glucocorticoid)
		  Observe for hypoglycemia
		  Monitor intake and output
		  Provide cortisone replacement before and after surgery
		Avoid coughing
		Avoid tooth brushing for 2 weeks

D. Evaluation

1. Have the child's growth and developmental needs been met?
2. Have the parents adjusted to child's condition?

▶ CANCER

A. Assessment

   1. American Cancer Society Warning Signs

      a. Change in bowel, bladder habits

      b. A sore that does not heal

      c. Unusual bleeding or discharge

      d. Thickening or a lump in the breast or elsewhere

      e. Indigestion or difficulty in swallowing

      f. Obvious change in a wart or mole

      g. Nagging cough or hoarseness

B. Diagnose

   1. Risk factors

      a. Immunosuppression

      b. Advancing age

      c. Genetic predisposition

   2. Causative factors

      a. Physical

         1) Radiation—excessive exposure to sunlight and radiation

         2) Chronic irritation

      b. Chemical

         1) Food additives—e.g., nitrites

         2) Industry—e.g., asbestos

         3) Pharmaceutical—e.g., stilbesterol

         4) Smoking

         5) Alcohol

      c. Genetic

      d. Viral—incorporated into cell genesis: Epstein-Barr virus, Burkitt's lymphoma

      e. Stress—co-causative factor

   3. Common cancer types

      a. Caucasian

         1) Lung

         2) Breast

         3) Colorectal

         4) Prostate

      b. African American

         1) Lung

         2) Prostate

         3) Breast

4) Colorectal

5) Uterine

c. Asian

1) Breast

2) Colorectal

3) Prostate

4) Lung

5) Stomach

d. Hispanic

1) Prostate

2) Breast

3) Colorectal

4) Lung

4. Classifications

a. Carcinoma—epithelial tissue

b. Sarcoma—connective tissue

c. Lymphoma—lymphoid tissue

d. Leukemia—blood-forming tissue (WBCs and platelets)

5. Potential nursing diagnoses

a. Skin integrity, impaired

b. Risk for infection

c. Fear/death anxiety

d. Grieving

e. Acute/chronic pain

f. Fatigue

C. Plan/Implementation

1. Cancer prevention

a. Avoid known carcinogens

1) Don't smoke

2) Wear sunscreen

3) Eliminate asbestos in buildings

b. Modify dietary habits

1) Avoid excessive intake of animal fat

2) Avoid nitrates found in prepared lunch meats, sausage, and bacon

3) Decrease intake of red meat

4) Limit alcohol intake to one or two drinks per day

5) Increase intake of bran, broccoli, cauliflower, brussels sprouts, cabbage, and foods high in vitamin A and C

2. Chemotherapy

3. Teletherapy (radiotherapy)

a. External radiation (e.g., cobalt)

1) Leave radiology markings intact on skin

2) Avoid creams , lotions, deodorants, and/or perfumes, unless prescribed

3) Use lukewarm water to cleanse area

4) Assess skin for redness, cracking

5) Administer antiemetics for nausea, analgesics for pain

6) Observe skin, mucous membranes, and hair follicles for adverse effects

7) No hot water bottle, tape; don't expose area to cold or sunlight

8) Wear cotton clothing

  b. Brachytherapy (internal radiation) (e.g., cesium, radium, gold)

    1) Sealed source (cesium)—mechanically positioned source of radioactive material placed in body cavity or tumor

      a) Lead container and long-handled forceps in room in event of dislodged source

      b) Save all dressings, bed linens until source is removed; then discard dressings and linens as usual

      c) Urine, feces not radioactive

      d) Do not stand close or in line with radioactive source

      e) Client on bedrest while implant in place

      f) Position of source verified by radiography

    2) Unsealed source of radiation—unsealed liquid given orally, or instilled in body cavity (e.g., ^{131}I)

      a) All body fluids contaminated

      b) Greatest danger from body fluids during first 24–96 hours

    3) Nursing care for internal radiation

      a) Assign client to private room

      b) Place "Caution: Radioactive Material" sign on door

      c) Wear dosimeter film badge at all times when interacting with client (offers no protection but measures amount of exposure; each nurse has individual badge)

      d) Do not assign pregnant nurse to client

      e) Rotate staff caring for client; limit close contact to 30 minutes per 8 hour shift

      f) Organize tasks so limited time is spent in client's room

      g) Limit visitors

      h) Encourage client to do own care

      i) Provide shield in room

      j) Use antiemetics for nausea

      k) Consider body image (e.g., alopecia)

      l) Provide comfort measures, analgesic for pain

      m) Provide good nutrition

4. Skin care

  a. Avoid use of soaps and powders

  b. Wear cotton, loose-fitting clothing

5. Mouth care

  a. Stomatitis—develops 5–14 days after chemotherapy begins

  b. Symptoms—erythema, ulcers, bleeding

      c. Rinse with saline or chlorhexidine; avoid hard-bristled toothbrush, dental floss, lemon glycerin swabs

      d. Avoid hot (temperature) or spicy foods

      e. Topical antifungals and anesthetics

6. Hair care

      a. Alopecia commonly seen, alters body image

      b. Assist with wig or hair piece

      c. Scarves, hats

7. Nutritional changes

      a. Anorexia, nausea, and vomiting commonly seen with chemotherapy

      b. Malabsorption and cachexia (wasting) common

      c. Make meals appealing to senses

      d. Conform diet to client preferences and nutritional needs

      e. Small, frequent meals with additional supplements between meals (high-calorie, high-protein diet)

      f. Encourage fluids but limit at meal times

      g. Perform oral hygiene and provide relief of pain before meal time

      h. PN as needed

8. Neutropenia precautions—prevent infection among clients with immunosuppression; absolute neutrophil count less than or equal to 1000 cells x $10^3/mm^3$

      a. Assess skin integrity every 8 hours; auscultate breath sounds, presence of cough, sore throat; check temperature every 4 hours, report if higher than 101° F (38°C); monitor CBC and differential daily

      b. Private room when possible

      c. Thorough hand hygiene before entering client's room

      d. Allow no staff with cold or sore throat to care for client

      e. No fresh flowers or standing water

      f. Clean room daily

      g. Low microbial diet; no fresh salads, unpeeled fresh fruits and vegetables

      h. Deep breathe every 4 hours

      i. Meticulous body hygiene

      j. Inspect IV site, meticulous IV site care

9. Pain relief—three-step ladder approach

      a. For mild pain—nonnarcotic medication used(acetaminophen) along with antiemetics, antidepressants, glucocorticoids

      b. For moderate pain—weak narcotics (codeine) and nonnarcotics are used

      c. For severe pain—strong narcotics are used (morphine)

      d. Give pain medications on regularly scheduled basis (preventative approach), additional analgesics given for breakthrough pain

10. Activity level

      a. Alternate rest and activity

      b. Maintain normal lifestyle

11. Psychosocial issues

    a. Encourage participation in self-care and decision-making

    b. Provide referral to support groups, organizations

    c. Hospice care

D. Evaluation

    1. Has client been assisted through stages of grief?

    2. Has client's comfort been maintained?

▶ LEUKEMIA

A. Assessment

    1. Ulcerations of mouth and throat

    2. Pneumonia, septicemia

    3. Altered leukocyte count ($15,000–500,000 \times 10^3/mm^3$)

    4. Anemia, fatigue, lethargy, bone and joint pain, hypoxia

    5. Bleeding gums, ecchymosis, petechiae, retinal hemorrhages

    6. Weakness, pallor, weight loss, hepatomegaly, splenomegaly

    7. Headache, disorientation, convulsions

B. Diagnose

    1. Neoplastic disease that involves the blood-forming tissues of the bone marrow, spleen, and lymph nodes; abnormal, uncontrolled, and destructive proliferation of one type of white cell and its precursors

    2. Diagnostic tests

        a. Bone marrow aspiration

            1) Informed consent required

            2) Done at iliac crest and sternum

            3) Local anesthetic used

            4) Apply sterile dressing to area after procedure; apply pressure to site if bleeding

            5) Complications

                a) Osteomyelitis

                b) Bleeding

                c) Puncture of vital organs

    3. Classification of the leukemias

        a. Acute leukemia—rapid onset and progresses to a fatal termination within days to months; more common among children and young adults

        b. Chronic leukemia—gradual onset with a slower, more protracted course; more common between ages 25 and 60

    4. Factors associated with development

        a. Viruses

        b. Ionizing radiation

        c. Genetic predisposition

        d. Absorption of certain chemicals, e.g., benzene, pyridine, and aniline dyes

C. Plan/Implementation

1. Assess for signs of bleeding, e.g., petechiae, bruising, bleeding, thrombocytopenia; follow bleeding precautions

2. Monitor for signs of infection, e.g., changes in vital signs, chills, neutropenia

3. Good mouth care

4. High-calorie, high-vitamin diet

5. Frequent feedings of soft, easy-to-eat food

6. Antiemetics

7. Neutropenia precautions, if necessary

8. Strict handwashing

9. Prevent skin breakdown, e.g., turning, positioning

10. Administer and monitor blood transfusions (whole blood, platelets)

11. Administer medications, treatments as ordered, and observe for adverse effects

    a. Chemotherapy

       1) Nausea, vomiting, diarrhea

       2) Stomatitis, alopecia, skin reactions

       3) Bone marrow depression

    b. Radiation or radioisotope therapy

    c. Bone marrow transplants

D. Evaluation

1. Is client in remission?

2. Does client exhibit minimal complications of the disease?

▶ SKIN CANCER

A. Assessment

1. Basal cell carcinoma—small, waxy nodule on sun-exposed areas of body (e.g., face); may ulcerate and crust

2. Squamous cell carcinoma—rough, thick, scaly tumor seen on arms or face

3. Malignant melanoma—variegated color (brown, black mixed with gray or white) circular lesion with irregular edges seen on trunk or legs

B. Diagnose

1. Major risk factor—overexposure to sun

2. Basal cell carcinoma—most common type of skin cancer; rarely metastasize but commonly reoccurs

3. Squamous cell carcinoma—may metastasize to blood or lymph

4. Malignant melanoma—most lethal of skin cancers; frequently seen 20–45 years old; highest risk persons with fair complexions, blue eyes, red or blond hair, and freckles; metastases to bone, liver, spleen, CNS, lungs, lymph

5. Diagnosed by skin lesion biopsy

C. Plan/Implementation

    1. Postop care following surgical excision

    2. Teach prevention

        a. Avoid exposure to sun 10 a.m. to 3 p.m.

        b. Use sunscreen with SPF (solar protection factor) to block harmful rays (especially important for children)

        c. Reapply sunscreen after swimming or prolonged time in sun

        d. Use lip balm with sunscreen protection

        e. Wear hat when outdoors

        f. Do not use lamps or tanning booths

        g. Teach client to examine skin surfaces monthly

    3. Teach how to identify danger signs of melanoma—change in size, color, shape of mole or surrounding skin

    4. Chemotherapy for metastases

D. Evaluation

    1. Is client knowledgeable about ways to prevent skin cancer?

    2. Is client knowledgeable about danger signs of malignant melanoma?

▶ INTRACRANIAL TUMORS

A. Assessment—signs and symptoms vary depending on location

    1. Motor deficits

    2. Language disturbances

    3. Hearing difficulties, visual disturbances (occipital lobe)

    4. Dizziness, paresthesia (cerebellum), coordination problems

    5. Seizures (motor cortex)

    6. Personality disturbances (frontal lobe)

    7. Papilledema

    8. Nausea and vomiting

    9. Drowsiness, changes in level of consciousness

B. Diagnose

    1. Types—classified according to location

        a. Supratentorial—incision usually behind hairline, surgery within the cerebral hemisphere

        b. Infratentorial—incision made at nape of neck around occipital lobe; surgery within brain stem and cerebellum

    2. Causes—unknown

    3. Medical/surgical management—intracranial surgery (burr holes, craniotomy, cranioplasty),and radiation

C. Plan/Implementation

    1. Preoperative care

        a. Detailed neurological assessment for baseline data

        b. Head shave—prep site

        c. Psychological support

        d. Prepare client for postoperative course

2. Postoperative care
   a. Maintain patent airway
   b. Elevate head of bed 30–45° after supratentorial surgery
   c. Position client flat and lateral on either side after infratentorial surgery
   d. Monitor vital and neurological signs
   e. Observe for complications—respiratory difficulties, increased intracranial pressure, hyperthermia, meningitis, wound infection
   f. Administer medications—corticosteroids, osmotic diurectics, mild analgesics, anticonvulsants, antibiotics, antipyretics, antiemetics, hormone replacement as needed; no narcotics postoperatively (masks changes in LOC), use acetaminophen

D. Evaluation
   1. Have postoperative complications been avoided?
   2. Has client adjusted to the change in body image?

▶ PANCREATIC TUMORS

A. Assessment
   1. Weight loss
   2. Vague upper or mid-abdominal discomfort
   3. Abnormal glucose tolerance test (hyperglycemia)
   4. Jaundice, clay-colored stools, dark urine

B. Diagnose
   1. Tumors may arise from any portion of the pancreas (head or tail); each has unique clinical manifestations
   2. Diagnostic tests—CT, CT-guided needle biopsy, MRI
   3. Risk factor—smoking, pancreatitis, exposure to environmental toxins

C. Plan/Implementation
   1. Medical
      a. High-calorie, bland, low-fat diet; small, frequent feedings
      b. Avoid alcohol
      c. Anticholinergics
      d. Chemotherapy, radiation therapy, stent placement
   2. Surgery (Whipple procedure)—removal of head of pancreas, distal portion of common bile duct, the duodenum, and part of the stomach
   3. Postop care
      a. Monitor for peritonitis and intestinal obstruction
      b. Monitor for hypotension
      c. Monitor for steatorrhea
      d. Administer pancreatic enzymes
      e. Monitor for diabetes mellitus

D. Evaluation
   1. Has client's comfort been maintained?
   2. Have postoperative complications been avoided?

▶ CARCINOMA OF THE LARYNX

A. Assessment

1. Pain radiating to the ears
2. Hoarseness, dysphagia, foul breath
3. Dyspnea
4. Enlarged cervical nodes
5. Hemoptysis

B. Diagnose

1. Diagnostic tests

   a. Laryngoscopy, Bronchoscopy

   b. Biopsy

   c. CT, MRI

   d. X-rays

2. Causes

   a. Industrial chemicals

   b. Cigarette smoking and alcohol use

   c. Straining of the vocal cords

   d. Chronic laryngitis

   e. Family predisposition

C. Plan/Implementation

1. Caring for the client with a laryngectomy

   a. Preoperative care

      1) Explain compensatory methods of communication

      2) Referral to speech therapy

   b. Postoperative care

      1) Laryngectomy care—stoma care, suction

      2) Place in semi-Fowler's position

      3) Turn, cough, and deep breathe

      4) Provide humidified oxygen

      5) Suction oral secretions

      6) Assess condition of skin flap

      7) Nasogastric, gastrostomy, or jejunostomy feeding tube

2. Observe for postoperative complications after laryngectomy

   a. Respiratory difficulties

   b. Fistula formation and wound breakdown

   c. Rupture of carotid artery

   d. Stenosis of trachea

3. Monitor weight, food intake, and fluid intake and output

4. Communication for total laryngectomy clients

   a. Esophageal speech

   b. Artificial larynx—commonly used mechanical device for speech

5. Radiation therapy—small, localized cancers; sore throat, increased hoarseness, dysphagia

D. Evaluation

1. Is client knowledgeable about compensatory methods of artificial speech?

2. Has client adjusted to altered body image?

Chapter 6

PHYSIOLOGICAL INTEGRITY: BASIC CARE AND COMFORT

Units

1. **Mobility and Immobility**

2. **Conditions Limiting Mobility**

3. **Interventions to Promote Comfort**

4. **Musculoskeletal Trauma**

5. **Rest and Sleep Disturbances**

6. **Nutrition**

7. **Elimination**

▶ MOBILITY

A. Assessment

1. Body build, height, weight—proportioned within normal limits
2. Posture, body alignment—erect
   a. Lumbar lordosis—exaggerated concavity in the lumbar region
   b. Kyphosis—exaggerated convexity in the thoracic region
   c. Scoliosis—lateral curvature of a portion of the vertebral column
3. Gait, ambulation—smooth
4. Joints—freely movable (see Table 1)
5. Skin integrity—intact
6. Muscle tone, elasticity, strength—adequate
7. Exercise level—appropriate
8. Rest and sleep patterns—adequate
9. Sexual activity—appropriate
10. Job-related activity—acceptable
11. Developmental mobility—within normal limits

Table 1 JOINT MOVEMENTS	
MOVEMENT	ACTION
Flexion	Decrease angle of joint, e.g., bending elbow
Extension	Increase angle of joint, e.g., straightening elbow
Hyperextension	Excessively increase angle of joint, e.g., bending the head backward
Abduction	Moving bone away from midline of body
Adduction	Moving bone toward midline of body ("add" to body)
Rotation	Moving bone around its central axis
Dorsiflexion	Flexion of the foot toward the trunk of the body ("toes toward the nose")
Plantar flexion	Flexion of the foot away from the trunk of the body ("pointing the toes")
Inversion	Turning the foot inward at the ankle
Eversion	Turning the foot outward at the ankle
Pronation	Rotation of the forearm so that the palm of the hand turns downward
Supination	Rotation of the forearm so that the palm of the hand turns upward

B. Diagnose

    1. Activity

        a. Maintains muscle tone and posture

        b. Serves as an outlet for tension and anxiety

    2. Exercise

        a. Maintains joint mobility and function

        b. Promotes muscle strength

        c. Stimulates circulation

        d. Promotes optimum ventilation

        e. Stimulates appetite

        f. Promotes elimination

        g. Enhances metabolic rate

    3. Potential nursing diagnoses

        a. Impaired walking

        b. Activity intolerance

        c. Risk for falls

        d. Risk for injury

C. Plan/Implementation

    1. Avoid injury

        a. Prevent motor vehicle accidents, use seat belts and helmets

        b. Avoid job-related accidents, follow safety procedures

        c. When engaging in contact sports, perform proper body conditioningand use protective devices

        d. For aged persons, rugs should be secure, stairways lit and clear of debris

        e. During pregnancy use bathtub grips, low-heeled shoes

        f. Assist client to sit on side of bed

            1) Place hand under knees and shoulders of client

            2) Instruct client to push elbow into bed; at the same time the nurse should lift the client's shoulders with one arm and swing the client's legs over edge of bed with the other arm

        g. Assist client to stand

            1) Face client with hands firmly grasping each side of his/her rib cage

            2) Push nurse's knee against one knee of the client

            3) Rock client forward as he/she comes to a standing position

            4) Pivot client to position him/her to sit in chair (placed on client's stronger side)

        h. Assist client out of bed

            1) If client has a weaker side, move the client toward the stronger side (easier for client to pull the weak side)

            2) Use the larger muscles of the legs to accomplish a move rather than the smaller muscles of the back

3) Drawsheets are a better method of moving a client than sliding a client across a surface

4) Always have an assistant standing by if there is any possibility of problems in completing a transfer

   i. Teach client ADLs

1) Observe what client can do and allow him/her to do it

2) Encourage client to exercise muscles used for activity

3) Start with gross functional movement before going to finer motions

4) Extend period of activity as much and as fast as the client can tolerate

5) Give positive feedback immediately after every accomplishment

D. Evaluation

1. Is the client's mobility within normal limits?

2. Has a safe transfer been accomplished?

▶ IMMOBILITY

A. Assessment

1. Gait, ambulation

2. Joint movement

3. Muscle tone

4. Skin integrity

Table 2 THERAPEUTIC EXERCISES		
EXERCISE	**DESCRIPTION**	**RATIONALE**
Passive range of motion	Performed by nurse without assistance from client	Retention of joint range of motion; maintenance of circulation
Active assistive range of motion	Performed by client with assistance of nurse	Increases motion in the joint
Active range of motion	Performed by client without assistance	Maintains mobility of joints and increases muscle strength
Active resistive range of motion	Performed by client against manual or mechanical resistance	Provision of resistance to increase muscle strength; 5-pound bags/ weights may be used
Isometric exercises	Performed by client; alternate contraction and relaxation of muscle without moving joint	Maintenance of muscle strength when joint immobilized

B. Diagnose

1. Activity intolerance

2. Impaired walking

3. Risk for Disuse syndrome

4. Fatigue

C. Plan/Implementation
1. Therapeutic exercises (see Table 2)
2. Prevent complication of immobility (see Table 3)
3. Maintain specific therapeutic positions (see Table 4)

D. Evaluation
1. Have complications of immobility been prevented?
2. Has client resumed normal functioning?

Table 3 COMPLICATIONS OF IMMOBILITY		
COMPLICATION	SEQUELAE	NURSING CONSIDERATIONS
Decubitus ulcer	Osteomyelitis Tissue maceration Infection	Frequently turn, provide skin care Ambulate as appropriate Use draw sheet when turning to avoid shearing force Provide balanced diet with adequate protein, vitamins, and minerals Use air mattress, flotation pads, elbow and heel pads, sheepskin Assist with use of Stryker frame or Circ-O-Lectric bed
Sensory input changes	Confusion, disorientation	Orient frequently Place clock, calendar within sight
Osteoporosis	Pathological fractures Renal calculi	Encourage weight-bearing on long bones Provide balanced diet Monitor estrogen therapy, if ordered
Negative nitrogen balance	Anorexia, debilitation, weight loss	Give high-protein diet and small, frequent feedings
Hypercalcemia	Impaired bone growth	Reduce calcium in diet, encourage fluids
Increased cardiac workload	Tachycardia	Use trapeze to decrease Valsalva maneuver when moving in bed Teach client how to move without holding breath
Contractures	Deformities	Frequent change of position Use pillows, trochanter rolls, foot board to promote proper body alignment Exercise as appropriate

Table 3 COMPLICATIONS OF IMMOBILITY *(CONTINUED)*		
COMPLICATION	**SEQUELAE**	**NURSING CONSIDERATIONS**
Thrombus formation	Pulmonary emboli	Leg exercises–flexion, extension of toes for 5 minutes every hour Ambulate as appropriate Frequent change of position Avoid using knee gatch on bed or pillows to support knee flexion Use TED or elastic hose Assess edema, warmth and pain
Orthostatic hypotension	Weakness, faintness, dizziness	Teach client to rise from bed slowly Increase activity gradually
Stasis of respiratory secretions	Hypostatic pneumonia	Teach client the importance of turning, coughing, and deep breathing Administer postural drainage as appropriate
Constipation	Fecal impaction	Ambulate as appropriate Increase fluid intake and fiber in diet Ensure privacy for use of bed pan or commode Administer stool softeners, e.g., Colace
Urinary stasis	Urinary retention Renal calculi	Have client void in normal position, if possible Increase fluid intake Low-calcium diet, increase acid ash residue to acidify urine and prevent formation of calcium stones
Boredom	Restlessness	Allow visitors, use of radio, television Schedule occupational therapy
Depression	Insomnia Restlessness	Encourage self-care Start with simple, gross activity before advancing to finer motor movements Increase period of activity as rapidly as client can tolerate Support client with positive feedback for effort/accomplishment

Table 4 SPECIFIC THERAPEUTIC POSITIONS	
POSITION	**FUNCTION**
Supine	Avoids hip flexion, which can compress arterial flow
Dorsal recumbent	Supine with knees flexed, more comfortable
Prone	Promotes extension of the hip joint Not well tolerated by persons with respiratory or cardiovascular difficulties
Side lateral or side-lying	Allows drainage of oral secretions
Knee-chest	Provides maximal visualization of rectal area
Side with upper leg bent (Sim's)	Allows drainage of oral secretions Decreases abdominal tension
Head elevated (Fowler's)	Increases venous return Allows maximal lung expansion High-Fowler's: 60–90° Fowler's: 45–60° Semi-Fowler's: 30–45° Low-Fowler's: 15–30°
Modified Trendelenburg (feet elevated 20°, knees straight, trunk flat, and head slightly elevated)	Increases blood return to heart Used for shock
Head elevated and knees elevated	Increases blood return to heart Relieves pressure on lumbosacral area
Elevation of extremity	Increases venous return Decreases blood volume to extremity
Lithotomy (Flat on back, thighs flexed, legs abducted)	Increases vaginal opening for examination

▶ ASSISTIVE DEVICES

A. Tilt table

1. Used for weight-bearing on long bones to prevent decalcification of bones and resulting bone weakness, renal calculi

2. Stimulates circulation to lower extremities

3. Use elastic stockings to prevent postural hypotension

4. Should be done gradually; board can be tilted in 5-10° increments

5. Blood pressure should be checked during the procedure

6. If blood pressure goes down and dizziness, pallor, diaphoresis, tachycardia, or nausea occur, stop procedure

B. Crutches (see Table 5)

1. Guideline for crutch height—measure two fingers below axilla

2. Client should support weight on handpiece, not on axilla—brachialas plexus may be damaged, producing "crutch palsy"

3. Crutches should be kept 8 to 10 inches out to side

4. Elbows should be flexed at 20–30° angle for correct placement of hand grips

5. Stop and rest if diaphoretic or short of breath

Table 5 CRUTCH WALKING GAITS		
GAIT	DESCRIPTION	USES
Four-point	Slow, safe; right crutch, left foot, left crutch, right foot	Use when weight-bearing is allowed for both legs
Two-point	Faster, safe; right crutch and left foot advance together; left crutch and right foot advance together	Use when weight-bearing is allowed for both legs
Three-point	Faster gait, safe; advance weaker leg and both crutches simultaneously; then advance good leg	Use when weight-bearing is allowed on one leg
Swing-to-swing-through	Fast gait but requires more strength and balance; advance both crutches followed by both legs (or one leg is held up)	Use when partial weight-bearing is allowed on both legs
NOTE: To go up stairs: advance good leg first, followed by crutches and affected leg. To go down stairs: advance crutches with affected leg first, followed by good leg. ("Up with the good, down with the bad.")		

C. Walker

1. Definition—metal frame with handgrips, four legs and an open side; used for clients who need greater stability than that provided by other ambulatory aids

2. Guidelines for use

   a. Elbows should be flexed at 20–30° angle when standing with hands on grips

   b. Lift and move walker forward 8–10 inches

   c. With partial or nonweight-bearing put weight on wrists and arms and step forward with affected leg, supporting self on arms, and follow with good leg

   d. Nurse should stand behind client, hold onto gait belt at waist as needed for balance

   e. Sit down by grasping armrest on affected side, shift weight to good leg and hand, lower self into chair

   f. Client should wear sturdy shoes

D. Cane

1. Types

   a. Straight cane—least stable type

   b. Quad cane—has four legs, provides more stability

2. Guideline for use

   a. Tip should have concentric rubber rings as shock absorber and to provide optimal stability

    b. Flex elbow 30° angle and hold handle; tip of cane should be 15 cm lateral to the base of the fifth toe

    c. Hold cane in hand opposite affected extremity

    d. Advance cane and affected leg

    e. Lean on cane when moving good leg

    f. To go up and down stairs, step up on good extremity, thenplace cane and affected extremity on step; reverse when goingdown ("up with the good, down with the bad")

E. Lift (Hoyer)

1. Used for clients who cannot help themselves and/or are too heavy for safe lifting by others

2. Mechanically operated metal frame with a sling usually made of canvas straps

3. Lock the bed; raise the bed to promote the use of good body mechanics by the nurse

4. Center canvas straps under client by rolling client side to side, one under the shoulders and one under the knees

5. Widen base-adjusting lever and lock

6. Position lift base under bed and center lift arm over the canvas sling; lock lift wheels

7. While holding onto arm, release valve to lower arm enough to attach sling

8. Attach sling to overhead arm using hook facing away from client

9. The shorter arm of the sling goes under the client's back; client should be centered in sling

10. Instruct client to cross arms over chest and lock lift wheels

11. Close release valve and pump using long, slow, even strokes; then unlock lift wheels

12. One person guides lift, second person lifts legs off the bed and steadies the sling

13. Position wheelchair between lift base legs; lock legs and lift wheels

14. One person slowly releases valve to lower arm while second person guides client into wheelchair

F. Sliding board

1. Place wheelchair close to bed, lock wheels, lock the bed

2. Remove arm rest from wheelchair

3. Powder the sliding board

4. Place one end of sliding board under client's buttocks; the other end on the surface of the wheelchair

5. Instruct client to push up with hands to shift buttocks, and then slide across board to wheelchair

6. Assist client to slide gently off the bed

G. Adaptive devices
1. Buttonhook—threaded through buttonhole to assist with buttoning shirts
2. Extended shoe horn—can also be used to turn light switches on and off from wheelchair
3. Gel pad—placed under plate or items to prevent shifting during use
4. Foam build-ups—applied to eating utensils, pen and pencils, buttonhook
5. Velcro straps—applied to utensils, pen, and pencil to stabilize in hand
6. Long-handled reacher—assists to obtain objects from high or low location

Unit 2

▶ **HERNIATED INTERVERTEBRAL DISK**

A. Assessment

1. Low back pain (knife-like)

2. Lack of muscle tone

3. Poor posture or body mechanics

4. Sensory changes

B. Diagnose

1. Diagnostic procedures

   a. Computerized tomography

   b. Magnetic resonance imaging

   c. Myelography—encourage fluids, keep head of bed elevated 30° to reduce risk of seizures

   d. Diskogram

2. Surgical procedures

   a. Laminectomy—excision of a portion of the lamina to expose the affected disk for removal

   b. Laminectomy with fusion—involves several disks; operation includes use of bone graft to strengthen the weakened vertebral column

   c. Minimally invasive surgery; microdiskectomy

   d. Interbody cage fusion

C. Plan/Implementation

1. Preoperative

   a. Apply moist heat

   b. Put client in Fowler's position with moderate hip and knee flexion

   c. Use firm mattress, bedboard, or floor for back support

   d. Isometric exercises for abdominal muscles

   e. Daily exercise program

   f. Assist with exercises initiated in physical therapy

   g. Medications—muscle relaxants, NSAIDs, analgesics

   h. Traction—separates vertebrae to relieve pressure on nerve

   i. TENS (transcutaneous electrical nerve stimulation)

2. Postoperative

   a. Maintain body alignment

   b. Log-roll every two hours with pillow between legs

   c. Calf exercises

   d. Assess for sensation and circulatory status, especially of lower extremities

   e. Monitor elimination

   f. Assist with ambulation

g. Support neck after cervical laminectomy

h. Straight back during ambulation

3. Client teaching

a. Exercise daily but avoid strenuous exercises

b. Correct posture at all times

c. Avoid prolonged sitting, standing, walking, driving

d. Rest at intervals

e. Use hardboard or firm mattress for bed

f. Avoid prone position

g. Avoid straining or lifting heavy objects

D. Evaluation

1. Have complications been prevented?

2. Does client understand teaching?

▶ DEVELOPMENTAL DYSPLASIA OF THE HIP (DDH)

A. Assessment

1. Uneven gluteal folds and thigh creases (deeper on affected side) (see Figure 1)

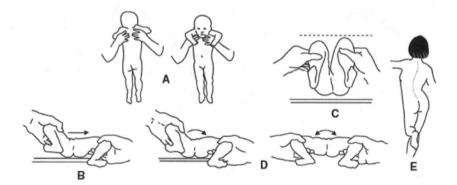

Figure 1. Congenital Hip Dislocation

2. Limited abduction of hip with pain, unequal knee height with thigh flexion

3. Ortolani's sign (seen in infants less than 4 weeks old) (see Figure 1)

a. Place infant on back, leg flexed

b. Click sound heard when affected hip is moved to abduction

4. Shortened limb on affected side in older infant and child

5. Delays in walking; limp, lordosis, and waddling gait with older child

B. Diagnose

1. Predisposition

a. Intrauterine position (breech)

b. Gender (female)

c. Hormonal imbalance (estrogen)

    d. Cultural and environmental influences—some cultures carry their children straddled against the hip joint, causing a decreased incidence (Far Eastern and African); cultures that wrap infants tightly in blankets or strap to boards have high incidence (Navajo Indian)

  2. Definition—acetabulum unable to hold head of femur

  3. Confirmed by x-ray

  4. Potential nursing diagnoses

    a. Physical mobility, impaired

    b. Body image disturbance

    c. Injury, risk for

C. Plan/Implementation

  1. Newborn to 6 months (intervention varies with age and extent)

    a. Reduced by manipulation

    b. Splinted with proximal femur centered in the acetabulum in position of flexion

    c. Pavlik harness—worn full-time for 3–6 months until hip stable for infants less than 3 months age (see Figure 2)

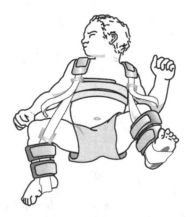

Figure 2. Pavlik Harness

    d. Encourage normal growth and development by allowing child to perform appropriate activities

    e. Teach parents: reapply harness and rationale for maintaining abduction

    f. Tell parents to move child from one room to another for environmental change

    g. Discuss modification in bathing, dressing, and diapering with parents

      1) Since harness is not to be removed, sponge bath is recommended

      2) Put undershirt under chest straps and knee sox under foot and leg pieces to prevent skin irritation

      3) Check skin areas 2–3 times a day

      4) Gently massage skin under straps daily to stimulate circulation

      5) Avoid use of lotions and powders

      6) Place diapers under straps

      7) Pad shoulder straps as needed

  h. Tell parents to touch and hold child to express affection and reinforce security

 2. 16–18 months

  a. Gradual reduction by traction (bilateral Bryant's traction)

  b. Cast for immobilization (see Figure 3)

 3. Older Child

  a. Preliminary traction

  b. Open reduction

  c. Hip spica cast (see Figure 3)

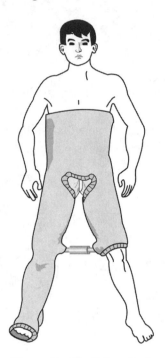

Figure 3. Hip Spica Cast

D. Evaluation

 1. Has hip joint alignment been re-established?

 2. Have child's growth and developmental needs been met?

▶ SCOLIOSIS

A. Assessment (see Figure 4)

 1. Poor posture

 2. Uneven hips or scapulae

 3. Kyphosis lump on back

 4. Uneven waistline

 5. Visualization of deformity—bend at waist 90°

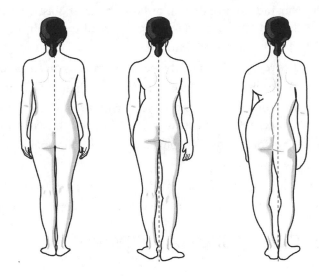

Figure 4. Scoliosis

B. Diagnose

1. Definition—lateral deviation of one or more vertebrae commonly accompanied by rotary motion

2. Types

   a. Functional—flexible deviation that corrects by bending

   b. Structural—permanent, hereditary deviation

3. Potential nursing diagnoses

   a. Disturbed body image

   b. Deficient knowledge

   c. Ineffective therapeutic regimen management

   d. Impaired physical mobility

C. Plan/Implementation

1. Exercise for functional type—teach isometric exercises to strengthen the abdominal muscles

   a. Sit-ups

   b. Pelvic tilt

   c. Push-ups with pelvic tilt

2. Electrostimulation

3. Surgery—spinal fusion with Harrington rod insertion; Dwyer instrumentation with anterior spinal fusion; screw and wire (Luque) instrumentation

4. Thoracolumbosacral orthotic (TLSO) brace

   a. Types effective for 30–40 degree curves not associated with extreme deformity

      1) Thoracolumbosacral orthotic (TSLO) brace

      2) Boston brace (TSLO) brace

      3) Milwaukee brace (cerico-throraco-lumbo-sacral orthotic)

      b. Nursing care: Underarm orthosis made of plastic custom molded to the body and shaped to correct or hold the deformity

        1) Skin care to pressure areas

        2) Wear t-shirt under brace to minimize skin irritation

        3) Teach isometric exercises to strengthen abdominal muscles

        4) Provide activities consistent with limitations, yet allow positive peer relationships to promote healthy self-concept

      c. Wear for 23 hours—removed 1 hour for personal hygiene

D. Evaluation

    1. Has child's lateral deviation of the spine been corrected?

    2. Have the child's growth and developmental needs been met?

▶ CLUB FOOT (TALIPES EQUINOVARUS)

A. Assessment

    1. Plantar flexion or dorsiflexion

    2. Inversion/adduction of forepart of foot

B. Diagnose

    1. Rigid abnormality of talus bone at birth

    2. Does not involve muscles, nerves, or blood vessels

C. Plan/Implementation

    1. Foot exercises—manipulation of foot to correct position every 4 hours regularly

    2. Casts and splints correct the deformity in most cases if applied early (see Figure 5); changed every few days for 1–2 weeks, then at 1–2-week intervals to accommodate infant's rapid growth

    3. Surgery is usually required for older child

    4. Denis-Browne—horizontal abduction bar with footplates

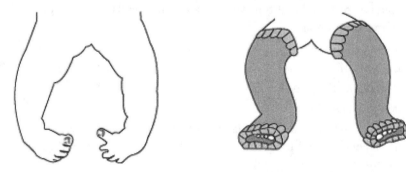

Figure 5. Casting of Talipes Equinovarus

D. Evaluation

    1. Has mobility of foot been maintained?

    2. Has structure of foot been corrected?

▶ **JOINT DISORDERS**

A. Assessment (see Table 1)

B. Diagnose (see Table 1)

  1. Risk factors

    a. Osteoarthritis

      1) Increased age

      2) Obesity

      3) Trauma to joints due to repetitive use

        a) Carpet installer

        b) Construction worker

        c) Farmer

        d) Sports injuries

    b. Rheumatoid arthritis

      1) Positive family history

    c. Gout

      1) Obesity

      2) Diuretics

      3) Family history

  2. Diagnostic tests

    a. Arthrocentesis—needle puncture of a joint space to remove accumulated fluid

      1) Strict asepsis is essential to avoid infection

      2) Usually elastic bandage wrap and joint rest for 24 hours to prevent hemorrhage

    b. Arthroscopy—direct visualization of a joint by use of arthroscope

      1) Local anesthesia given

      2) Teach breathing exercises to reduce discomfort

      3) Post-test bulky pressure dressing applied

  3. Potential nursing diagnoses

    a. Acute/chronic Pain

    b. Impaired physical mobility

    c. Self-care deficit

    d. Disturbed body image

    e. Ineffective role performance

C. Plan/Implementation

  1. Nursing care (see Table 1)

  2. Medications: analgesics, anti-inflammatory medication

D. Evaluation

  1. Has joint mobility been maintained?

  2. Has client comfort been maintained?

Table 1 JOINT DISORDERS				
TYPE	ASSESSMENT	DIAGNOSE	DIAGNOSTIC TESTS	NURSING CONSIDERATIONS
Rheumatoid arthritis Juvenile rheumatoid arthritis (JRA)	Joint pain, swelling, and limitation of movement Contracture deformities Nodules over bony prominences Ulnar deviation High fever and rheumatoid rash, particularly seen in JRA Salmon-pink macular rash on chest, thighs, and upper arms	Systemic; pannus formation Bony ankylosis Progressive Remissions and exacerbations	Rheumatoid factor (may be negative) C-reactive protein ESR, ANA Aspiration of synovial fluid X-rays	Pain management, rest, activity, exercise Weight control if obese Heat (e.g., warm tub baths; warm, moist compresses; paraffin dips) Splints for joints Analgesics, anti-inflammatory drugs Disease-modifying antirheumatic drugs Immunosuppressive drugs Antitumor necrosis drugs
Osteoarthritis	Joint pain, swelling, and limitation of movement Contracture deformities Joint stiffness after rest Heberden's and Bouchard's nodes of the fingers	Nonsystemic; spur formation; closure of joint spaces Degenerative No remissions	X-rays of joints show narrowing of joint spaces	Pain management, rest, activity, exercise Weight control if obese Analgesics, anti-inflammatory drugs Heat application
Gout	Joint pain, swelling, limitation of movement Contracture deformities Tophi	Nonsystemic Disturbed purine metabolism Elevated uric acid in blood Tophi formation (deposits of urates in joints) Exacerbations	X-rays Blood tests—WBC, ESR, uric acid level Synovial aspiration	Pain management Diet: avoid meats rich in purines (e.g., organ meats, sardines, fish), alcohol, ketoacidosis, dehydration Analgesics—aspirin Medications for gout

▶ PAGET'S DISEASE

A. Assessment

   1. Pain

   2. Bowed legs, decreased height

   3. Shortened trunk with long-appearing arms

   4. Enlarged skull

   5. Long bone, spine, and rib pain

   6. Labored, waddling gait

   7. Kyphosis

   8. Pathologic fractures

B. Diagnose

   1. Unknown etiology

   2. Excessive bone resorption (loss)

   3. Occurs more often in older adults

C. Plan/Implementation

1. Administer analgesics

2. Encourage rest

3. Prevent pathological fractures by using safety precautions

4. Administer medications: calcitonin, biphosphonates, e,g., alendronate; pamidronate.

D. Evaluation

1. Has client comfort been maintained?

2. Have complications been prevented?

▶ BURSITIS

A. Assessment

1. Pain due to inflammation

2. Decreased mobility, especially on abduction

B. Diagnose

1. Definition—inflammation of connective tissue sac between muscles, tendons, and bones, particularly affecting shoulder, elbow, and knee

2. Potential nursing diagnoses

a. Acute/chronic pain

b. Impaired physical mobility

c. Self-care deficit

C. Plan/Implementation

1. Rest

2. Immobilize affected joint with pillows, splints, slings

3. Administer pain medication, muscle relaxants (diazepam), steroids

4. Apply heat/cold packs to decrease swelling

5. Promote exercise (ROM)

6. Assist in performance of ADL by modifying activities relative to limitations

7. Assist with cortisone injection, draining of bursae

D. Evaluation

1. Has client's pain been minimized?

2. Has client's mobility been maintained?

▶ OSTEOPOROSIS

A. Assessment

1. Decreased height

2. Low back pain, especially hips and spine

3. Kyphosis

B. Diagnose

1. Reduction in bone mass with no changes in mineral composition

2. Degenerative disease characterized by generalized loss of bone density and tensile strength

3. Diagnosed by bone mineral density (BMD) T-scores—BMD T-score less than or equal to 2.5 indicates osteoporosis

4. Risk factors

   a. Age greater than 60 years

   b. Small-framed and lean body build

   c. Caucasian or Asian race

   d. Inadequate intake of calcium or vitamin D

   e. Postmenopausal

   f. Immobility and sedentary lifestyle

   g. History of smoking

   h. High alcohol intake

   i. Prolonged use of steroids

5. Potential nursing diagnoses

   a. Acute/chronic pain

   b. Self-care deficit

   c. Risk for trauma

C. Plan/Implementation

   1. Diet high in calcium, protein, and vitamin D

   2. Teach about medications

   3. Encourage weight-bearing on the long bones (walking)

   4. Fall prevention

   5. ROM exercises

   6. Physiotherapy

   7. Safety precautions to prevent pathological fractures

      a. Use back brace or splint for support

      b. Use bedboards or hard mattress

   8. Administer medications: calcitonin; biphosphonates, e.g., alendronate; selective receptor modulators, e.g., raloxifene; estrogen replacement therapy

D. Evaluation

   1. Has client's mobility been maintained?

   2. Is client knowledgeable about dietary requirements?

▶ **OSTEOMYELITIS**

A. Assessment

   1. Pain

   2. Swelling, redness, warmth on affected area

   3. Fever, leukocytosis

   4. Elevated sedimentation rate

   5. Positive culture and sensitivity

   6. X-ray of affected part

B. Diagnose

1. Infection of the bone, usually caused by *Staphylococcus aureus*, carried by the blood from a primary site of infection or from direct invasion, e.g., orthopedic surgical procedures or fractures

2. Risk factors

   a. Poorly nourished

   b. Elderly

   c. Obesity

   d. Impaired immune system

   e. Long-term corticosteroid therapy

3. Potential nursing diagnoses

   a. Acute pain

   b. Ineffective bone tissue perfusion

   c. Risk for injury

   d. Deficient knowledge

C. Plan/Implementation

1. Teach about risk factors for osteomyelitis, e.g., joint prosthesis

2. Medications: analgesics, antibiotics, antipyretics

3. Support affected extremity with pillows, splints to maintain proper body alignment

4. Provide cool environment and lightweight clothing

5. Avoid exercise and heat application to the affected area

6. Encourage fluid intake, monitor intake and output

7. Asepsis with wound care

8. Provide diversionary activities

9. High-protein diet with sufficient carbohydrates, vitamins, and minerals

10. Instruct about home wound care and antibiotic administration

D. Evaluation

1. Has client comfort been maintained?

2. Have complications been prevented?

▶ OSTEOMALACIA

A. Assessment

1. Bone pain and tenderness

2. Muscle weakness

3. Bowed legs, kyphosis

4. X-ray (porous bones)

B. Diagnose

1. Decalcification of bones due to inadequate intake of vitamin D, absence of exposure to sunlight, or intestinal malabsorption, chronic kidney disease

2. Potential nursing diagnoses

    a. Injury, risk for

    b. Delayed growth and development

    c. Body image disturbance

C. Plan/Implementation

1. Administration of analgesics

2. Increase sun exposure

3. Instruct about high vitamin D foods (milk, eggs, vitamin D enriched cereals and bread products)

4. Administer vitamin D, calcium, and expose to sunlight and/or ultraviolet irradiation

5. Assist with performance of ADL to prevent pathological fractures

D. Evaluation

1. Has client mobility been maintained?

2. Has client's pain been minimized?

▶ SPINA BIFIDA/NEURAL TUBE DEFECTS

A. Assessment (see Figure 6)

1. Dimpling at the site (spina bifida occulta)

2. Bulging, saclike lesion filled with spinal fluid and covered with a thin, atrophic, bluish, ulcerated skin (meningocele)

3. Bulging, saclike lesion filled with spinal fluid and spinal cord element (myelomeningocele)

4. Hydrocephalus increases risk

5. Paralysis of lower extremities

6. Musculoskeletal deformities—club feet, dislocated hips, kyphosis, scoliosis

7. Neurogenic bladder and bowel, prolapsed rectum

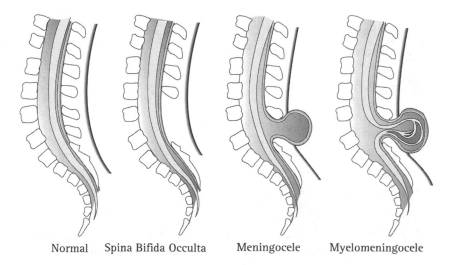

Normal   Spina Bifida Occulta   Meningocele   Myelomeningocele

Figure 6. Types of Spina Bifida

B. Diagnose

1. Congenital anomaly of the spinal cord characterized by nonunion between the laminae of the vertebrae

2. Risk factors

   a. Maternal folic-acid deficiency

   b. Previous pregnancy affected by neural tube defect

3. Etiology

   a. Combination of unknown genetic/environmental factors

   b. Advanced maternal age

   c. High levels of alpha-fetoprotein at amniocentesis

C. Plan/Implementation

1. Occulta: no treatment

2. Meningocele/myelomeningocele: surgical repair at 24–48 hours

3. Observe for irritation, CSF leakage, and signs of infection

4. Maintain optimum asepsis; cover lesion with moist sterile dressings

5. Position client on abdomen or semiprone with sandbags

6. Provide optimum skin care, especially to perineal area

7. Check for abnormal movement of extremities, absent or abnormal reflexes, incontinence, fecal impaction, flaccid paralysis of lower extremities

8. Observe for increased intracranial pressure (headache, changes in LOC, motor functions, and vital signs)

9. Observe for symptoms of meningeal irritation or meningitis

10. Provide frequent sources of stimulation appropriate for child's age level

11. Provide postoperative care—vertebral fusion or surgical repair

12. Focus postoperative observation on detecting signs of meningitis, shock, increased intracranial pressure, and respiratory difficulty

13. Foster parental bonding

14. Perform family teaching on how to care for child at home

15. Discuss with family referrals for PT, orthopedic procedures, bladder and bowel management

D. Evaluation

1. Have complications been prevented?

2. Have infant's physical needs been met?

▶ HYDROCEPHALUS

A. Assessment

1. Fronto-occipital circumference increases at abnormally fast rate (see Figure 7)

2. Split sutures and widened, distended, tense fontanelles

3. Prominent forehead, dilated scalp veins

4. Sunset eyes, nystagmus

5. Irritability, vomiting

6. Unusual somnolence

7. Convulsions

8. High-pitched cry

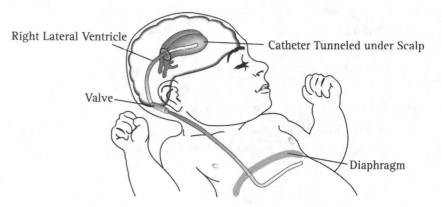

Figure 7. Ventriculoperitoneal Shunt for Hydrocephalus

B. Diagnose

1. Congenital or acquired condition characterized by an increase in the accumulation of CSF within the ventricular system and subsequent increase in ventricular pressure

2. Causes

   a. Neoplasm

   b. Aqueductal stenosis—stenosis/obstructions in ventricular system

   c. Spina bifida

   d. Congenital cysts/vascular malformations

3. Types

   a. Communicating—due to increased production of CSF or impaired absorption of CSF

   b. Noncommunicating—due to obstruction/blockage of CSF circulation between ventricles and subarachnoid space

C. Plan/Implementation

1. Operative management

   a. Ventriculoperitoneal shunt—connection between ventricles and peritoneal cavity (see Figure 7)

   b. Ventricular atrial shunt—connection between ventricles and right atrium

   c. Ventricular drainage—provides external drainage of fluid

2. Observation of shunt functioning

3. Observe for increased intracranial pressure and for signs of shunt infection (irritability, high pitched cry, lethargy)

4. Postoperative positioning—on unoperated side in flat position; do not hold infant with head elevated

5. Shunt needs to be modified as child grows

6. Continual testing for developmental abnormalities/intellectual delay

7. Discharge planning/community referral

8. Teach parents about increased risk for allergies if myelomeningocele present

D. Evaluation

1. Has child attained optimal growth and development?

▶ NEUROMUSCULAR DISORDERS

A. Assessment (see Table 2)

B. Diagnose (see Table 2)

Table 2 NEUROMUSCULAR DISORDERS		
	CEREBRAL PALSY	MUSCULAR DYSTROPHY
Assessment	Athetosis, spasticity, rigidity, ataxia, atonicity; repetitive, involuntary, slow, gross movements Neonate: cannot hold head up, feeble cry, inability to feed, body noticeably arched or limp Infant: failure-to-thrive syndrome Toddler/preschooler: intellectual delay, delayed physical development	Muscle weakness, lordosis/scoliosis, waddling gait, joint contractures Stumbling and falling
Analysis	Voluntary muscles poorly controlled due to brain damage Etiology: unclear Predisposition: prematurity, existing prenatal brain abnormalities, trauma, anoxia, or infection at time of birth Treatment: ambulation devices, surgical lengthening of heel cord to promote stability and function Medications: muscle relaxants, tranquilizers, anticonvulsants, baclofen, intrathecal pump	Progressive muscular weakness, atrophy of voluntary muscles, no nerve effect Etiology: genetic Diagnostic tests: CPK (creatinine phosphokinase), abnormal electromyogram, abnormal muscle biopsy Predisposition: heredity Progressive/terminal Treatment: intensive physical therapy, active and passive stretching and ROM Light spinal braces or long leg braces may help ambulation
Potential nursing diagnosis	Nutrition: less than body requirements Compromised family coping Self-care deficit Impaired physical mobility Delayed growth and development	Self-care deficit Compromised family coping Body image disturbance Impaired physical mobility Ineffective breathing pattern Impaired swallowing Delayed growth and development

C. Plan/Implementation
1. Cerebral palsy
   a. Assist with early diagnosis
   b. Assist with physical and occupational therapy
   c. Give referrals to appropriate agencies
   d. Provide emotional support to parents and client
   e. Assist with feeding, place food at back of mouth or on either side of tongue toward cheek, apply slight downward pressure with the spoon
   f. Never tilt head backward when feeding (leads to choking)
   g. High-calorie diet
2. Muscular dystrophy
   a. Promote safety to avoid slips and falls due to gait and movement disturbances; use braces or wheelchair
   b. Assist with diagnostic tests
   c. Client/parent education on nature of the disease
   d. Provide emotional support to child and family
   e. Discuss balance between activity and rest for the child
   f. Prevent contractures
   g. Referrals to appropriate agencies

D. Evaluation
1. Has child's mobility been maintained?
2. Have the child's nutritional needs been met?

▶ DISTURBED TRANSMISSION OF NERVE IMPULSES

A. Assessment (see Table 3)
B. Diagnose (see Table 3)

Table 3 DISORDERS OF NERVE IMPULSE TRANSMISSION			
	PARKINSON'S DISEASE	MYASTHENIA GRAVIS	MULTIPLE SCLEROSIS
Assessment	Tremors (pill-rolling motion), akinesia (loss of automation), rigidity, weakness "Motorized" propulsive gait, slurred monotonous speech, dysphagia Salivation, masklike expression, drooling Constipation Depression Dementia	Muscular weakness produced by repeated movements soon disappears following rest Diplopia, ptosis, impaired speech, dysphagia Respiratory distress Periods of remissions and exacerbations	Early—vision, motor sensation changes Late—cognitive and bowel changes Muscular incoordination, ataxia, spasticity, intention tremors, nystagmus, chewing and swallowing difficulties, impaired speech Incontinence, emotional instability, sexual dysfunction
Analysis	Deficiency of dopamine; increased acetylcholine levels Etiology unclear; chronic and progressive; intellect intact Does not lead to paralysis	Deficiency of acetylcholine at myoneural junction Etiology unclear; chronic and progressive; intellect intact Diagnosis—based on administration of anticholinesterase; positive result evidenced by a striking increase in muscular strength 5-10 minutes after administration No muscular atrophy No loss of sensation	Demyelination of white matter throughout brain and spinal cord Etiology unclear; chronic and progressive; intellect intact Leads to paraplegia or complete paralysis
Nursing diagnosis	Self-care deficit Nutrition, altered Body image disturbance Caregiver rule strain Communication, impaired verbal Impaired walking Impaired swallowing	Self-care deficit Airway clearance, ineffective Physical mobility, impaired Impaired swallowing Anxiety/fear	Self-care deficit Nutrition, altered Urinary elimination, altered Physical mobility, impaired Fatigue Disturbed visual, Kinesthetic, Tactile, Sensory perception Powerlessness Compromised/Disabled Family coping

C. Plan/Implementation

  1. Parkinson's disease

    a. Encourage finger exercises, e.g., typing, piano-playing

    b. ROM as appropriate

    c. Teach client ambulation modification, refer to physical therapy

      1) Goose-stepping walk

      2) Walk with wider base

      3) Concentrate on swinging arms while walking

      4) Turn around slowly using small steps

    d. Promote family understanding of the disease

      1) Client's intellect is not impaired

      2) Sight and hearing are intact

      3) Disease is progressive but slow

      4) Does not lead to paralysis

    e. Refer for speech therapy, potential stereotactic surgery

    f. Administer dopaminergics, e.g., levodopa–carbidopa; dopamineagonists, e.g., pramipexole; anticholinergics, e.g., benztropine, trihexyphenidyl; antivirals, e.g., amantadine

2. Myasthenia gravis

    a. Promote family understanding of the disease

      1) It is neither a central nervous system nor a peripheral nervous system disease

      2) There is no muscular atrophy or loss of sensation

      3) It is not hereditary

    b. Administer medications before eating

      1) Anticholinesterases

      2) Corticosteroids

      3) Immunosuppressants

    c. Good eye care (artificial tears, eye patch for diplopia)

    d. Maintain optimal mobility

    e. Provide environment that is restful and free of stress

    f. Client teaching

      1) Importance of taking medications on time; dosage depends on physiological needs and living patterns

      2) Wear Medic-Alert band

      3) Avoid factors that may precipitate myasthenia crisis, e.g., infections, emotional upsets, use of streptomycin or neomycin (they produce muscular weakness), surgery

      4) Be alert for myasthenia crisis—sudden inability to swallow, speak, or maintain a patent airway

3. Multiple sclerosis (MS)

    a. Teach relaxation and coordination exercises

    b. Teach progressive resistance exercises, ROM

    c. Encourage fluid intake 2000 mL/day

    d. Warm baths and packs

    e. Administer medications–immunosuppressants; corticosteroids;antispasmodics; interferon beta-1a; monoclonal antibodies

    f. Wide-based walk, use of cane or walker

    g. Use weighted bracelets and cuffs to stabilize upper extremities

    h. Bladder and bowel training (care of Foley catheter if appropriate)

    i. Self-help devices

    j. Eye patch for diplopia

    k. No tetracycline or neomycin because they increase muscle weakness with MS

    l. Occupational therapy

    m. Provide emotional support

    n. Referrals—National Multiple Sclerosis Society

D. Evaluation

1. Is client able to maintain independent functioning?

2. Have client's physical needs been met?

▶ AMYOTROPHIC LATERAL SCLEROSIS (LOU GEHRIG'S DISEASE)

A. Assessment

1. Tongue fatigue, atrophy with fasciculations (brief muscle twitching)

2. Nasal quality to speech, dysarthria

3. Dysphagia, aspiration

4. Progressive muscular weakness, muscular wasting, atrophy, spasticity

   a. Usually begins in upper extremities

   b. Distal portion affected first

   c. Fasciculations

5. Emotional lability, cognitive dysfunction

6. Respiratory insufficiency (usual cause of death)

7. No alteration in autonomic, sensory, or mental function

B. Diagnose

1. Progressive, degenerative disease involving the lower motor neurons of the spinal cord and cerebral cortex; the voluntary motor system is particularly involved with progressive degeneration of the corticospinal tract, leads to a mixture of spastic and atrophic changes in cranial and spinal musculature

2. No specific pattern exists—involvement may vary in different parts of the same area

3. Possible etiologies

   a. Genetic, familial

   b. Chronic (slow) viral infection

   c. Autoimmune disease

   d. Environmental factors (toxic, metabolic)

C. Plan/Implementation

1. Apply principles of care of client with progressive, terminal disease

2. Treat self-care deficits symptomatically

3. Maintain adequate nutrition

4. Physical therapy/speech therapy

5. Adaptive home equipment

6. Provide psychosocial support

D. Evaluation

1. Is client able to maintain optimal physical functioning for as long as possible?

2. Has client comfort been maintained?

INTERVENTIONS TO PROMOTE COMFORT Unit 3

▶ PAIN

A. Assessment
1. The fifth vital sign
2. History
   a. P–precipitating factors
   b. Q–quality
   c. R–region/radiation
   d. S–severity
   e. T–timing
3. Potential responses to pain (see Table 1)

Table 1 POTENTIAL RESPONSES TO PAIN	
ASSESSMENT	RESULT
Increased BP and heart rate leads to increased blood flow to brain and muscles Rapid, irregular respirations leads to increased O_2 supply to brain and muscles	Enhanced alertness to threats Preoccupation with painful stimulus
Increased pupillary diameter leads to increased eye accommodation to light	Increased visual perception of threats
Increased perspiration	Removal of excess body heat
Increased muscle tension leads to increased neuromuscular activity	Musculoskeletal system ready for rapid motor activity and responsiveness
Altered GI motility leads to nausea and vomiting	Altered metabolic processes
Apprehension, irritability, and anxiety Verbalizes pain	Enhanced mental alertness to threats Communication of suffering and pleas for help

B. Diagnose
1. Definition—"Whatever the person says it is, and it exists whenever the person says it does"
2. Types
   a. Acute—an episode of pain that lasts from a split second to about 6 months; causes decreased healing, vital sign changes, diaphoresis
   b. Chronic—an episode of pain that lasts for 6 months or longer; causes fatigue, depression, weight gain, immobility
3. Factors influencing pain experiences
   a. Individual's responses or reactions to pain are generally dependent on what is expected and accepted in his/her culture
   b. Past experiences with pain generally make the individual more sensitive to the pain experience

4. Potential nursing diagnoses

 a. Acute/chronic pain

 b. Activity intolerance

 c. Ineffective therapeutic regimen management

 d. Social isolation

 e. Readiness for enhanced comfort

 f. Imbalanced nutrition: less than body requirements

C. Plan/Implementation

1. Establish a therapeutic relationship

 a. Tell client you believe what he/she says about his/her pain experience

 b. Listen and allow client to verbalize

 c. Allow client to use own words in describing pain experience

2. Establish a 24-hour pain profile

 a. Location

   1) External

   2) Internal

   3) Both external and internal

   4) Area of body affected

 b. Character and intensity

   1) Acute/chronic

   2) Mild/severe

 c. Onset

   1) Sudden

   2) Insidious

 d. Duration

 e. Precipitating factors

 f. Identify associated manifestations, as well as alleviating or aggravating factors

3. Teach client about pain and pain relief

 a. Explain quality and location of impending pain, (e.g., before uncomfortable procedure)

 b. Help client learn to use slow, rhythmic breathing to promote relaxation

 c. Explain effects of analgesics and benefits of preventative approach

 d. Demonstrate splinting techniques that help reduce pain

4. Reduce anxiety and fears

 a. Give reassurance

 b. Offer distraction

 c. Spend time with client

5. Provide comfort measures

 a. Proper positioning

 b. Cool, well ventilated, quiet room

 c. Back rub

 d. Allow for rest

6. Administer pain medications
   a. Use preventive approach
      1) If pain is expected to occur throughout most of a 24-hour period, a regular schedule is better than prn
      2) Usually takes a smaller dose to alleviate mild pain or prevent occurrence of pain
      3) Pain relief is more complete and client spends fewer hours in pain
      4) Helps prevent addiction
   b. PCA (client-controlled analgesia) pumps—a portable device that delivers predetermined dosage of intravenous narcotic (e.g., dose of 1 mg morphine with a lock-out interval of 5–15 minutes for a total possible dose of 5 mg per hour)
   c. Non-opioid analgesics
   d. Nonsteroidal anti-inflammatory drugs (NSAIDs)
   e. Opioids
   f. Anticonvulsants
   g. Alpha-2 adrenergics
7. Other methods of pain relief
   a. Neurectomy/sympathectomy
   b. TENS (transcutaneous electric nerve stimulation)—produces tingling, buzzing sensation in area of pain; used for chronic and acute pain
8. Complementary and alternative methods of pain control
   a. Relaxation techniques
   b. Meditation
   c. Progressive relaxation
   d. Yoga/exercise
   e. Distraction
   f. Guided imagery
   g. Herbal remedies
   h. Biofeedback
   i. Acupuncture
   j. Heat/cold application
   k. Therapeutic touch; consider cultural factors
   l. Massage
   m. Hypnosis
D. Evaluation
   1. Has client comfort been maintained?
   2. Is client able to demonstrate splinting techniques to reduce pain?

MUSCULOSKELETAL TRAUMA

▶ ## CONTUSIONS, SPRAINS, JOINT DISLOCATIONS

A. Assessment

1. Contusions
   a. Ecchymosis
   b. Hematoma

2. Strains/sprains
   a. Pain
   b. Swelling

3. Joint dislocations
   a. Pain
   b. Deformity

B. Diagnose

1. Contusions—injury of soft tissue
2. Strains—muscle and/or tendon pull or tear
3. Sprains—torn ligament or stretched ligament
4. Dislocation—displacement of joint bones so their articulating surfaces lose all contact

C. Plan/Implementation

1. Contusions—treated with cold application for 24 hours followed by moist heat; apply elastic bandage
2. Strains/sprains—treated with rest and elevation of affected part; intermittent ice compresses for 24 hours, followed by heat application; apply elastic pressure bandage; minimize use
3. Dislocations—considered an orthopedic emergency; treated with immobilization and reduction, e.g., the dislocated bone is brought back to its normal position, usually under anesthesia; bandages and splints are used to keep affected part immobile until healing occurs

D. Evaluation

1. Is client comfort restored?
2. Have complications been prevented?

▶ ## FRACTURES

A. Assessment

1. Swelling, pallor, ecchymosis of surrounding subcutaneous tissue
2. Loss of sensation to body parts
3. Deformity
4. Pain and/or acute tenderness
5. Muscle spasms
6. Loss of function, abnormal mobility
7. Crepitus (grating sound on movement of ends of broken bone)

8. Shortening of affected limb

9. Decreased or absent pulses distal to injury

10. Affected extremity colder than contralateral part

B. Diagnose

1. Fractures—break in continuity of bone

2. Types (see Figure 1, panels A–D)

3. Complications of fractures

   a. Fat emboli—caused after fracture of long bones when fat globules move into bloodstream; may occlude major vessels

   b. Hemorrhage

   c. Delayed union—healing of fracture is slowed; caused by infection or distraction of fractured fragments; will see increase in bone pain

   d. Malunion—improper alignment of fracture fragments; may develop with premature weight-bearing

   e. Nonunion—healing has not occurred 4–6 months after fracture; insufficient blood supply, repetitive stress on fracture site, infection, inadequate internal fixation; treated by bone grafting, internal fixation, electric bone stimulation

   f. Sepsis

   g. Compartment syndrome—high pressure within a muscle compartment of an extremity compromises circulation; pressure may be internal (bleeding) or external (casts); if left untreated neuromuscular damage occurs within 4–6 hours; limb can become permanently useless within 24–48 hours; will see unrelenting pain out of proportion to injury and unrelieved by pain medication, decreased pulse strength, numbness and tingling of extremity, possible cyanosis, and pale cool extremity

   h. Peripheral nerve damage

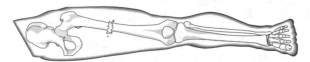

A. Complete: break across entire cross-section of bone

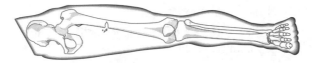

B. Incomplete: break through portion of bone

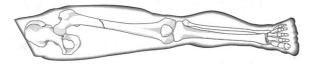

C. Closed: no external communication

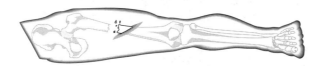

D. Open: extends through skin

Figure 1 Types of Fractures

C. Plan/Implementation

1. Provide emergency care

   a. Immobilization before client is moved by use of splints; immobilize joint below and above fracture

   b. In an open fracture, cover the wound with sterile dressings or cleanest material available; control bleeding by direct pressure

   c. Check temperature, color, sensation, capillary refill distal to fracture

   d. Emergency room—give narcotic adequate to relieve pain (except in presence of head injury)

2. Treatment

   a. Splinting—immobilization of the affected part to prevent soft tissue from being damaged by bony fragments

   b. Internal fixation—use of metal screws, plates, nails, and pins to stabilize reduced fracture

   c. Open reduction—surgical dissection and exposure of the fracture for reduction and alignment

   d. Closed reduction—manual manipulation or of fracture

3. Traction (see Figures 2–6)

    a. Purposes

        1) Reduce the fracture

        2) Alleviate pain and muscle spasm

        3) Prevent or correct deformities

        4) Promote healing

    b. Types of traction

        1) Skin (Buck's extension, Russell's, pelvic traction)– pulling force applied to skin

        2) Skeletal (halo, Crutchfield tongs)–pulling force applied to bone

    c. Care

        1) Maintain straight alignment of ropes and pulleys

        2) Assure that weights hang free

        3) Frequently inspect skin for breakdown areas

        4) Maintain position for countertraction

        5) Encourage movement of unaffected areas

        6) Investigate every report of discomfort/difficulty immediately and thoroughly

        7) Maintain continuous pull

        8) Clean pins with half-strength peroxide or saline and sterile swabs 1–2 times a day, if ordered

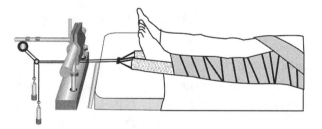

Figure 2 Buck's Traction

Relieves muscular spasm of legs and back; if no fracture, may turn to either side; with fracture, turn to unaffected side. 8–20 lb used; 40 lb for scoliosis. Elevate foot of bed for countertraction. Use trapeze for moving. Place pillow beneath lower legs, not heel. Don't elevate knee gatch.

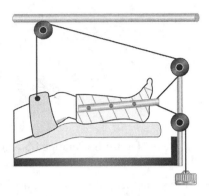

Figure 3   Russell's Traction

"Pulls" contracted muscles; elevate foot of bed with shock blocks to provide countertraction; sling can be loosened for skin care; check popliteal pulse. Place pillows under lower leg. Make sure heel is off the bed. Must not turn from waist down. Lift client, not leg, to provide assistance.

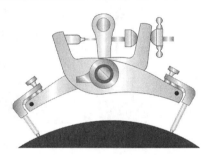

Figure 4   Cervical (skull tongs)

Realigns fracture of cervical vertebrae and relieves pressure on cervical nerves; never lift weights—traction must be continuous. No pillow under the head during feeding; hard to swallow, may need suctioning.

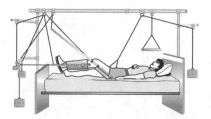

Figure 5 Balanced Suspension

Realigns fractures of the femur; uses pulley to create balanced suspension by countertraction to the top of the thigh splint. Thomas splint (positioned under anterior thigh) with Pearson attachment (supports leg from knee down) frequently used.

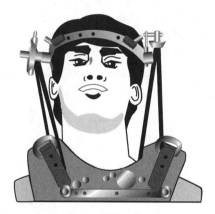

Figure 6 Halo Fixation Device (vest)

Provides immobilization of cervical spine; pins are used to maintain traction; care of insertion site includes cleansing area around pins using sterile technique. If prescribed by health care provider, clean with half-strength peroxide or saline and sterile swabs 1–2 times/day.

4. Casting—provides rigid immobilization of affected body part for support and stability, may be plaster or fiberglass (lighter, stronger, water-resistant, porous; diminishes skin problems, does not soften when wet, thus allowing for hydrotherapy)

   a. Immediate care

   1) Avoid covering cast until dry (48 hours or longer); handle with palms, not fingertips (plaster cast)

   2) Avoid resting cast on hard surfaces or sharp edges

   3) Keep affected limb elevated above heart on soft surface until dry; don't use heat lamp or cover with heavy blankets

        4) Watch for danger signs, e.g., blueness or paleness, pain, numbness, or tingling sensations on affected area; if present, elevate casted area; if it persists, contact health care provider

        5) Elevate arm cast above level of heart

   b. Intermediate care

        1) When cast is dry, client should be mobilized

        2) Encourage prescribed exercises (isometrics and active ROM of joints above and below cast)

        3) Report to health care provider any break in cast or foul odor from cast

        4) Tell client not to scratch skin underneath cast, skin may break and infection can set in; don't put anything underneath cast

        5) If fiberglass cast gets wet, dry with hair dryer on cool setting

   c. After-cast care

        1) Wash skin gently

        2) Apply baby powder, cornstarch, or baby oil

        3) Have client gradually adjust to movement without support of cast

        4) Inform client that swelling is common

        5) Elevate limb and apply elastic bandage

   d. Complications

        1) Impaired circulation

        2) Peripheral nerve damage

        3) Pressure necrosis

D. Evaluation

   1. Has fracture healed without complications?

   2. Has client mobility been restored?

▶ FRACTURED HIP

A. Assessment

   1. Leg shortened, adducted, externally rotated

   2. Pain

   3. Hematoma, ecchymosis

   4. Confirmed by x-rays

B. Diagnose

   1. Commonly seen with elderly women with osteoporosis

   2. Potential nursing diagnoses

     a. Impaired physical mobility

     b. Risk for peripheral neurovascular dysfunction

     c. Risk for impaired gas exchange

     d. Acute pain

C. Plan/Implementation

1. Total hip replacement—acetabulum, cartilage, and head of femur replaced with artificial joint (see Figure 7)

2. Abduction of affected extremity (use splints, wedge pillow, or 2 or 3 pillows between legs)

3. Turn client as ordered; keep heels off bed

4. Ice to operative site

5. Over bed trapeze to lift self onto fracture bedpan

6. Prevention of thromboembolism–low molecular weight heparin (LMWH) and warfarin; do not sit for prolonged periods

7. Initial ambulation with walker

8. Crutch walking—three-point gait

9. Chair with arms, wheelchair, semireclining toilet seat

10. Medications—anticoagulants to prevent pulmonary embolism, antibiotics to prevent infection

11. Don't sleep on operated side

12. Don't flex hip more than 90°

13. Continuous passive motion device—used after knee replacement to prevent development of scar tissue; extends and flexes knee

14. Use adaptive devices for dressing–extended handles, shoe horns

15. Report increased hip pain to health care provider immediately

16. Cleanse incision daily with mild soap and water; dry thoroughly

17. Teach client to inspect hip daily for redness, heat, drainage; if present, call health care provider immediately

18. Complications

    a. Dislocation of prosthesis

    b. Excessive wound drainage

    c. Thromboembolism

    d. Infection

19. Postoperative discharge teaching

    a. Maintain abduction

    b. Avoid stooping

    c. Do not sleep on operated side until directed to do so

    d. Flex hip only to 90°

    e. Never cross legs

    f. Avoid position of flexion during sexual activity

    g. Walking is excellent exercise; avoid overexertion

    h. In 3 months, will be able to resume ADLs, except strenuous sports

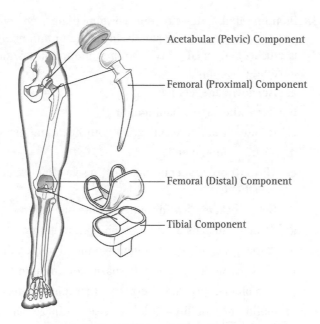

Figure 7 Total Hip and Knee Replacement

D. Evaluation

1. Is client knowledgeable about restrictions of activity?

2. Have complications of total hip replacement been prevented?

▶ AMPUTATION

A. Assessment

1. Trauma

2. Peripheral vascular disease

3. Osteogenic sarcoma

B. Diagnose

1. Disarticulation—resection of an extremity through a joint

2. Above-knee amputation (AKA)

3. Below-knee amputation (BKA)

4. Guillotine or open surface

5. Closed or flap

C. Plan/Implementation (see Table 1)

1. Delayed prosthesis fitting—residual limb covered with removable cast or residual limb sock; note if penrose drain is inserted follow orders for dressing changes

2. Immediate prosthesis fitting—residual limb covered with dressing and rigid plastic dressing; Penrose drain usually not inserted; rigid dressing helps prevent bleeding by compressing residual limb

3. Phantom limb pain—experienced immediately postop up to 2-3 months postop; occurs more frequently in AK amputations; feeling that extremity is crushed, cramped, or twisted into abnormal position; may be intense burning or cramping

   a. Acknowledge feelings

   b. Early intensive rehabilitation

   c. Residual limb desensitization with kneading massage

   d. Distraction and activity

   e. TENS (transcutaneous electrical nerve stimulation), ultrasound, local anesthetic

   f. Beta blockers used for dull, burning sensations

   g. Anticonvulsants used for stabbing and cramping sensations

   h. Antidepressants used to improve mood and coping ability

   i. Antispasmodics for muscle spasms or cramping

   j. Complementary and alternative therapies—biofeedback and hypnosis

4. Promotion of mobility—ROM exercises; trapeze with overhead frame; firm mattress; prone position every 3 hours for 20 to 30 minutes

Table 1 POST-OPERATIVE AMPUTATION CARE		
TYPE OF CARE	DELAYED PROSTHESIS FITTING	IMMEDIATE PROSTHESIS FITTING
Residual limb care	Observe dressings for signs of excessive bleeding; keep large tourniquet on hand to apply around residual limb in event of hemorrhage; dressings changed daily until sutures removed; wrap with elastic bandage to shape, reduce edema, and keep dressing in place; figure-eight because it prevents restriction of blood flow	Observe rigid dressing for signs of oozing; if blood stain appears, mark area and observe every 10 minutes for increase; report excessive oozing immediately to health care provider; provide cast care; guard against cast slipping off
Positioning	If ordered by health care provider, elevate residual limb by elevating foot of bed to hasten venous return and prevent edema.	Elevation of residual limb for 24 hours usually sufficient; rigid cast acts to control swelling
Turning	Turn client to prone position for short time first postop day, then 30 min 3 times daily to prevent hip contracture; have client roll from side to side	Same; rigid cast, however, acts to prevent both hip and joint contractures
Exercises	Have client start exercises to prevent contractures 1st or 2nd day postop, including: active range of motion, especially of remaining leg, strengthening exercises for upper extremities, hyperextension of residual limb	Exercises not as essential because rigid dressing prevents contractures; early ambulation prevents immobilization disabilities

TYPE OF CARE	DELAYED PROSTHESIS FITTING	IMMEDIATE PROSTHESIS FITTING
Ambulation	Dangle and transfer client to wheelchair and back within 1st or 2nd day postop; crutch walking started as soon as client feels sufficiently strong	Dangle and assist client to ambulate with walker for short period 1st day; increase length of ambulation each day; in physical therapy client uses parallel bars, then crutches, then cane
Psychological support	Observe for signs of depression or despondency; remind depressed client that he/she will receive prosthesis when wound heals	Observe for signs of depression; clients usually less depressed if they awaken with prosthesis attached
Discharge	Teach residual limb care—inspect daily for abrasions, wash, expose to air, do not apply lotions, use only cotton or wool residual limb socks	Same

Table 1 POST-OPERATIVE AMPUTATION CARE *(CONTINUED)*

D. Evaluation

1. Has client's mobility been maintained?

2. Have complications been prevented?

REST AND SLEEP DISTURBANCES Unit 5

▶ **HOSPITALIZED CLIENTS**

A. Assessment

1. Restlessness
2. Fatigue
3. Inability to concentrate
4. Irritability
5. Depression
6. Hallucinations after extended periods of sleeplessness

B. Diagnose

1. Rest—basic physiological need
   a. Allows body to repair its own damaged cells
   b. Enhances removal of waste products from the body
   c. Restores tissue to maximum functional ability before another activity is begun
2. Sleep—basic physiological need, although the purpose and reason for it is unclear; possible theories include:
   a. To restore balance among different parts of the central nervous system
   b. To mediate stress, anxiety, and tension
   c. To help a person cope with daily activities
3. Causes of disturbances
   a. Stress
   b. Drugs, e.g., hypnotics, barbiturates
   c. Unfamiliar environment
4. Potential nursing diagnoses
   a. Sleep pattern disturbance
   b. Activity intolerance
   c. Injury, risk for

C. Plan/Implementation

1. Establish database on client's pattern of rest and sleep
2. Give care in blocks of time to allow uninterrupted periods of rest and sleep
3. Remove unpleasant odors
4. Avoid unnecessary light and noises
5. Avoid excessively warm or cool temperatures
6. Reposition client as appropriate
7. Spend time with client
8. Give unhurried backrub
9. Straighten and replace wrinkled or soiled linens

10. Give warm, nonstimulating beverages

11. Give pain medication—preferable to sleep medications, which interfere with REM stage of sleep

12. Provide diversionary and occupational activities during the day to relieve boredom and utilize nighttime for sleep

13. Listen actively to client's concerns

14. Explain treatments ahead of time

15. Give a thorough orientation to the hospital setting

D. Evaluation

1. Is client able to fall asleep and stay asleep?

2. Has client's comfort been maintained?

▶ ELDERLY CLIENTS

A. Assessment

1. Difficulty getting to sleep

2. Waking early in the morning

3. Brief periods of wakefulness during the night

B. Diagnose

1. Sleep patterns change with advancing age

2. Levels of deep sleep occur less frequently

C. Plan/Implementation

1. Establish regular schedule for sleeping, go to bed at same time and wake up at same time

2. Avoid caffeinated beverages late in the evening

3. Establish bedtime ritual

   a. Warm bath

   b. Warm milk

4. Exercise regularly

5. If unable to sleep, perform quiet activity or read

6. Bedroom should be well ventilated and humidified

7. Reduce daytime napping and inactivity

8. Evaluate for sleep apnea

9. Evaluate for nocturia

D. Evaluation

1. Is client able to wake refreshed?

2. Is client able to perform ADLs?

▶ SLEEP APNEA SYNDROME

A. Assessment

1. Client snores loudly, stops breathing for 10 seconds or more, then awakens abruptly with loud snort; multiple nighttime awakenings

2. Excessive daytime sleepiness and fatigue

3. Morning headache

4. Sore throat

5. Personality and behavioral changes

6. Dysrhythmias, hypertension, increased risk of stroke, myocardial infarction and heart failure

B. Diagnose

1. Occurs in older, overweight men, elderly, people with thick necks, smokers

2. Polysomnography (PSG)—EEG, EMG, ECG, oxygen saturation levels; diaphragmatic movement monitored during sleep

3. Types

   a. Obstructive—lack of airflow due to occlusion of pharynx

   b. Central—cessation of airflow and respiratory movements

   c. Mixed—combination of central and obstructive apnea within an episode

C. Plan/Implementation

1. Avoid alcohol and medications that depress upper airway

2. Weight-reduction diet and activity

3. For severe cases, if client is hypoxic and hypercapnic, will use continuous positive airway pressure (CPAP) or bilevel positive airway pressure (BIPAP) with additional oxygen

4. Position-fixing devices used to prevent tongue obstruction and subluxation of neck

5. Surgery to correct obstruction

6. Low-flow oxygen

7. Tracheostomy if life-threatening dysrhythmias are present; unplugged only during sleep

D. Evaluation

1. Has client's sleeping pattern been restored?

2. Is client knowledgeable about how to use home equipment?

► ALZHEIMER'S DISEASE

A. Assessment

1. Forgetfulness progressing to inability to recognize familiar faces, places, objects

2. Depression, paranoia, combativeness

3. Unable to formulate concepts and think abstractly

4. Impulsive behavior

5. Short attention span

6. Agitation and increase in physical activity

7. Night wandering

8. Inability to perform ADLs (unkempt appearance)

9. Dysphasia

10. Incontinence

B. Diagnose

1. Progressive, irreversible, degenerative neurological disease characterized by loss of cognitive function and disturbance in behavior

2. Risk factors

   a. Age

   b. Family history

3. Potential nursing diagnoses

   a. Self-care deficit

   b. Communication, impaired verbal

   c. Incontinence, total

4. Death occurs due to complications

   a. Pneumonia

   b. Malnutrition

   c. Dehydration

C. Plan/Implementation

1. Support cognitive function

   a. Provide calm, predictable environment and present change gradually

   b. Establish regular routine

   c. Give clear and simple explanations and repeat information

   d. Display clock and calendar

   e. Color-code objects and areas

2. Provide for safety

   a. Use night light, call light, and low bed with half-bed rails

   b. Allow smoking only with supervision

   c. Monitor medications and food intake

   d. Secure doors leading from house

   e. Gently distract and redirect during wandering behavior

   f. Avoid restraints (increases combativeness)

   g. Client should wear identification bracelet or neck chain

   h. Frequent reorientation

3. Reduce anxiety and agitation

   a. Reinforce positive self-image

   b. Encourage to enjoy simple activities (e.g., walking, exercising,socializing)

   c. Keep environment simple, familiar, noise-free

   d. If client experiences catastrophic reaction (overreaction to excessive stimulation), remain calm and stay with client; provide distraction such as listening to music, rocking, or therapeutic touch to quiet client

4. Improve communication

   a. Reduce noise and distractions

   b. Use clear, easy-to-understand sentences

   c. Provide lists and simple written instructions

5. Promote independence in ADLs
    a. Organize daily activities into short, achievable steps
    b. Allow client to make choices when appropriate
    c. Encourage to participate in self-care activities
6. Provide for socialization
    a. Encourage letters, visits (one or two persons at a time), phone calls
    b. Provide a pet
7. Promote good nutrition
    a. Simple, calm environment
    b. Offer one dish at a time to prevent playing with food
    c. Cut food into small pieces to prevent choking
    d. Check temperature of foods to prevent burns
    e. Use adaptive equipment as needed for feeding self
    f. Provide apron or smock instead of bib to respect dignity
8. Promote balance of activity and rest
    a. Allow client to walk in protected environment
    b. Provide music, warm milk, back rub to encourage sleep
    c. Discourage long naps during the day
9. Provide teaching and support to caregivers
    a. Refer to Alzheimer's Association, family support groups, respite care, adult day care
10. Complementary/alternative therapy
    a. Ginkgo biloba
    b. Fish high in omega-3 fatty acids
    c. 1000 international units vitamin E twice daily
11. Administer medications—cholinesterase inhibitors; NMDA-receptor antagonists antidepressants

D. Evaluation
1. Has client's independence been maintained as much as possible?
2. Are caretakers knowledgeable about how to care for client at home?

▶ THYROID DISORDERS

A. Assessment (see Table 1)

B. Diagnose (see Table 1)

Table 1 THYROID DISORDERS		
	MYXEDEMA/HYPOTHYROIDISM	GRAVES' DISEASE/HYPERTHYROIDISM
Assessment	Diagnostic tests: ↓ BMR (basal metabolic rate) ↓ T3 ↓ T4 ↑ TSH Decreased activity level Sensitivity to cold Potential alteration in skin integrity Decreased perception of stimuli Obesity, weight gain Potential for respiratory difficulty Constipation Alopecia Bradycardia Dry skin and hair Decreased ability to perspire Reproductive problems	Diagnostic tests: ↑ BMR ↑ T3 ↑ T4 High titer anti-thyroid antibodies Hyperactivity Sensitivity to heat Rest and sleep deprivation Increased perception of stimuli Weight loss Potential for respiratory difficulty Diarrhea Tachycardia Exophthalmus Frequent mood swings Nervous, jittery Fine, soft hair
Analysis	Hyposecretion of thyroid hormone Slowed physical and mental functions	Hypersecretion of thyroid hormone Accelerated physical and mental functions
Predisposing factors	Inflammation of thyroid Iatrogenic—thyroidectomy, irradiation, overtreatment with antithyroids Pituitary deficiencies Iodine deficiency Idiopathic	Thyroid-secreting tumors Iatrogenic–overtreatment for hypothyroid Pituitary hyperactivity Severe stress, e.g., pregnancy
Treatment and management	Hormone replacement (levothyroxine sodium)	Antithyroid drugs (SSKI methimazole, propylthiouracil) Irradiation (^{131}I) Surgery
Potential nursing diagnosis	Disturbed body image Imbalanced nutrition: more than body requirements Activity intolerance Constipation Hypothermia Deficient knowledge Decreased cardiac output	Activity intolerance Altered body temperature Social interaction, impaired Imbalanced nutrition: less than body requirements Hyperthermia Fatigue Risk for impaired tissue integrity

C. Plan/Implementation

   1. Myxedema/hypothyroidism

     a. Pace activities

     b. Allow client extra time to think, speak, act

     c. Teaching should be done slowly and in simple terms

     d. Frequent rest periods between activities

     e. Maintain room temperature at approximately 75°F

     f. Provide client with extra clothing and bedding

     g. Restrict use of soaps and apply lanolin or creams to skin

     h. High-protein, low-calorie diet

     i. Small, frequent feedings

     j. Prevent constipation—high-fiber, high-cellulose foods

     k. Increase fluid intake

     l. Cathartics or stool softeners as ordered

     m. Explain to client that symptoms are reversible with treatment

     n. Explain to family that client's behavior is part of the condition andwill change when treatment begins

     o. Administer drug replacement therapy (e.g., levothyroxine;dose gradually increased and adjusted.)

     p. Administer sedatives carefully–risk of respiratory depression

     q. Instruct about causes of myxedema coma (acute illness, surgery, chemotherapy, discontinuation of medication)

   2. Graves' disease/hyperthyroidism

     a. Limit activities to quiet ones (e.g., reading, knitting)

     b. Provide for frequent rest periods

     c. Restrict visitors and control choice of roommates

     d. Keep room cool; advise light, cool clothing

     e. Avoid stimulants, (e.g., coffee)

     f. Accept behavior

     g. Use calm, unhurried manner when caring for client

     h. Interpret behavior to family

     i. Administer antithyroid medication, irradiation with ^{131}I PO (short-term)

     j. Provide post-thyroidectomy care

       1) Low or semi-Fowler's position

       2) Support head, neck, and shoulders to prevent flexion or hyperextension of suture line; elevate head of bed 30°

       3) Tracheostomy set and suction supplies at bedside

       4) Give fluids as tolerated

  5) Observe for complications
    a) Laryngeal nerve injury—detected by hoarseness
    b) Thyroidtoxicosis—increased temperature, increased pulse, hypertension, abdominal pain, diarrhea, confusion, agitation, seizures; treatment—hypothermia blanket, O$_2$, potassium iodine, propylthiouracil (PTU), propranolol, hydrocortisone, acetaminophen; also caused by trauma, infection, palpation, RAI therapy
    c) Hemorrhage; check back of neck and upper chest for bleeding
    d) Respiratory obstruction
    e) Tetany (decreased calcium from parathyroid involvement—check Chvostek's and Trousseau's signs
    f) Have IV calcium gluconate or IV calcium chloride available
  6) Analgesics, cold steam inhalations for sore throat
  7) Adjust diet to new metabolic needs
  k. Antithyroid medications—methimazole; propylthiouracil; potassium iodide (SSKI); radioactive iodine
D. Evaluation
  1. Is client knowledgeable about the dietary considerations?
  2. Have complications been prevented?

▶ PARATHYROID DISORDERS

A. Assessment (see Table 2)
B. Diagnose (see Table 2)
C. Plan/Implementation (see Table 2)
D. Evaluation
  1. Has client's mobility been maintained?
  2. Have complications been prevented?

Table 2 PARATHYROID DISORDERS ·		
	HYPOPARATHYROIDISM	HYPERPARATHYROIDISM

Assessment	Tetany
	
	Muscular irritability (cramps, spasms)
	
	Carpopedal spasm, clonic convulsions
	
	Dysphagia
	
	Paresthesia, laryngeal spasm
	
	Anxiety, depression, irritability
	
	Tachycardia
	
	    + Chvostek's sign
	
	    + Trousseau's sign
		Fatigue, muscle weakness
		
		Cardiac dysrhythmias
		
		Emotional irritability
		
		Renal calculi
		
		Back and joint pain, pathological fractures
		
		Pancreatitis, peptic ulcer

Diagnose	Decreased secretion of parathyroid hormone
	
	Introgenic–post thyroidectomy
	
	Hypomagnesemia
	
	Diagnostic tests:
	
	    Serum calcium ↓
	
	    Serum phosphorus ↑
	
	    ↓ parathyroid hormone (PTH)
	
	    X-ray–bones appear dense
		Oversecretion of parathyroid hormone
		
		Benign parathyroid tumor
		
		Parathyroid carcinoma
		
		Neck trauma
		
		Neck radiation
		
		Diagnostic tests:
		
		    ↑ Serum calcium
		
		    ↓ Serum phosphorus
		
		    X-ray–bones appear porous
		
		    ↑ serum parathyroid hormone

Potential nursing diagnosis	Risk for injury Deficient knowledge	Risk for injury Impaired urinary elimination Nutrition: less than body requirements Constipation
Plan/Implementation	Emergency treatment–calcium chloride or gluconate over 10–15 minutes Calcitriol 0.5–2 mg daily for acute hypocalcemia Ergocalciferol 50,000–400,000 units daily Observe for tetany Low-phosphorus, high-calcium diet	Relieve pain Prevent formation of renal calculi increase fluid intake Offer acid-ash juices (improves solubility of calcium) Administer appropriate diet Prevent fractures Safety precautions Monitor potassium levels (counteracts effect of calcium on cardiac muscles) Provide postparathyroidectomy care (essentially same as for thyroidectomy) IV Furosemide and saline promote calcium excretion IV phosphorus is used only for rapid lowering of calcium level Surgery–parathyroidectomy

▶ **NUTRITION**

A. Assessment

1. Physical signs (see Table 1)
2. Laboratory values: hemoglobin, hematocrit, serum albumin

Table 1 PHYSICAL SIGNS OF ADEQUATE NUTRITIONAL STATUS	
BODY AREA	NORMAL APPEARANCE
Hair	Shiny, firm, intact scalp without areas of pigmentation
Teeth	Evenly spaced, straight, no cavities, shiny
Tongue	Deep red in color
Gums	Firm, without redness, even-colored
Skin	Smooth, moist, even shading
Nails	Firm, without ridges
Extremities	Full range of motion
Abdomen	Flat, non-tender
Legs	Good color
Skeleton	No malformations
Weight	Normal for height
Posture	Erect
Muscles	Firm
GI	Good appetite and digestion
Vitality	Good endurance, good sleep patterns

3. Health history
   a. Chronic diseases—dietary alteration may be necessary because of disease entity, e.g., low-sodium diet for heart disease
   b. Therapies—treatment modalities may alter food intake, e.g., adverse effects of chemotherapy and radiation therapy, such as nausea and vomiting, may cause a decrease in intake
   c. Surgeries—some surgeries may alter actual intake, e.g., head and neck surgery, and/or absorption concurrent with digestion, e.g., GI surgery
   d. Usual eating habits (takes 1–2 weeks for malnutrition to develop)
   e. Recent changes in appetite or food history
   f. Level of growth and development (increased needs)

B. Diagnose

1. Caloric requirement—a calorie is a measurement unit of energy; person's height and weight, as well as level of activity, determine energy need; average adult requires anywhere from 1,500 kcal to 3,000 kcal a day

2. Fluid requirement—average fluid requirement for normal healthy adult is approximately 1,800–2,500 ml/day

3. Nutrient requirements

   a. Carbohydrates—first substance used for energy production in starvation; only source of energy production for the brain

   b. Fats—second source of energy production used by the body in starvation; waste products are ketone bodies, which can create an acidic environment in the blood

   c. Proteins—last energy source used in starvation; depletion of protein leads to muscle wasting as well as loss of oncotic pressure in the vascular space; low albumin level in the blood indicates protein malnutrition

   d. Vitamins—organic substances found in foods; essential in small quantities for growth and for transformation of food substances into tissue

      1) Fat-soluble vitamins (see Table 2)

      2) Water-soluble vitamins (see Table 3)

      3) Minerals (see Table 4)

Table 2 FAT-SOLUBLE VITAMINS			
VITAMINS	FUNCTION(S)	PRIMARY SOURCE(S)	CLINICAL MANIFESTATION(S)
A	Visual acuity Adaptation to light and dark	Beta-carotene Liver Egg yolk Cream, milk, margarine Yellow fruits, and orange and green leafy vegetables (carrots, squash, peaches) Butter, cheese	D: Night blindness, skin infection, xerophthalmia, corneal ulceration T: CNS changes (lethargy, headache) GI (portal hypertension)
D	Calcification of bones Absorption of Ca, phosphorus	Fish oils Fortified milk/dairy products, egg yolks Sunlight's irradiation of body cholesterol	D: Rickets, poor bone growth T: Hypercalcemia, renal calculi
E	Antioxidant Growth	Green leaf vegetables Fats, oils Liver Grains, nuts	D: Breakdown of red blood cells Hemolytic anemia T: Fatigue, headache, blurred vision, diarrhea
K	Blood clotting	Leafy vegetables Eggs, cheese Synthesized by intestinal bacteria	D: Bleeding, bruises T: Anemia, liver/renal damage, and intestinal bacterial infection
D: DEFICIENCY T: TOXICITY			

Table 3 WATER-SOLUBLE VITAMINS			
VITAMINS	**FUNCTION(S)**	**PRIMARY SOURCES**	**CLINICAL MANIFESTATION(S)**
Thiamine (B_1)	Normal growth Carbohydrate metabolism	Legumes, meat Enriched grains Eggs, fish	D: Beriberi (numbness, decreased reflexes fatigue) Wernicke-Korsakoff syndrome T: Shock
Riboflavin (B_2)	Coenzyme in protein and energy metabolism	Milk Liver (organ meats)	D: Ariboflavinosis Tissue inflammation
Niacin (nicotinic acid)	Normal growth	Meat Grains	D: Pellagra (rough, scaly skin, glossitis, decreased weight) T: Vasodilation, flushing
Pyridoxine (B_6)	Amino acid metabolism	Corn and soy Meat and liver Yeast, egg yolk, sunflowers	D: Anemia, CNS changes (seizures) Peripheral neuropathy T: Diminished proprioceptive sensory function
Folic acid	RBC formation	Liver Oranges Broccoli	D: Anemia T: Diminished proprioceptive and sensory function
Cyanocobalamin (B_{12})	Nerve function RBC formation	Meat Milk, eggs	D: Pernicious anemia
Ascorbic acid (C)	Collagen synthesis	Fruits, esp. citrus Vegetables Tomatoes	D: Scurvy (joint pain and weakness) Anemia (in infants) T: Oxalate hypersensitivity
D: DEFICIENCY T: TOXICITY			

Table 4 MINERALS			
MINERAL	**PRIMARY FUNCTION(S)**	**PRIMARY SOURCE(S)**	**DEFICIENCY SYMPTOM(S)**
Calcium	Bone formation Muscle contraction Thrombus formation	Milk products Green leafy vegetables Eggs	Rickets Porous bones Tetany
Phosphorus	Bone formation Cell permeability	Milk, eggs Nuts	Rickets
Fluoride	Dental health	Water supply	Dental caries
Iodine	Thyroid hormone synthesis	Seafood Iodized salt	Goiter
Sodium	Osmotic pressure Acid-base balance Nerve irritability	Table salt Canned vegetables Milk, cured meats Processed foods	Fluid and electrolyte imbalance

Table 4 MINERALS *(CONTINUED)*			
MINERAL	PRIMARY FUNCTION(S)	PRIMARY SOURCE(S)	DEFICIENCY SYMPTOM(S)
Potassium	Water balance in cells Protein synthesis Heart contractility	Grains, meats Vegetables	Arrhythmias Fluid and electrolyte imbalance
Iron	Hemoglobin synthesis	Liver, oysters Leafy vegetables Apricots	Anemia Lethargy

Table 5 FOOD GUIDELINES		
GROUP	FOOD EXAMPLES	RECOMMENDED DAILY INTAKE
Grains	Bread, cereals, cooked cereals, popcorn, pasta, rice, tortillas Half of all grains should be whole grains	Children—3–5 ounce equivalents Teens—5–7 ounce equivalents Young adults—6–8 ounce equivalents Adults—6–7 ounce equivalents Older adults—5–6 ounce equivalents
Vegetables	Dark green vegetables (broccoli, spinach, greens, leafy vegetables), orange vegetables (carrots, pumpkin, sweet potatoes), dried beans and peas (split peas, pinto, kidney, black, soy [tofu]), starchy vegetables (corn, peas, white potatoes)	Children—1–1½ cups Teens—2–3 cups Young adults—2½–3 cups Adults—2½–3 cups Older adults—2–2½ cups
Fruits	Apple, bananas, strawberries, blueberries, orange, melons, dried fruits, fruit juices	Children—1–1½ cups Teens—1½–2 cups Young adults—2 cups Adults—1½–2 cups Older adults—1½–2 cups
Oils	Nuts, butter, margarine, cooking oils, salad dressings	Children—3–4 teaspoons Teens—5–6 teaspoons Young adults—6–7 teaspoons Adults—5–6 teaspoons Older adults—5–6 teaspoons
Milk	Milk, yogurt, cheese, puddings	Children—2 cups Teens—3 cups Young adults—3 cups Adults—3 cups Older adults—3 cups
Meat and beans	Meat, poultry, fish, dry beans, eggs, peanut butter, nuts, seeds	Children—2–4 ounce equivalents Teens—5–6 ounce equivalents Young adults—5½–6½ ounce equivalents Adults—5–6 ounce equivalents Older adults—5–5½ ounce equivalents

C. Plan/Implementation

1. General diet—eat a variety of foods (see Table 5)

2. Vegetarian diet

   a. Types

      1) Vegan diet includes fruits, vegetables, nuts, beans, and seeds; excludes all sources of animal protein, fortified foods, and nutritional supplements of animal origin; risk of vitamin B_{12} deficiency

      2) Lacto-vegetarian diet includes all foods on a vegan diet, along with milk, cheese, yogurt, and other milk products as the only source of animal protein; avoids meat, fish, poultry and eggs

      3) Ovo-vegetarian diet includes all foods on a vegan diet, along with eggs as the only source of animal protein

      4) Lacto–ovo-vegetarian diet includes all foods on a vegan diet, along with milk, cheese, yogurt, other milk products, and eggs as only sources of animal protein

      5) "Red-meat abstainers" consider themselves vegetarians and eat animal products with the exception of red meat

   b. Analysis

      1) Become vegetarians due to religion (Seventh Day Adventists), ecology, economic reasons, health reasons

      2) Risk deficiency of vitamin B_{12} associated with megaloblastic anemia; vitamin B_{12} is found only in animal products

      3) Risk toxic levels of vitamin A causing anorexia, irritability, dry skin, hair loss

   c. Plan/Implementation

      1) Increase intake of legumes, beans, nuts, seeds, tofu, dark green leafy vegetable

      2) Eat fortified cereals, soy beverages, and meat analogs

      3) Must eat adequate amounts of protein, calcium, zinc, vitamin D, and vitamin B_{12}

      4) During pregnancy should take supplements to meet increased nutritional needs

      5) Children may experience mild anemia due to the poor availability of iron from grains and legumes; should include source of vitamin C with meals; diet should include nonmeat animal proteins such as milk, cheese, and eggs; vegan diet is unable to sustain growth needs of children

      6) Vegetarian diet often causes weight loss due to elimination of meat which is a major source of fat; fat has twice the number of kilocalories per gram than carbohydrates or proteins

3. Choose My Plate—recommendations by the U.S. Department of Agriculture; includes diet choices for vegetarians and members of ethnic/cultural groups (see Figure 1)

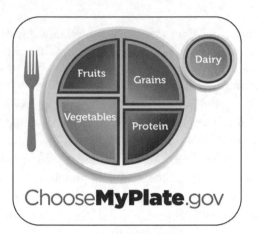

Figure 1   ChooseMyPlate.gov

4. Common therapeutic diets (see Table 6)
5. Complementary/Alternative therapies
   a. General guidelines for herbal and dietary supplements
      1) Supplements do not compensate for an inadequate diet
      2) Recommended daily amounts (RDA) should not be exceeded due to the potential for toxicity
      3) Multivitamin-mineral products recommended for certain age or gender groups contain different amounts of some minerals
      4) Iron supplements beyond those contained in multivitamin-mineral combinations are intended for short-term or special-need (e.g., pregnancy) use and should not be taken for longer periods of time because of potential for toxicity
      5) Most adolescent and adult females should consume calcium 1,000 to 1,300 mg daily
      6) Supplementing with selenium as an antioxidant and zinc to prevent colds and promote wound healing is not proven
6. Herbals used to lower cholesterol:
   a. Flax or flaxseed
      1) Decreases the absorption of other medications
      2) Nausea, vomiting, increased flatulence
      3) May decrease absorption of other medications
   b. Garlic
      1) Increases the effects of anticoagulants and antiplatelets
      2) Increases the hypoglycemic effects of insulin
      3) May stimulate labor

    c. Green tea

        1) Produces a stimulant effect when the tea contains caffeine

        2) Multiple drug interactions—anticoagulants, antiplatelets, beta blockers

    d. Soy

        1) Multiple drug interactions—estrogens, tamoxifen

D. Evaluation

    1. Have client's nutritional needs been met?

    2. Have any nutritional deficiencies been corrected?

Table 6 COMMON THERAPEUTIC DIETS		
CLEAR LIQUID DIET	**FULL LIQUID DIET**	**LOW–FAT, CHOLESTEROL–RESTRICTED DIET**
Sample meal items: Gelatin dessert, popsicle, tea with lemon, ginger ale, bouillon, fruit juice without pulp	Sample meal items: Milkshakes, soups, custard; all clear liquids	Sample meal items: Fruit, vegetables, cereals, lean meat
Common medical diagnoses: Postoperative; acute vomiting or diarrhea	Common medical diagnoses: GI upset (diet progression after surgery)	Common medical diagnoses: Atherosclerosis, cystic fibrosis (CF)
Purpose: To maintain fluid balance	Purpose: Nutrition without chewing	Purpose: To reduce calories from fat and minimize cholesterol intake
Not allowed: Fruit juices with pulp, milk	Not allowed: Jam, fruit, solid foods, nuts	Not allowed: Marbled meats, avocados, milk, bacon, egg yolks, butter
SODIUM-RESTRICTED DIET	**HIGH-ROUGHAGE, HIGH-FIBER DIET**	**LOW-RESIDUE DIET**
Sample meal items: Cold baked chicken, lettuce with sliced tomatoes, applesauce	Sample meal items: Cracked wheat bread, minestrone soup, apple, brussel sprouts	Sample meal items: Roast lamb, buttered rice, sponge cake, "white" processed foods
Common medical diagnoses: Heart failure, hypertension, cirrhosis	Common medical diagnoses: Constipation, large bowel disorders	Common medical diagnoses: Temporary GI/elimination problems (e.g., lower bowel surgery)
Purpose: To lower body water and promote excretion	Purpose: To maximize bulk in stools	Purpose: To minimize intestinal activity
Not allowed: Preserved meats, cheese, fried foods, cottage cheese, canned foods, added salt	Not allowed: White bread, pies and cakes from white flour, "white" processed foods	Not allowed: Whole wheat, corn, bran

Table 6 COMMON THERAPEUTIC DIETS *(CONTINUED)*		
HIGH–PROTEIN DIET	**KIDNEY DIET**	**LOW PHENYLALANINE DIET**
Sample meal items: 30 grams powdered skim milk and 1 egg in 100 ml water *or* Roast beef sandwich and skim milk	Sample meal items: Unsalted vegetables, white rice, canned fruits, sweets	Sample meal items: Fats, fruits, jams, low-phenylalanine milk
Common medical diagnoses: Burns, infection, hyperthyroidism	Common medical diagnoses: Chronic/Acute renal failure	Common medical diagnoses: Phenylketonuria (PKU)
Purpose: To re-establish anabolism to raise albumin levels	Purpose: To keep protein, potassium, and sodium low	Purpose: Low-protein diet to prevent brain damage from imbalance of amino acids
Not allowed: Soft drinks, "junk" food	Not allowed: Beans, cereals, citrus fruits	Not allowed: Meat, eggs, beans, bread

▶ **CULTURAL FOOD PATTERNS**

Not all members of a culture choose to follow all dietary traditions.

A. Orthodox Jewish

1. Dietary laws based on Biblical and rabbinical regulations

2. Laws pertain to selection, preparation, and service of food

3. Laws

   a. Milk/milk products never eaten at same meal as meat (milk may not be taken until 6 hours after eating meat)

   b. Two meals contain dairy products and one meal contains meat

   c. Separate utensils are used for meat and milk dishes

   d. Meat must be kosher (drained of blood)

   e. Prohibited foods

      1) Pork

      2) Diseased animals or animals who die a natural death

      3) Birds of prey

      4) Fish without fins or scales (shellfish—oysters, crab, lobster)

B. Muslim

1. Dietary laws based on Islamic teachings in Koran

2. Laws

   a. Fermented fruits and vegetables prohibited

   b. Pork prohibited

   c. Alcohol prohibited

    d. Foods with special value: figs, olives, dates, honey, milk, buttermilk

    e. Meat must be Halal (drained of blood)

    f. Follow humane process of slaughter of animals for meat

  3. 30-day period of daylight fasting required during Ramadan

C. Hispanic

  1. Basic foods: dried beans, chili peppers, corn

  2. Use small amounts of meat and eggs

  3. Saturated fat use in food preparation common

D. Puerto Rican

  1. Main type of food is viandos—starchy vegetables and fruits (plantain and green bananas)

  2. Diet includes large amounts of rice and beans

  3. Coffee main beverage

E. Native American

  1. Food has religious and social significance

  2. Diet includes meat, bread (tortillas, blue corn bread), eggs, vegetables (corn, potatoes, green beans, tomatoes), fruit

  3. Frying common method of food preparation

F. African American

  1. Minimal use of milk in diet

  2. Frequent use of leafy greens (turnips, collards, and mustard)

  3. Pork, fat, cholesterol, and sodium common in diet

G. French American

  1. Foods are strong-flavored and spicy

  2. Frequently contains seafood (crawfish)

  3. Food preparation starts with a roux made from heated oil and flour, vegetables and seafood added

H. Chinese

  1. Uses freshest food available; cooked at a high temperature in a wok using a small amount of fat and liquid

  2. Meat used in small amounts

  3. Eggs and soybean products used for protein

I. Japanese

  1. Rice is basic food

  2. Soy sauce is used for seasoning

  3. Tea is main beverage

  4. Seafood frequently used (sometimes raw fish—sushi)

J. Southeast Asian

  1. Rice is basic food, eaten in separate rice bowl

  2. Soups frequently used

  3. Fresh fruits and vegetables frequently part of diet

  4. Stir-frying in wok is common method of food preparation

K. Italian

1. Bread and pasta are basic foods

2. Cheese frequently used in cooking

3. Food seasoned with spices, wine, garlic, herbs, olive oil

L. Greek

1. Bread is served with every meal

2. Cheese (feta) frequently used for cooking

3. Lamb and fish frequently used

4. Eggs used in main dish, but not breakfast food

5. Fruit used for dessert

▶ PREMATURE INFANTS

A. Assessment

1. Body composition—premature infant has more water, less protein and fat per pound than full-term infant

2. Poor temperature control due to little subcutaneous fat

3. Bones are poorly calcified

4. Sucking reflexes are poor

5. Gastrointestinal and renal function are poor

6. Prone to infection

7. Immature development of lungs

B. Diagnose

1. Less than 2,500 g and less than 37 weeks gestation

2. Nutritional requirements

   a. 100–200 cal/kg/day

   b. Higher sodium, calcium, and protein requirements than full-term infant

C. Plan/Implementation

1. Feeding

   a. Parenteral nutrition—usually required until oral feedings can be established

   b. Gavage feedings—usually given because of poor sucking coordination

   c. Soft (preemie) nipples are usually effective for very small infants

2. Supplements

   a. Vitamins A, C, D, and iron are usually given orally

   b. Occasionally, vitamin E is needed to prevent oxidation of RBCs

   c. Long-chain fats are not well tolerated; medium-chain triglycerides (MCTs) are often used

   d. Glucose is often substituted for lactose in premature formulas because of its passive absorption in GI tract

   e. Vitamin K prophylaxis to prevent clotting problems

D. Evaluation

    1. Has infant gained weight?

    2. Have complications been prevented?

▶ FULL-TERM INFANTS

A. Assessment

    1. Energy requirements are high; 120 cal/kg/day

    2. Rooting and sucking reflexes are well developed

    3. Six to eight wet diapers per day and at least 1 stool daily

B. Diagnose

    1. Weighs more than 2,500 g and greater than 37 weeks gestation

C. Plan/Implementation

    1. Breastfeeding

        a. Human milk is ideal food; recommended for first 6 to 12 months of life

        b. Colostrum is secreted at first

            1) Clear and colorless

            2) Contains protective antibodies

            3) High in protein and minerals

        c. Milk is secreted after day 2 to 4

            1) Milky white appearance

            2) Contains more fat and lactose than colostrum

    2. Formula feeding

        a. Formula is cow's milk modified to resemble human milk more closely; avoid cow's milk first year (deficient in vitamins and iron)

            1) Diluted to reduce protein content

            2) Sugar is added to increase carbohydrate content

            3) Home preparation from evaporated milk is most economical

            4) Formula is necessary for first 12 months of life; then, unmodified cow's milk is acceptable

            5) If problems with diarrhea, change formula to prevent profound dehydration

        b. Feeding technique

            1) Child should be cradled when fed

            2) Child should be regulator of milk volume

    3. Introduction to solid foods (see Table 7)

        a. Introduce only one at a time for each two–week period

        b. Least allergenic foods are given in first half of the first year; more allergenic foods (e.g., egg, orange juice) are offered in last half of first year; usual order: cereal, fruit, vegetables, potatoes, meat, egg, orange juice

        c. No honey should be given during first year due to high risk of botulism

Table 7 INTRODUCTION TO SOLID FOODS	
AGE	FOOD
1–4 months	Liquid vitamins only—A, D, C, fluoride (if indicated)
4–5 months	Cereal—usually rice is first; strained fruit
5–6 months	Strained vegetables; strained meat
7–9 months	Chopped meat; hard breads and "finger foods"; potato baked, mashed

▶ TODDLERS

A. Assessment

    1. Six to eight teeth have erupted

    2. Begins to use large muscles and bones

B. Diagnose

    1. 12 to 36 months

C. Plan/Implementation

    1. Allow choice of foods from food pyramid to prevent struggle over eating; may prefer one type of food over another

    2. Needs fewer calories in diet but more protein and calcium than infant

    3. Give 32 ounces or less of formula to decrease risk iron-deficiency anemia

D. Evaluation

    1. Have toddler's nutritional needs been met?

▶ PRESCHOOLER AND SCHOOL-AGE

A. Assessment

    1. Growth rate slows

    2. Protein and calcium needs remain high

B. Diagnose

    1. Growth rate is gradual until adolescence; then spurts occur

C. Plan/Implementation

    1. Nutritional intake (see Table 8)

Table 8 NUTRIENT INTAKE FOR CHILDREN	
FOOD	**SERVINGS**
Fruits and vegetables	4–8
Vitamin C type	1–2
Vitamin A type	1–2
Fruit type	1–2
Other vegetables	1–2
Cereals (bread, etc.)	4
Fats and carbohydrates	To meet caloric needs
Meats (proteins, peanuts, eggs)	3
Milk (cheese, yogurt)	2–3

D. Evaluation

    1. Have the nutritional needs of the school-age child been maintained?

▶ ADOLESCENT NUTRITION

A. Assessment

    1. Rapid growth spurts occur

    2. Acne develops

B. Diagnose

    1. Caloric, calcium, and protein needs are high

    2. Females experience menstrual losses of iron; require increased intake

    3. Mineral and vitamin needs are high because of rapid tissue growth

C. Plan/Implementation

    1. High-calorie, high-protein diet

    2. High intake of iron for menstruating adolescents

    3. High minerals and vitamins in diet

D. Evaluation

    1. Have adolescent's nutritional needs been met?

▶ ADULT AND ELDERLY POPULATION

A. Assessment

    1. Balanced diet continues to be important

    2. Calorie limitation with decreasing physical activity

    3. Declining ability to chew and changing taste perception can cause impaired nutrition in the elderly

B. Diagnose

    1. With increased age, reduction in calories needed, improved food quality

    2. Need same level of minerals and vitamins as in early adulthood

C. Plan/Implementation
   1. Goal is to decrease calories but to ensure food consumed is high in minerals and vitamins
   2. Prevent osteoporosis in postmenopausal women
   3. Complementary/Alternative Therapy
      a. To reduce all-cause mortality, older adults should consume oral protein and energy supplements
D. Evaluation
   1. Have the nutritional needs of the elderly been met?
   2. Has weight gain been controlled?

▶ NUTRITION DURING PREGNANCY AND LACTATION

A. Assessment
   1. Pre-pregnancy weight
   2. Maternal age
   3. Labs: hemoglobin and hematocrit
   4. Pre-existing health problems
B. Diagnose
   1. Age and parity of mother varies
   2. Preconception nutrition influences overall requirements
   3. Individual needs vary; recommended weight gain is 24–28 pounds
   4. Folic acid needed to prevent neural tube defects and megaloblastic and macrocytic anemia
C. Plan/Implementation
   1. Diet plan for pregnancy and lactation (see Table 9)
   2. High-risk pregnancies
      a. Adolescence
         1) Must meet own nutritional requirements (high protein and calcium)
         2) Tendency to deliver low-birthweight babies

Table 9 DIET PLAN FOR PREGNANCY AND LACTATION		
FOOD	PREGNANCY	LACTATION
Protein (meat, 1 egg, cheese)	3 servings	4 servings
Vegetable—yellow or green (includes vitamin C foods)	5 servings	5–6 servings
Bread and cereal (whole grain or enriched)	5 servings	5 servings
Milk products (cheese, ice cream, milk, cottage cheese)	4 cups	5 cups
Calories over maintenance	+300/day	+500/day
Folic acid	400 mcg	280 mcg

    b. Diabetes

        1) Glucose levels must be monitored closely

        2) Prevent postmature deliveries

        3) C-section may be necessary because mother may not be able to handle the glucose requirements of labor

    c. Sickle cell—stress of labor and pregnancy must be considered in relation to oxygenation capabilities of these mothers; C-section is usually indicated

    d. Cardiac—myocardial stress specifically related to delivery may require decreased activity, as well as C-section, to decrease demand on heart

D. Evaluation

    1. Have the nutritional needs of the pregnant woman been met?

    2. Have the nutritional needs of the lactating woman been met?

▶ ENTERAL NUTRITION

A. Alternative feeding (required because of inability to use gastrointestinal route)

B. Liquid food delivered to the stomach, distal duodenum, or proximal jejunum via a nasogastric, percutaneous endoscopic gastrostomy (PEG), or percutaneous endoscopic jejunostomy (PEJ) tube

C. Conditions requiring enteral feeding (see Table 10)

Table 10 CONDITIONS REQUIRING ENTERAL FEEDING	
CONDITION	**CAUSE**
Preoperative need for nutritional support	Inadequate intake preoperatively, resulting in poor nutritional state
Gastrointestinal problems	Fistula, short-bowel syndrome, Crohn's disease, ulcerative colitis, nonspecific maldigestion or malabsorption
Adverse effects of oncology therapy	Radiation, chemotherapy
Alcoholism, chronic depression, eating disorders	Chronic illness, psychiatric, or neurological disorder
Head and neck disorders or surgery	Disease or trauma

D. Complications of enteral feeding (see Table 11)

Table 11 COMPLICATIONS OF ENTERAL FEEDINGS	
COMPLICATION	NURSING CONSIDERATIONS
Mechanical Tube displacement	Replace tube
Aspiration	Elevate head of bed, check residual before feeding
Gastrointestinal Cramping, vomiting, diarrhea	Decrease feeding rate Change formula to more isotonic Administer at room temperature
Metabolic Hyperglycemia	Monitor glucose, serum osmolality Monitor glucose, give insulin if needed Reduce infusion rate
Dehydration	Flush tube with water according to hospital policy
Formula–drug interactions	Check compatibility Flush tubing prior to and after medication

▶ PARENTERAL NUTRITION

A. Assessment

    1. Conditions requiring enteral feeding (see Table 10)

B. Diagnose

    1. Method of supplying nutrients to the body by the intravenous route (see Figure 2)

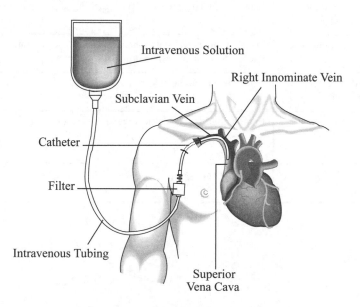

Figure 2 Parenteral Nutrition (PN)

2. Types of solutions

    a. PN—amino acid-dextrose formulas; 2–3 liters of solution given over 24 h; 500 ml of 10% fat emulsions (Intralipid) given with PN over 6 h 1–3 times/week; fine bacterial filter used

    b. TNA (Total Nutrient Admixture)—amino acid-dextrose-lipid, "3-in-1" formula; 1-liter solution given over 24 h; no bacterial filter used

    c. Lipids—provides fatty acids

3. Methods of administration

    a. Peripheral—used to supplement oral intake; should not administer dextrose concentrations above 10% due to irritation of vessel walls; usually used for less than 2 weeks

    b. Central—catheter inserted into subclavian vein

        1) Peripherally inserted catheters (PICC)—catheter threaded through central vein; dextrose solution ≥10% basilic or cephalic vein to superior vena cava; usually ≤4 weeks

        2) Percutaneous central catheters through subclavian vein

        3) Triple lumen central catheter often used; distal lumen (16-gauge) used to infuse or draw blood samples, middle lumen (18-gauge) used for PN infusion, proximal lumen (18-gauge) used to infuse or draw blood and administer medications

        4) If single lumen catheter used, cannot use to administer medications (may be incompatible) or give blood (RBCs coat catheter lumen); medications and blood must be given through peripheral IV line, not piggyback to the PN IV line

    c. Atrial

        1) Right atrial catheters—Hickman/Biovac and Groshong

        2) Subcutaneous port—Huber needle used to access port through skin

C. Plan/Implementation

1. Initial rate of infusion 50 ml/h and gradually increased (100–125 ml/h) as client's fluid and electrolyte tolerance permits

2. Infuse solution by pump at constant rate to prevent abrupt change in infusion rate

    a. Increased rate results in hyperosmolar state (headache, nausea, fever, chills, malaise)

    b. Slowed rate results in "rebound" hypoglycemia caused by delayed pancreatic reaction to change in insulin requirements; do not discontinue suddenly

3. Client must be carefully monitored for signs of complications; infection and hyperglycemia are common (see Table 12)

° Table 12 COMPLICATIONS OF PN	
COMPLICATION	NURSING CONSIDERATIONS
Infection/Sepsis	Maintain closed intravenous systems with filter No blood drawn or medications given through PN line Dry sterile occlusive dressing applied to site
Pneumothorax because of line placement	PN to be started only after chest x-ray validates correct placement Monitor breath sounds and for presence of shortness of breath
Hyperglycemia Hyperosmolar coma	Monitor glucose level and serum osmolality Administer insulin according to sliding scale insulin
Hypoglycemia	Hang 10% dextrose solution if PN discontinued suddenly
Fluid overload	Monitor breath sounds, weight and peripheral perfusion Do not "catch up" if PN behind
Air embolism	Monitor for respiratory distress Valsalva maneuver during tubing and cap change

4. Change IV tubing and filter every 24 hours

5. Keep solutions refrigerated until needed; allow to warm to room temperature before use

6. If new solution unavailable, use 10% dextrose and water solution until available

7. Monitor daily weight, glucose, temperatures, intake and output; three times a week check BUN, electrolytes (calcium, magnesium); check CBC, platelets, prothrombin time, liver function studies (AST, ALT), prealbumin, serum albumin once a week

8. Do not increase flow rate if PN behind scheduled administration time

9. Discontinuation

   a. Gradually tapered to allow client to adjust to decreased levels of glucose

   b. After discontinued, isotonic glucose solution administered to prevent rebound hypoglycemia (weakness, faintness, diaphoresis, shakiness, confusion, tachycardia)

D. Evaluation

   1. Is the client receiving PN free from infection?

   2. Is the client receiving PN well hydrated?

▶ **URINARY ELIMINATION**

A. Assessment

    1. Characteristics of urine

        a. Color—yellow

        b. Consistency—clear, transparent

        c. Specific gravity—1.010–1.030

        d. pH—4.5–8.0

        e. 24-hour production—1,000–2,000 mL (approximately 1 mL/Kg/hr)

    2. Serum changes

        a. BUN (normal 10–20 mg/dL) (3.6–7.1 mmol/L)

        b. Creatinine (normal 0.7–1.4 mg/dL)(62–124 µmol/L)

B. Diagnose

    1. Potential nursing diagnoses

        a. Impaired urinary elimination

        b. Readiness for enhanced urinary elimination

        c. Fluid volume deficit

        d. Urinary retention

        e. Urinary incontinence

    2. Definitions

        a. Anuria—total urinary output less than 100 mL/24 hours

        b. Oliguria—total urinary output 100–400 mL/24 hours

        c. Polyuria—total urinary output greater than 2000 mL/24 hours

        d. Dysuria—painful or difficult voiding

    3. Predisposing factors

        a. Bedrest

        b. Tumors

        c. Prostatic hypertrophy, anticholinergic medications

        d. Decreased bladder tone—previous use of indwelling catheter, childbirth

        e. Cancer

        f. Neurogenic—CVA, spinal injuries

        g. Calculi

        h. Stress

        i. Urinary tract infection

C. Plan/Implementation

    1. Hydration—adequate intake 1,500–2,000 mL/day

    2. Voiding habits

        a. Know client's pattern

        b. Provide time and privacy

3. Teach Kegel exercises—strengthen muscles of pelvic floor; tighten pelvic muscles for count of 3, then relax for count of 3; perform lying down, sitting and standing for total of 45

4. Teach bladder retraining

   a. Triggering techniques—stroking medial aspect of thigh, pinching area above groin, pulling pubic hair, providing digital anal stimulation (used with upper motor neuron problem); Valsava and Credé maneuvers (used with lower motor neuron problem)

   b. Intermittent catheterization every 2–3 hours after attempting to void and Valsalva or Credé maneuver; if volume is less than 150 mL, time interval is increased to 3–4 hours, then 4–6 hours; never more than 8 hours

   c. Toileting schedule—first thing in a.m., before and after meals, before and after physical activity, bedtime

   d. Bladder training—drink a measured amount of fluid every 2 hours, then attempt to void 30 minutes later; time between voiding should be gradually increased

5. Catheterization

6. Respond immediately to call

7. Avoid diuretics such as caffeine

8. Encourage fluid intake to 2,000 mL

9. Clamp indwelling catheters intermittently before removal

10. Toilet training

    a. Never begin before 18th month of life

    b. 2–3 years: bladder reflex control achieved

    c. 3 years: regular voiding habits established

    d. 4 years: independent bathroom activity

    e. 5 years: nighttime control expected

11. Enuresis—bed-wetting in a child at least 5 years old

    a. Usually have small bladder capacity

    b. More common in males

    c. Tend to be deep sleepers

D. Evaluation

1. Is client's voiding pattern adequate?

2. Has toilet training been successfully completed?

▶ BOWEL ELIMINATION

A. Assessment

1. Abdomen nontender and symmetrical

2. High-pitched gurgles indicate normal peristalsis

3. Stool light to dark brown in color

4. Negative guaiac for occult blood

5. Negative for fat, mucus, pus, pathogens

B. Diagnose—potential nursing diagnoses

   1. Bowel incontinence

   2. Constipation

   3. Perceived constipation

   4. Risk for constipation

   5. Diarrhea

C. Plan/Implementation

   1. Promote normal elimination

     a. Teach client to respond to urge to defecate

     b. Provide facilities, privacy, and allow sufficient time

     c. Fluids—encourage adequate intake; 8 or more glasses of fluid daily; hot liquids and fruit juices

     d. Foods—encourage fiber, fruits, vegetables, grains

     e. Activity—encourage exercise and ambulation to maintain muscle tone

     f. Emotional state—teach client that stress affects autonomic nervous system, which controls peristalsis

     g. Positioning

       1) For ambulatory client—teach that optimal posture is with feet flat on floor, hips and knees flexed

       2) For bedrest client—place in Fowler's position on bedpan

D. Evaluation

   1. Has the client maintained a normal pattern of bowel elimination?

   2. Is client's diet adequate to promote normal bowel elimination?

▶ CONGENITAL MALFORMATIONS OF THE URINARY TRACT

A. Assessment (see Table 1)

B. Diagnose (see Table 1)

C. Plan/Implementation (see Table 1)

Table 1 CONGENITAL MALFORMATIONS OF THE URINARY TRACT		
ASSESSMENT	ANALYSIS	NURSING CONSIDERATIONS
Epispadias	Urethral opening on dorsal surface of the penis	Surgical correction No circumcision—foreskin used in surgical repair
Hypospadias	Male urethral opening on the ventral surface of penis, or female urethral opening in vagina	Surgical reconstruction No circumcision—foreskin used in surgical repair
Bladder exstrophy	Posterior and lateral surfaces of the bladder are exposed	Reconstructive surgery to close bladder and abdominal wall

D. Evaluation

   1. Have parents adjusted to the altered body image of their infant?

   2. Has reconstructive surgery been successful?

▶ KIDNEY AND URETERAL CALCULI (UROLITHIASIS)

A. Assessment

1. Pain (renal colic)—depends on location of stone (flank pain with renal calculi, radiating flank pain with ureter or bladder stones); pain often severe

2. Diaphoresis

3. Nausea and vomiting

4. Fever and chills

5. Hematuria, WBCS and bacteria in urine

B. Diagnose

1. Nephrolithiasis—kidney stones; ureterolithiasis—stones in ureter

2. Causes

   a. Obstruction and urinary stasis

   b. Hypercalcemia, dehydration, immobility, gout, increased intake of oxalates (spinach, Swiss chard, wheat germ, peanuts)

3. Diagnostic tests—intravenous pyelogram, renal ultrasound, CT scan, cystoscopy, MRI, x-ray of kidneys, ureter and bladder (KUB)

C. Plan/Implementation

1. Monitor I and O and temperature

2. Avoid overhydration or underhydration to decrease pain when passing stone

3. Strain urine and check pH of urine

4. Monitor temperature

5. Analgesics

6. Diet for prevention of stones—most stones contain calcium, phosphorus, and/or oxalate

   a. Low in calcium if stones are due to excessive dietary calcium—avoid milk, cheeses, dairy products

   b. Low in sodium—sodium increases calcium in urine

   c. Low in oxalates to prevent increased calcium absorption (avoid: spinach, cola, tea, chocolate)

   d. Avoid vitamin D-enriched foods (increases calcium absorption)

   e. Decrease purine sources—organ meats

   f. To make urine alkaline, restrict citrus fruits, milk, potatoes

   g. To acidify urine increase consumption of eggs, fish, cranberries

7. Drug therapy

   a. Antibiotics (broad spectrum)

   b. Thiazide diuretics, orthophosphate, sodium cellulose phosphase—decrease calcium reabsorption

   c. Allopurinol and vitamin B6 (pyridoxine)—decrease oxalic acid levels

   d. Allopurinol—decrease uric acid levels

8. Surgery (see Table 2)

Table 2	COMMON SURGERIES OF THE URINARY TRACT	
NAME	PROCEDURE	NURSING CONSIDERATIONS
Stenting	Stent placed in ureter during ureteroscopy	Indwelling catheter may be placed
Retrograde ureteroscopy	Ureteroscope used to remove stone	Indwelling catheter may be placed
Percutaneous ureterolithotomy or nephrolithotomy	Lithotripter inserted through skin	Ureterostomy tube may be left in place
Nephrolithotomy	Incision into kidney to remove stones	Ureteral catheter Incisional drain Don't irrigate nephrostomy tube Indwelling catheter
Pyelolithotomy	Flank incision into kidney to remove stones from renal pelvis	Incisional drain Surgical dressing Ureteral catheter
Ureterolithotomy	Incision into ureter to remove stones	Do not irrigate ureteral catheter Check incisional drain Check surgical dressing
Nephrectomy	Removal of kidney due to tumor, infection, anomalies	Penrose drain Indwelling catheter Surgical dressing Check urine output closely "Last resort" intervention
Nephrostomy	Flank incision and insertion of nephrostomy tube into renal pelvis	Penrose drain Surgical dressing

9. Mechanical intervention (cystoscopy with catheter insertion)
10. Extracorporeal shock-wave lithotripsy (ESWL)
    a. Strain urine following procedure
    b. Voided parts of stones sent to lab for analysis
    c. Encourage to increase fluid intake to facilitate passage of broken stones
    d. Teach to report fever, decreased urinary output, pain
    e. Hematuria expected but should clear in 24 hours

D. Evaluation
1. Is client knowledgeable about dietary restrictions?
2. Has client comfort been maintained?

▶ CYSTITIS

A. Assessment
1. Urgency, frequency
2. Burning on urination, cloudy urine, strong odor to urine

B. Diagnose

1. Inflammation of bladder
2. Predisposing factors
   a. Females more prone
   b. Catheterization, instrumentation

C. Plan/Implementation

1. Obtain clean-catch midstream urine specimen for urinalysis, urine culture, colony count, and possibly Gram stain
2. Encourage fluids 3,000 mL/day
3. Cranberry juice or other urinary acidifiers
4. Culture and sensitivity (C and S)
5. Medications: antibiotics (e.g., sulfamethoxazole-trimethoprim), urinary tract analgesics (e.g., phenazopyridine)
6. Teach females to void before and after intercourse
7. Clean properly after defecation (wipe front to back)
8. Void every 2–3 hours

D. Evaluation

1. Have client's symptoms subsided?
2. Is client knowledgeable about ways to prevent a recurrence of cystitis?

▶ PYELONEPHRITIS

A. Assessment

1. Chills, fever
2. Malaise
3. Flank pain
4. Urinary frequency, dysuria
5. CVA tenderness

B. Diagnose

1. Definition—inflammation of kidney caused by bacterial infection
2. Predisposing factors
   a. Urinary tract infection
   b. Pregnancy
   c. Tumor
   d. Urinary obstruction
   e. Usually caused by *E. coli*
3. Diagnostic tests—urinalysis (RBCs, bacteria, leukocyte casts)

C. Plan/Implementation

1. Bedrest during acute phase
2. Antibiotic therapy, antiseptics, analgesics
3. Encourage fluid intake 3000 mL/day

D. Evaluation

1. Is client compliant with medication regimen?
2. Have client's symptoms subsided?

▶ GLOMERULONEPHRITIS

A. Assessment

1. Fever, chills

2. Hematuria, red cell casts, proteinuria, urine dark-colored

3. Weakness, pallor

4. Dyspnea, weight gain, lung rales, fluid overload

5. Anorexia, nausea, vomiting (uremia)

6. Generalized and/or facial and periorbital edema

7. Moderate-to-severe hypertension

8. Headache, decreased level of consciousness, confusion

9. Abdominal or flank pain

10. Oliguria with fixed specific gravity (indicates impending renal failure)

11. Antistreptolysin-O titers, decreased serum complement levels, renal biopsy

B. Diagnose

1. Damage to glomerulus caused by an immunological reaction that results in proliferative and inflammatory changes within the glomerular structure

2. Acute glomerulonephritis (most common) usually caused by *Group A beta hemolytic streptococcal* infection elsewhere in the body (URI, skin infection); *Chlamydia, pneumococcal, mycoplasma* or *klebsiella* pneumonia; autoimmune diseases, e.g., SLE, *beta-hemolytic streptococcal* infection elsewhere in the body

3. Occurs 10 days after a skin or throat infection

C. Plan/Implementation

1. Administer medications to eliminate infection; alter immune balance to alleviate inflammation; treat volume overload and hypertension

   a. Antibiotics

   b. Corticosteroids

   c. Antihypertensives

   d. Immunosuppressive medications

   e. Diuretics

2. Restrict sodium intake; restrict water if oliguric

3. Daily weights

4. Assess I and O and serum potassium

5. Bedrest

6. High-calorie, low-protein diet

7. Dialysis (uremia) or plasma electrophoreses if renal failure develops (antibody removal)

D. Evaluation

1. Have complications been prevented?

2. Is client knowledgeable about dietary/fluid restrictions?

▶ PROSTATIC HYPERTROPHY (BENIGN PROSTATIC HYPERPLASIA)

A. Assessment

1. Hesitancy (dribbling, weak urinary stream)
2. Frequency, urgency, dysuria, nocturia
3. Hematuria before or after voiding
4. Retention

B. Diagnose

1. Enlargement of the prostate gland; causes urinary flow obstruction, incontinence, possible infection
2. Benign hypertrophy, increase in size with age (over 50)
3. BUN and creatinine
4. Prostate-specific antigen (PSA)—normal is less than 4 mg/mL; may be increased in prostatitis, prostatic hypertrophy, prostate cancer
5. Trans-abdominal or trans-rectal ultrasound
6. Prostate biopsy

C. Plan/Implementation

1. Conservative—urinary antiseptics and follow-up
2. Administer medications
   a. 5-alpha reductive inhibitor
   b. Alpha-blocking medications
3. Suprapubic cystostomy—opening into bladder, drainage via catheter through abdominal wall (temporary measure to divert urine)
   a. Covered with sterile dressing
   b. Connected to sterile closed drainage system
   c. To test ability to void, clamp catheter for 4 hours, have client void, unclamp catheter and measure residual urine; if residual is less than 100 mL on 2 occasions (morning and evening), catheter is removed
   d. After removal of catheter, sterile dressing placed over site
4. Prostatectomy
   a. Transurethral (TURP)
   b. Suprapubic resection (through bladder)
   c. Retropubic resection (through abdomen)
5. Assess for shock and hemorrhage—check dressing and drainage: urine may be reddish-pink initially, monitor continuous bladder irrigation (CBI); monitor vital signs
6. Monitor intake and output after catheter removed; expect dribbling and urinary leakage around wound
7. Avoid long periods of sitting and strenuous activity until danger of bleeding is over
8. Complementary and alternative therapies
   a. Saw palmetto
   b. Lycopene

9. Avoid consumption of large amounts of fluids, caffeine

10. Avoid anticholinergic, antihistamine, decongestant medication

D. Evaluation

1. Has normal urinary elimination been restored?

2. Is client knowledgeable about postoperative care?

▶ URINARY DIVERSIONS

A. Assessment

1. Bladder tumors requiring cystectomy

2. Birth defects

3. Strictures and trauma to ureters and urethra

4. Neurogenic bladder

5. Interstitial cystitis

B. Diagnose

1. Types (see Table 3 and Figure 1)

Table 3 URINARY DIVERSIONS		
NAME	PROCEDURE	NURSING CONSIDERATIONS
Nephrostomy	Flank incision and insertion of nephrostomy tube into renal pelvis	Penrose drain Surgical dressing
Ureterosigmoidostomy	Ureters detached from bladder and anastomosed to sigmoid colon	Urine and stool are evacuated through anus Encourage voiding via rectum every 2–4 h; no enemas or cathartics Monitor complications—fluid and electrolyte imbalance, pyelonephritis, obstruction
Cutaneous ureterostomy	Single or double-barreled stoma, formed from ureter(s) excised from bladder and brought out through the skin into the abdominal wall	Stoma usually constructed on right side of abdomen below waist Extensive nursing intervention required for alteration in body image
Ileal conduit	Portion of terminal ileum is used as a conduit; ureters are replanted into ileal segment; distal end is brought out through skin and forms a stoma	Most common urinary diversion Check for obstruction (occurs at the anastomosis) Postop mucus threads normal
Kock pouch Continent ileal conduit	Ureters are transplanted to an isolated segment of ileum (pouch) with a one-way valve; urine is drained by a catheter	Urine collects in pouch until drained by catheter Valve prevents leakage of urine Drainage of urine by catheter is under control of client Pouch must be drained at regular intervals

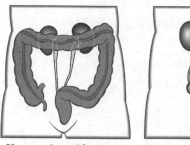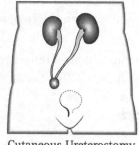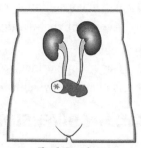

Ureterosigmoidostomy   Cutaneous Ureterostomy   Ileal Conduit

Figure 1. Types of Urinary Diversions

C. Plan/Implementation (see Table 3)

D. Evaluation

   1. Is client knowledgeable about how to care for urinary diversion equipment?

   2. Has client adjusted to change in body image?

▶ ACUTE KIDNEY DISORDERS

A. Assessment

   1. Oliguric phase of acute kidney injury (AKI)

      a. Urinary output less than 0.5 mL/kg/hr

      b. Nausea, vomiting

      c. Irritability, drowsiness, confusion, coma

      d. Restlessness, twitching, seizures

      e. Increased serum K^+, BUN, creatinine

      f. Increased Ca^+, Na^+, decreased pH

      g. Anemia

      h. Pulmonary edema, CHF

      i. Hypertension

      j. Albuminuria

   2. Diuretic or recovery phase of acute kidney injury

      a. Urinary output 4–5 liter/day

      b. Increased serum BUN

      c. Na^+ and K^+ loss in urine

      d. Increased mental and physical activity

   3. Chronic

      a. Anemia

      b. Acidosis

      c. Azotemia

      d. Fluid retention

      e. Urinary output alterations

B. Diagnose

    1. Causes of acute kidney injury

        a. Prerenal

            1) Circulating volume depletion

            2) Vascular obstruction

            3) Vascular resistance

        b. Acute kidney injury (see Table 4)

            1) Acute tubular necrosis (ATN)

                a) Nephrotoxic drugs

                b) Transfusion reaction

            2) Trauma

            3) Glomerulonephritis

            4) Severe muscle exertion

            5) Genetic conditions—polycystic kidney disease

        c. Postrenal failure

            1) Obstruction—benign prostatic hyperplasia, tumors, renal or urinary calculi

    2. Causes of chronic kidney disease

        a. Hypertension

        b. Diabetes mellitus

        c. Lupus erythematosus

        d. Sickle cell disease

        e. Chronic glomerulonephritis

        f. Repeated pyelonephritis

        g. Polycystic kidney disease

        h. Nephrotoxins

Table 4 ACUTE KIDNEY INJURY	
LOW-OUTPUT STAGE	**HIGH-OUTPUT STAGE**
Limit fluids	Fluids as needed to replace output
Diet adjustment	Diet adjustment
Specific medications as needed, e.g., Kayexalate for high potassium	Replacement for potassium
Treatment: dialysis (hemodialysis or peritoneal dialysis)	Treatment: dialysis (hemodialysis or peritoneal dialysis)

C. Plan/Implementation

1. Dialysis (see Tables 5 and 6)

Table 5 HEMODIALYSIS AND PERITONEAL DIALYSIS		
	HEMODIALYSIS	**PERITONEAL DIALYSIS**
Circulatory access	Subclavian catheter AV fistula, AV graft	Catheter in peritoneal cavity (Tenckoff, Gore-Tex)
Dialysis bath	Electrolyte solution similar to that of normal plasma	Similar to hemodialysis
Dialyzer	Artificial kidney machine with semipermeable membrane	Peritoneum is dialyzing membrane
Procedure	Blood shunted through dialyzer for 3–5 h 2 to 3 times/wk	Weigh client before and after dialysis Repeated cycles can be continuous Catheter is cleansed and attached to line leading to peritoneal cavity Dialysate infused into peritoneal cavity to prescribed volume Dialysate is then drained from abdomen after prescribed amount of time

Complications	Hemorrhage
	Hepatitis
	Nausea and vomiting
	Disequilibrium syndrome (headache, mental confusion)
	Muscle cramps
	Air embolism
	Sepsis
		Protein loss
		Peritonitis
		  Cloudy outflow, bleeding
		  Fever
		  Abdominal tenderness, lower back problems
		  Nausea and vomiting
		  Exit site infection
		  Hypotension and hypovolemia

Nursing considerations	Check "thrill" and bruit every 8 h Don't use extremity for BP or to obtain blood specimens Monitor BP, apical pulse, temperature, respirations, breath sounds, weight Monitor for hemorrhage during dialysis and 1 h after procedure	Constipation may cause problems with infusion and outflow; high-fiber diet, stool softener If problems with outflow, reposition client (supine or low-Fowler's, side to side) Monitor BP, apical pulse, temperature, respirations, breath sounds, weight Clean catheter insertion site and apply sterile dressing

2. Monitor potassium levels; sodium polystyrene sulfonate (orally or retention enema) for elevated levels

3. Daily weight, I and O

4. Diet

    a. Oliguric phase—limit fluids; restriction of protein, potassium, and sodium

    b. After diuretic phase—high carbohydrate diet; restriction of protein, potassium, and sodium

    c. Chronic failure—regulate protein intake, fluid intake to balance fluid losses, some restriction of sodium and potassium, vitamin supplements; more protein allowed with dialysis

Table 6 PERITONEAL DIALYSIS	
TYPES	**NURSING CONSIDERATIONS**
Continuous ambulatory (CAPD)	Client performs self-dialysis 7 days/wk for 24 h/day Dialysate warmed (use heating pad), infused, dwell time 4–8 h Tubing and bag disconnected or rolled up and worn under clothing After dwell time, fluid drained back into bag and process repeated
Automated	Uses machine with warming chamber for dialysate infusion, dwell, and outflow Times and volumes preset; 30-minute exchanges (10 minutes for infusion, 10 min for dwell, 10 min for outflow) for 8–10 h
Intermittent	4 days a week for 10 h/day Can be automated or manual
Continuous	Automated machine used at night Final exchange is left in place during the next day and then drained that night

5. Monitor IV fluids

6. Use of diuretics controversial

7. Aluminum hydroxide used for elevated phosphate levels

8. Bedrest during acute phase

9. Good skin care

10. Monitor for infection; antibiotics if needed

11. Kidney transplant

    a. Donor selection: cadaver, identical twin, tissue match, histocompatible

    b. Preop: client education

        1) Explain surgical procedure and follow-up care to client

        2) Show client where the donated kidney will be located (iliac fossa anterior to iliac crest)

        3) Use of immunosuppressive drugs (e.g., prednisone, imuran, cyclosporine)

        4) Need for infection prevention (gingival disease and cavities)

    c. Postop

        1) Monitor vital signs, intake and output—expect scant urine production for several weeks postop

        2) Daily weight

        3) Vascular access care—may need hemodialysis until transplanted kidney functions well (2–3 weeks for kidney from cadaver)

    4) Psychological support for donor and recipient

    5) Monitor for complications

       a) Hemorrhage

       b) Shock

       c) Rejection—Acute (days to months; decreased urine output, increased BUN and creatinine, fever, tenderness and swelling over graft site); chronic (months to years; gradual decrease in renal function, proteinuria, gradual increase in BUN and creatinine)

       d) Infection

       e) Pulmonary complications

       f) Adverse effects of immunosuppressive and steroid medications

D. Evaluation

    1. Has normal kidney function been re-established?

    2. Have complications of acute renal failure been avoided?

Chapter 7

SAFE AND EFFECTIVE CARE ENVIRONMENT

Units

1. **Management of Care**

2. **Safety and Infection Control**

MANAGEMENT OF CARE Unit 1

▶ NURSE/CLIENT RELATIONSHIP

A. Professionalism

1. Specific knowledge and skills—foundation of nursing science

2. Person-centered

3. Autonomy and accountability—adheres to standards of practice and is responsible for care given

4. Nurse practice act

5. Ethical standards

   a. Respect for human dignity—give respectful service regardless of client's personal characteristics

   b. Confidentiality—does not discuss condition with anyone not involved with care

   c. Competence—has knowledge and skills to provide care

   d. Advocacy—protects client from incompetent or unethical practice

   e. Research—participates in process of scientific inquiry

   f. Promotion of public health—committed to local and global goals for health of community

B. Therapeutic nature of the nurse/client relationship

1. Professional

   a. Client-centered

   b. Responsible

   c. Goal-oriented

   d. Ethical

2. Characterized by genuineness

3. Nurse acts as a role model

4. Nurse copes with own feelings

5. Protected relationship—nurse or client (client) cannot be forced to reveal communication between them unless person who would benefit from relationship agrees to reveal it

▶ CLIENT'S BILL OF RIGHTS

A. Privacy

1. Right to be left alone without unwarranted or uninvited publicity

2. Right to make personal choices without interference (e.g., contraception, abortion, right to refuse treatment)

3. Right to have personal information kept confidential and distributed only to authorized personnel (consider the Health Insurance Portability and Accountability Act—HIPAA)

   a. Violated when confidential information revealed to unauthorized person(s), or unauthorized personnel directly or indirectly observes client without permission

   b. Authorized personnel—people involved in diagnosis and treatment(related to care of client)

   c. Health care team can't use data, photographs, videotapes, research data without explicit permission of client

   d. Be cautious about release of information on the phone (difficult to identify caller accurately)

   e. Necessary to obtain client's permission to release information to family members or close friends

   f. For employees, can only verify employment and comply with a legal investigation

B. Respectful care

C. Current information

D. Informed consent

   1. Requirements

      a. Capacity—age (adult), competence (can make choices and understand consequences)

      b. Voluntary—freedom of choice without force, fraud, deceit, duress, coercion

      c. Information must be given in understandable form (lay terminology)

      d. Cannot sign informed consent if client has been drinking alcohol or has been premedicated

      e. Informed consent may not be required in emergency situations

   2. Minors who can provide own consent for treatment

      a. Married minors

      b. Over a specific age (e.g., 12) for STIs, HIV testing, AIDS treatment, drug and alcohol treatment

      c. Emancipated and mature minors

      d. Minors seeking birth control services

      e. Minors seeking outpatient psychiatric services or inpatient voluntary admissions to a psychiatric facility

      f. Pregnant minor

         1) Can sign consent for themselves and the fetus

         2) After delivery

            a) The mother retains right to provide consent for infant

            b) Mother cannot give own consent unless she fits into one of other exemptions

   3. Includes

      a. Explanation of treatment and expected results

      b. Anticipated risks and discomforts

c. Potential benefits

d. Possible alternatives

e. Answers to questions

f. Statements that consent can be withdrawn at any time

4. Legal responsibility

a. Rests with individual who will perform treatment

b. When nurse witnesses a signature, it means that there is reason to believe that the client is informed about upcoming treatment

E. Confidentiality

1. Right to privacy of records

2. Information used only for purpose of diagnosis and treatment

3. Not released to others without permission; verify identity of persons asking for information

F. Refusal of treatment

1. Self-determination act—federal law requiring health care facilities to provide written information to adult clients about their rights to make health care decisions

2. Aggressive treatment

a. Extraordinary support measures used to maintain individual's physiologic processes

b. May be withheld to avoid prolonging life without dignity

c. Supportive care is provided to promote comfort and reduce suffering

3. Advanced directives

a. Living wills

1) Legal document signed by competent individual indicates treatment or life-saving measures (e.g., surgery, CPR, antibiotics, dialysis, respirator, tube feedings) to be used if individual's ability to make decisions is lost due to terminal illness or a permanently unconscious state

2) Indicates who is authorized to make health care decisions if individual becomes incapacitated

3) Legally binding in most states

b. Durable power of attorney for health care

1) Permits a competent adult to appoint surrogate or proxy in the event that the adult becomes incompetent

2) Health care provider must follow decisions stated in documents

3) In most states proxy can perform all legal actions needed to fulfill adult's wishes

G. Reasonable response to a request for services

H. Right to know hospital/clinic regulations

▶ **RESTRAINTS**

A. Restraints

1. Omnibus Budget Reconciliation Act provides clients with the right to be free from physical and chemical restraints imposed for the purpose of discipline or convenience and not required to treat medical symptoms

2. Mechanical restraint

   a. Needed to meet the client's therapeutic needs or ensure safety

   b. Least restrictive type of restraint to meet needs

   c. Accurate and thorough documentation needed

3. Chemical restraint

   a. Psychotropic drugs cannot be used to control behavior

   b. Can be used only for diagnoses-related conditions

   c. Inappropriate use causes deep sedation, agitation, combativeness

4. Informed consent is needed to use restraints

5. If client is unable to consent to use of restraints, then consent of proxy must be obtained after full disclosure of risks and benefits

6. Restraint of client without informed consent or sufficient justification is false imprisonment

B. Nursing considerations

1. Assess and document need for restraints (risk for falls, risk of injury to others, potential for removal of IV lines or other equipment)

2. Consider and document use of alternative measures

3. Health care provider's order is required specifying duration and circumstances under which restraints should be used

4. Cannot order restraints to be used PRN

5. Monitor client closely, periodically reassess for continued need for restraints, document

6. Remove for skin care and range of motion exercises

7. Use alternative measures prior to use of restraints (reorientation, family involvement, frequent assistance with toileting)

▶ **ADVOCACY**

A. Nurse as client advocate should

1. Actively support clients' rights

2. Defend clients' participation in decisions affecting them

3. Communicate clients' needs to interdisciplinary team (health care provider, RN, PT, dietitian, social worker, psychologist)

4. Safeguard clients' autonomy and independence

5. Provide clients with information about needs and available options so that clients can make informed decisions about health care

▶ LEGAL ISSUES

A. Negligence—unintentional failure of individual to perform an act that a reasonable person would or would not perform in similar circumstances; can be act of omission or commission

B. Malpractice—professional negligence involving misconduct or lack of skill in carrying out professional responsibilities

1. Required elements

   a. Duty—relationship between nurse and client

   b. Breach of duty

   c. Causation—nurse conduct causes injury

   d. Injury

C. Invasion of privacy—release of information to an unauthorized person without the client's consent

D. Assault—intentional threat to cause harm or offensive unwanted contact; battery—intentional touching without consent

E. False imprisonment

1. Client is denied discharge from a health care facility

2. Client is denied discharge after signing an against medical advice (AMA) document

3. Client is placed in restraints without appropriate medical need

F. Laws

1. Rules of conduct established and enforced by authority

2. Reflect public policy

3. Indicates what society views as good and bad, right and wrong behavior

G. Accountability

1. Nurse is responsible for using reasonable care in practicing nursing

2. To remain competent, nurse needs to participate in lifelong learning programs

H. State laws

1. Nurse practice acts—define "reasonable care" in each state; scope of nursing practice, roles, rules, educational requirements

2. Licensure requirements—differ slightly in requirements among states

3. Good Samaritan laws—limit the liability of professionals in emergency situations

4. Tarasoff Act—duty to warn of threatened suicide or harm to others

I. Need to assess health care provider's orders—must be safe and correct

J. Notify supervisor if more nurses are needed for safe client care

▶ ORGAN/TISSUE DONATION/TRANSPLANT

1. Clients have a right to decide to become an organ donor

2. Clients have a right to decide to refuse organ donation or transplant

3. Clients 18 years or older may choose to donate organs

4. Requests to the family are usually completed by the health care provider or a specially trained nurse

5. Religious beliefs should be taken into consideration when approaching the family

▶ **MANAGED CARE**

A. Health care focuses on individual client needs along the health continuum (wellness to illness)

B. Managed care

1. Goal is reduced health care costs
2. Focuses on client outcomes and maintenance of quality
3. Uses an interdisciplinary approach
4. Emphasizes costs; approval needed for diagnostic tests
5. Critical pathways (care maps) used as foundations for activities and guide services that clients receive for specific health conditions

C. Continuous quality improvement (CQI; previously called quality assurance)

1. Quality improvement is essential for all providers of client health care
2. Prevention-focused approach provides basis for managing risk
3. Involves organized incident reporting
4. Focused team: group of 5–10 people
5. Process
    a. Senior management establishes policy
    b. Coordinator provides for process and management health care team training
    c. Team, headed by a team leader, evaluates and improves the process

D. Risk management

1. Planned program of loss prevention and liability control
2. Problem-focused
3. Identifies, evaluates, develops plan, and takes corrective action against potential risks that would injure clients, staff, visitors
4. Focuses on noncompliance, informed consent, right to refuse treatment

E. Collaborative practice team

1. Consists of clinical experts: nursing, medicine, physical therapy, social work
2. Determines expected outcomes
3. Determines appropriate interventions with a specified time frame
4. Involves specific client diagnoses that are high-volume (frequently seen), high-cost, high-risk (frequently develop complications)

F. For managed care to be successful, need

1. Support from health care providers, nurses, administrators
2. Qualified nurse managers
3. Collaborative practice teams
4. Quality management system
5. All professionals are equal members of the team (one discipline doesn't determine interventions for another discipline)

6. Members agree on final draft of critical pathways, take ownership of client outcomes, accept responsibility and accountability for interventions and client outcomes

G. Critical pathways

1. Reduce complications

2. Reduce cost

3. Increase collaboration

4. Improve quality of care

5. Provide direction for care

6. Orient staff to expected outcomes for each day

7. If outcomes not achieved, case manager is notified and situation is analyzed to determine how to modify critical path

8. Alteration in time frame or interventions is a "variance"

9. All variances are tracked to note trends

10. Variance—change in established plan that includes more, different, or fewer services to client to achieve desired outcome

11. Interventions presented in modality groups (medications, nursing activities)

12. Include

a. Specific medical diagnoses

b. Expected length of stay

c. Client identification data

d. Appropriate time frames (days, hours, minutes, visits) for interventions

e. Clinical outcomes

f. Client outcomes

H. Variances

1. Deviations from specific plans (individual receives more, less, or different services)

2. Information is included in a database and is used to evaluate services provided

3. Continuous quality improvement (CQI) strategies are used to monitor variances

I. Case manager—usually has advanced degree and considerable experience

1. Doesn't provide direct client care

2. Supervises care provided by licensed and unlicensed personnel

3. Coordinates, communicates, collaborates, solves problems

4. Facilitates client care for a group of clients (10–15)

5. Follows client through the system from admission to discharge

6. Notes "variances" from expected progress

J. Case management

1. Identifies, coordinates, monitors implementation of services needed to achieve desired outcomes within specified period of time

2. Involves principles of CQI

3. Promotes professional practice

▶ ASSIGNMENT VERSUS DELEGATION

A. Assignment—allocating to health care team members work required to care for groups of individuals

1. Process

   a. Determine nursing care required to meet clients' needs (take into account time required, complexity of activities, acuity of clients, and infection control)

   b. Consider knowledge and abilities of staff members

   c. Decide which staff person is best able to provide care

   d. Take into account continuity of care

   e. Determine assignments to increase efficiency

   f. Describe assignments in measurable terms

   g. Be specific about expected results

   h. Give assignments to staff members (assign total responsibility for total client care, avoid assigning only procedures)

   i. Provide additional help as needed

B. Delegation

1. Responsibility and authority for performing a task (function, activity, decision) is transferred to another individual who accepts that responsibility and authority

2. Depending on state Nurse Practice Acts, LPN/PNs may delegate tasks to nursing assistive personnel (NAP), (NAP includes the nursing providers excluding RNs, such as UAP, NAs, CNAs, etc.)

3. Delegator remains accountable for task

4. Delegatee is accountable to delegator for responsibilities assumed

5. Can only delegate tasks for which that nursing care level is responsible

6. Definitions

   a. Responsibility—obligation to accomplish a task

   b. Accountability—accept ownership for results or lack of results

7. In delegation, responsibility is transferred; in accountability, it is shared

8. Guidelines

   a. Can delegate only those tasks for which you are responsible

   b. Responsibility is determined by

      1) Nurse practice acts (defines scope of nursing practice)

      2) Standards of care (established by organization)

      3) Job description (defined by organization)

      4) Policy statement (from organization)

   c. Must transfer authority (the right to act) along with the responsibility to act

   d. Empowers delegatee to accomplish task

9. Steps for delegation

   a. Define task to be delegated

      1) Can delegate only work for which you have responsibility and authority

       2) Delegate what you know best so you can provide guidance and feedback

         a) Routine tasks

         b) Tasks you don't have time to accomplish

         c) Tasks with lower priority

    b. Determine who should receive delegated task

    c. Identify what the task involves, determine its complexity

    d. Match task to individual by assessing individual skills and abilities

       1) Evaluate capacity of individual to perform task

       2) Consider availability, willingness to assume responsibility

    e. Provide clear communication about your expectations regarding the task, answer questions

10. To delegate

    a. Assume face-to-face position

    b. Establish eye contact

    c. Describe task using "I" statements

    d. Provide what, when, where, how of the task to be delegated

    e. State if delegatee needs to provide written or verbal report after the task is completed

    f. If written report is needed, inform delegatee where to put the report (e.g., table, chart, form)

    g. Identify what changes or incidents need to be brought to delegator's attention (e.g., "If client's BP is greater than 140/90, let me know immediately.")

    h. Provide reason for task, give incentive for accepting responsibility and authority

    i. Tell delegatee how and how often task will be evaluated

    j. Describe expected outcome and timeline for completion of task

11. Identify constraints for completing task and risks

12. Identify variables that would change authority and responsibility (e.g., "Feed client if coherent and awake; if client is confused, do not feed and notify me immediately.")

13. Obtain feedback from delegatee to make sure he/she understands task to be performed and your expectations; ask for questions, give additional information

14. Reach mutual agreement on task

15. Monitor performance and results according to established goals

16. Give constructive feedback to delegatee

17. Confirm that delegated tasks are performed as agreed

18. Delegator must remain accessible during performance of task

19. Don't delegate

    a. Total control

    b. Discipline issues

    c. Confidential tasks

    d. Technical tasks

    e. Controversial tasks

    f. During a crisis

20. Levels of delegation (in ascending order)

    a. Gather information for delegatee so you can decide what needs to be done

    b. List alternate courses of action and allow delegatee to choose course of action

    c. Have delegatee perform part of task and obtain approval before proceeding with the rest of the task

    d. Have delegatee outline entire course of action for the task and approve it before proceeding

    e. Allow delegatee to perform entire task using any preferred method, and report only results

21. Rule for determining delegatee—delegate to lowest person on hierarchy who has the required skills and abilities and who is allowed to do the task legally and according to the organization

22. Obstacles to delegation

    a. Nonsupportive environment—rigid organizational culture, lack of resources (limited personnel)

    b. Insecure delegator

    c. Fear of competition

    d. Fear of liability

    e. Fear of loss of control

    f. Fear of overburdening others

    g. Fear of decreased personal job satisfaction

    h. Unwilling delegatee

    i. Fear of failure

    j. Inexperience or incompetence

23. Ineffective delegation

    a. Under delegation

       1) Doesn't transfer full authority

       2) Takes back responsibility

       3) Fails to equip or direct delegatee

       4) Questions competence of delegatee

    b. Reverse delegation—lower person on hierarchy delegates to person higher on hierarchy

    c. Over delegation—delegator loses control of the situation by delegating too much authority and responsibility to delegatee

24. Rights of delegation

    a. Right task

    b. Right person (knowledge, skills, ability

    c. Right time (not in a crisis)

    d. Right information

    e. Right supervision (is task being performed correctly?)

    f. Right follow-up

25. Delegation empowers others, builds trust, enhances communication and leadership skills, develops teamwork, increases productivity

26. Failure to delegate and supervise properly can result in liability; need to consider delegatee's competence and qualifications

27. Nurses have a legal responsibility to make sure persons under their supervision perform consistently with established standards of nursing practice

▶ CRITICAL THINKING

A. Involves creativity, problem-solving, decision-making

B. Nursing responsibilities

1. Observe

2. Decide what data are important

3. Validate and organize data

4. Look for patterns and relationships

5. State problem

6. Transfer knowledge from one situation to another

7. Decide on criteria for evaluation

8. Apply knowledge

9. Evaluate according to criteria established

▶ DECISION MAKING

A. Purposeful and goal-directed; nurse identifies and selects options and alternatives

B. Types of decision making

1. Prescriptive

   a. Involves routine decisions with objective information

   b. Options are known and predictable

   c. Decisions made according to standard procedures or analytical tools

2. Behavioral

   a. Involves the nonroutine and unstructured information

   b. Options are unknown or unpredictable

   c. Decisions made by obtaining more data, using past experiences, using creative approach

3. Satisficing

   a. Solution minimally meets objectives

   b. Expedient; use when time is an issue

4. Optimizing

   a. Goal is to select ideal solution

   b. Best decision comes from this process but is the most time consuming

C. Phases

1. Define objectives

2. Generate options

3. Analyze options

       a. Identify advantages and disadvantages

       b. Rank options

    4. Select option that will successfully meet the defined objective

    5. Implement the selected option

    6. Evaluate the outcome

▶ PROBLEM SOLVING

A. Focus is trying to solve immediate problems; includes decision making

B. Methods

    1. Trial and error

       a. Repeated attempts at different solutions until it is identified that one solution works best

       b. Used by inexperienced staff

    2. Experimentation

       a. Study problem using trial periods or pilot projects to determine best outcome

       b. Will have greater probability of achieving best outcome if sufficient time devoted to the process

    3. Purposeful inaction

       a. Do-nothing approach

       b. Use when problem is judged to be insignificant or outside a person's control

C. Steps

    1. Define the problem

    2. Gather data

    3. Analyze data

    4. Develop solutions

    5. Select and implement a solution

    6. Evaluate the results

▶ DISTRIBUTION OF RESOURCES

A. Distributive justice

    1. Gives an individual what he/she deserves regardless of race, color, creed, gender, or socioeconomic status

    2. Provides equal access to care for all

    3. Designed to manage health care according to need rather than provide care for everyone

B. Resources—staff, time, equipment, supplies, knowledge

C. Allocation of resources

    1. Decision regarding how resources will be distributed

    2. There is a finite number of resources in health care that must be used wisely and efficiently

    3. Primary principle is to provide the greatest good for the greatest number of people

  a. Approval for inpatient admissions or emergency room visits required by insurance companies

  b. Early discharge from inpatient settings

  c. Stimulus for managed care—model of service delivery that focuses on client outcomes

  d. Is interdisciplinary and emphasizes cost

D. Rationing—decision about how limited resources (e.g., transplants) will be used

E. Nursing management

  1. Judiciously use resources to achieve identified client goals

  2. Coordinate the services received by a group of clients over a specific time period

  3. Identify client needs

  4. Identify resources available to meet needs

  5. Organize and direct use of available resources

  6. Evaluate the extent to which desired client outcomes are met controlling the process of client care

F. Standard of care and practice

  1. Guide nursing activities

  2. Used to evaluate quality of care

G. Resolution of conflict

  1. Determine the facts

  2. Identify the problem

  3. Ask for suggestions for resolution from those involved

  4. Determine solutions

  5. Evaluate results

  6. Evaluate conflict resolution

▶ DOCUMENTATION

A. Purpose

  1. Promotes communication

  2. Maintains a legal record

  3. Meets requirements of regulatory agencies

  4. Required for third-party reimbursement

B. Characteristics of good documentation

  1. Legible

  2. Accurate, factual, no summarizing data

  3. Timely

  4. Thorough

  5. Well organized and concise (follow chronological order of events)

  6. Confidential

  7. Proper grammar and spelling

  8. Authorized abbreviations

C. Documenting changes in client conditions

1. Assess
   a. Client's vital signs, symptoms, behaviors, reports from client, responses to treatments (PRN medications, dietary changes, I and O)
   b. Interdisciplinary team information
   c. Information from family members or significant other
2. Notify health care provider if client's physiological status and functional abilities change significantly
3. Notify interdisciplinary team of changes in medical plan (RN is responsible for coordinating interdisciplinary team for client)
4. Notify family or significant other about changes in client's condition and plan of care
   a. Nature of change
   b. Why changes were made
   c. Actions undertaken to provide needed care for client
   d. List of revisions on medical plan of care
   e. Help family to take active part in client's care and management
   f. Follow policy for privacy and confidentiality
5. Document in timely manner
   a. Date and time
   b. Nursing assessment
   c. Name of health care provider informed
   d. Date, time, method (e.g., telephone)
   e. Information provided about client
   f. Actions taken (revisions in plan of care)
   g. Information given and to whom (client, name of family, significant other)
   h. Responses by client and family members or significant other
6. Considerations
   a. If an error is made in charting, use a single line through the error and doc your initials, date, and time—do not erase, white out, or scratch out an error
   b. Do not chart for anyone else
   c. Keep your electronic access private
   d. Do not leave your electronic chart open when you are not in attendance

▶ INCIDENT REPORTS

A. Definition
   1. Agency record of unusual occurrence or accident and physical response
   2. Accurate and comprehensive report on any unexpected or unplanned occurrence that affects or could potentially affect a client, family member, or staff person
B. Purpose
   1. Documentation and follow-up of all incidents
   2. Used to analyze the severity, frequency, and cause of occurrences

    3. Analysis is the basis for intervention

C. Charting

    1. Don't include a reference to the incident report

    2. Don't use words such as "error" or "inappropriate"

    3. Don't include inflammatory words or judgmental statements

    4. If there are adverse reactions to incident, chart follow-up note updating client's status

    5. Documentation of client's reactions should be included as status changes and should be continued until client returns to original status

D. Sequence

    1. Person discovers and reports actual or potential risk

    2. Risk manager receives report within 24 hours

    3. Investigation of incident is conducted

    4. Referring health care provider and risk management committee consult together

E. Risk manager

    1. Clarifies misinformation for client and family

    2. Explains what happened to client and family

    3. Client is referred to appropriate resources

    4. Care is provided free of charge

    5. All records, incident reports, follow-up actions taken are filed in a central location

F. Common situations that require an incident report

    1. Medication errors—omitted medication, wrong medication, wrong dosage, wrong route

    2. Complications from diagnostic or treatment procedures (e.g., blood sample stick, biopsy, x-ray, LP, invasive procedure, bronchoscopy, thoracentesis)

    3. Incorrect sponge count in surgery

    4. Failure to report change in client's condition

    5. Falls

    6. Client is burned

    7. Break in aseptic technique

    8. Medical—legal incident

        a. Client or family refuses treatment as ordered and refuses to sign consent

        b. Client or family voices dissatisfaction with care and situation cannot be or has not been resolved

▶ **CHANGE OF SHIFT REPORT**

A. Regularly scheduled, structured exchange of information

B. Focuses on anticipated needs of individual clients in next 24 hours

C. Enables health care workers to

1. Organize work for specified time period

2. Communicate concerns

3. Provide continuity of care or consistent follow-through

D. Included

1. Client's status

2. Current care plan

3. Responses to current care

4. Things needing further attention

E. Reporting nurse describes

1. Actual or potential client needs

2. How these needs were addressed during previous shift by nursing and interdisciplinary team

3. Information about laboratory studies, diagnostic tests, treatments, and nursing activities anticipated during next shift

4. Reporting nurse must legally communicate all facts relevant to continuity of care of assigned clients

5. Information must be pertinent, current, and accurate

F. Change-of-shift reports should not contain

1. Information already known by the oncoming shift

2. Descriptions of routines (am or pm care)

3. Rumors or gossip

4. Opinions or value judgments (about client's lifestyle)

5. Client information that does not relate to health condition, needs, or treatments (e.g., idiosyncrasies)

G. To give change-of-shift report

1. Gather data to be discussed (flow sheets, work sheets, Kardex, progress notes, chart)

2. Avoid copying data in order to prevent errors and reduce time required

3. Use outline to organize report

4. Provide in logical, uniform manner

H. To deliver change-of-shift report, include

1. Client information

a. Name, room, and bed number

b. Note if off the unit (recovery room, diagnostic test, etc.)

2. Medical plan

a. Admitting diagnosis

b. Attending health care provider

c. Major diagnostic or surgical procedures with dates

      d. Health care provider's orders that have been discontinued or affect next shift

      e. IV solutions, flow rates, when current bag is scheduled to be completed, amount of solution remaining to be infused

      f. Medications

      g. Response to treatment (expected and untoward effects)

      h. Client's emotional response to condition

      i. Use of and response to PRN medications

      j. Completion of special procedures

  3. Nursing plan

      a. Personalized nursing approaches

      b. Special equipment, supplies, or pacing of activities

      c. Response to diet

      d. Behavioral response to treatment and health status (e.g., denial, frustration)

      e. Nursing assessments (e.g., vital signs, I and O, activity level)

      f. New concerns

      g. Changing client needs

      h. Client outcomes

      i. Interdisciplinary plans

      j. Referrals

      k. Teaching plans

      l. Discharge plans

I. Nurse receiving report should learn

  1. Individual client's symptoms

  2. Discomforts

  3. What has been done

  4. What remains to be done

  5. How client has responded to treatments and activities so changes can be made to meet client needs

J. To receive change-of-shift report

  1. Determine

      a. Number of clients

      b. Number of staff available for client care

      c. Anticipated admissions, transfers, discharges

      d. Clients in critical condition

      e. Clients with specific needs (e.g., blood transfusions, returning from surgery)

  2. Complete assignment sheets for staff under your supervision

  3. Write assignment on client care worksheets

  4. Make a "to do" list identifying tasks to be performed during shift (helps to organize activities)

K. During change-of-shift report

1. Determine appropriateness of client care assignments

2. Note key information about client condition, progress, response to treatments

L. Types of change-of-shift reports

1. Face-to-face

   a. Reporting nurse answers questions from oncoming staff

   b. Provides flexibility to report to a number of different oncoming staff

   c. Provides flexibility in pacing and sequencing of report

   d. Nurses listen to report only on their clients

2. Taped

   a. Less time-consuming because of lack of interruptions

   b. Nurse is frequently more systematic and thorough

   c. Gives nurse more sense of control over the process

   d. Reporting nurse can perform nursing activities while next shift is listening to report

   e. Reporting nurse returns to clarify information, answer questions,update information that changed since report was recorded

M. Organization of change-of-shift report

1. Computerized client care summary or Kardex—current summary of client's needs, status, goals or desired outcomes, care plans, nursing interventions, medications, medical treatments; updated during change-of-shift report

2. Assignment work sheet—uses chart for detailed information about individual clients

3. Progress notes or flow sheets provide detailed information about symptoms and effectiveness of treatments

N. Method of service delivery and change-of-shift reports

1. Functional method

   a. RN of previous shift reports to RN of oncoming shift

   b. Other staff may attend report or be given report according to assignments from RN

2. Team nursing method

   a. All members of oncoming shift attend report

   b. Reduces amount of time and communication needed to make changes in nursing care for client

3. Primary nursing method

   a. RN assigned to direct care of individual clients reports to RN assigned to direct care of same individual clients

4. Case management method

   a. Scheduled structured discussions with nursing team and interdisciplinary team in addition to change-of-shift reports

▶ CULTURAL NORMS

A. Cultural norms—group of individuals' values and beliefs that strongly influence individual's actions and behaviors

B. Values—personal preferences, commitments, motivations, patterns of using resources, objects, people, or events that have special meaning and influence individual's choices, behaviors, actions

C. Beliefs

1. Basic assumptions or personal convictions that the individual thinks are factual or takes for granted

2. Used to determine values

3. Handed down from generation to generation

4. Include cultural traditions

▶ ETHICS

A. Definition

1. Principles of right and wrong, good and bad

2. Governs our relationship with others

3. Used to identify solutions to problems arising from conflicts

4. Based on personal beliefs and cultural values that guide decision- making and determine conduct

5. As cultural diversity increases, need to understand ethical principles increases

B. ANA Code of Ethics—decision-making framework for solving ethical problems

1. Nurse provides care with respect for human dignity and uniqueness of individual without consideration of social or economic status, personal attributes, or nature of health problems

2. Nurse safeguards the client's right to privacy

3. Nurse acts to safeguard client and public when health care and safety are at risk from incompetent, unethical, or illegal practice of an individual

4. Nurse assumes responsibility and accountability for own individual actions and judgments

5. Nurse maintains competence in nursing

6. Nurse uses informed judgment, competence, and qualifications in accepting responsibilities and delegating nursing activities to others

7. Nurse participates in activities contributing to the development of the profession's body of knowledge

8. Nurse participates in profession's efforts to implement and improve standards of care

9. Nurse participates in profession's efforts to establish and maintain conditions of employment conducive to high-quality nursing care

10. Nurse participates in profession's efforts to protect the public from misinformation and misrepresentation and to maintain the integrity of nursing

11. Nurse collaborates with members of the health professions and others to promote community and national efforts to meet the health care needs of the public

C. Ethical principles of nursing

1. Autonomy—support of client's independence to make decisions and take action for themselves

2. Beneficence—duty to help others by doing what is best for them; client advocacy for refusal of care, autonomy overrides beneficence

3. Nonmaleficence—"do no harm"; act with empathy toward client and staff without resentment or malice; violated by acts performed in bad faith or with ill will, or when making false accusations about client or employee

4. Justice—use available resources fairly and reasonably

5. Veracity—communicate truthfully and accurately

6. Confidentiality—safeguard the client's privacy

7. Fidelity—following through on what the nurse says will be done; carefully attending to the details of the client's care

D. Ethical reasoning process

1. Recognize a moral issue

2. Analyze facts and identify the dilemma

3. Decide on possible alternative actions

4. Select specific action

5. Evaluate the effectiveness of the action

E. Behaviors for handling reports of dissatisfaction

1. Use active listening without interrupting or arguing

2. Don't get defensive

3. Ask person what is expected for solution to problem

4. Explain what you can and cannot do to solve the problem

5. Agree on specific steps that will be taken and determine a timeline

▶ **CLIENT EDUCATION**

A. Assessment

1. Definition—process of learning

2. Type of information needed

   a. Specific knowledge

   b. Type of learning

      1) Cognitive

      2) Psychomotor

      3) Affective

3. Client's motivation

   a. Client may need help to see need for learning

   b. Important to remove barriers to learning readiness, if possible

4. Client's needs

   a. Health behavior desired

   b. Current level of knowledge/understanding

  c. Skill level

  d. Client's attitudes and beliefs

  e. Social, cultural, and environmental factors influence health behavior

B. Diagnose

  1. Client education process requires skilled communication

   a. Mutual goals set

   b. Client feedback critical

  2. Factors influencing compliance with health regimen

   a. Duration—shorter duration increases compliance

   b. Complexity—greater complexity causes greater noncompliance

   c. Adverse effects—the greater the adverse effects, the greater the noncompliance

C. Plan/Implementation

  1. Set priorities

  2. Set realistic goals

  3. Consider involving family and significant other

  4. Use nonjudgmental, empathetic approach

  5. Use demonstration and return-demonstration for teaching skills

  6. Allow for practice periods

  7. Ensure, by observation, that knowledge has been incorporated

  8. Point out any success/benefits

  9. Recognize the difficulty of changing behavior

D. Evaluation

  1. Is the client able to verbalize an understanding of the health plan?

  2. Can the client demonstrate the required skills?

  3. Have identified health outcomes been reached?

▶ DISCHARGE PLANNING/HOME CARE

A. Assessment

  1. Begins with first encounter

  2. Potential effects of health problems identified

  3. Family and other social supports identified

  4. Client's functional level assessed

  5. Environmental factors identified

  6. Community agencies identified

  7. Client's preferences are always considered

  8. Mutually agreeable and appropriate plan is the goal of thorough assessment

B. Diagnose

  1. Goal is as much independence for client as safely possible

  2. Client's strengths as well as limitations are considered

  3. Community care between hospital and home maintained through appropriate referrals

  4. Appropriate level of care is determined

C. Plan/Implementation

1. Collaborate with interdisciplinary team and client to identify feasible, safe, humane plan

2. Make referrals to appropriate community services

3. Plan ways to adapt the home environment to client's current functional ability

4. Implement client education plan

5. Home care nurse continues this process

   a. Monitors health status

   b. Assesses client's needs in home environment

   c. Facilitates implementation of services

   d. Coordinates care

   e. Continues client education

D. Evaluation

1. Is the client's health status relatively stable at home?

2. Is the client safe at home?

3. Have services been implemented in a timely fashion and are they consistent with client's needs?

4. Is the client making the expected progress in terms of rehabilitation?

5. Have the client's and family's psychosocial needs been recognized and addressed?

SAFETY AND INFECTION CONTROL

▶ INFECTIONS AND INFECTION CONTROL

A. Assessment

1. Local (focal point)—heat, redness, pain/tenderness, swelling, possible drainage (bloody, serous, purulent), abscess (localized collection of pus), cellulitis (involving cellular and connective tissue)

2. Systemic (generalized)—fever, malaise, weakness

3. White blood cell count (WBC)—normally 4,500–11,000 x 10^3/mm3 (4.5 11 x 10^9/L); increase indicates the presence of disease or injury; differential of 30–40% lymphocytes; increased number immature neutrophils ("shift to left")

4. Erythrocyte sedimentation rate (ESR)—elevations greater than 15–20 mm/h indicate the presence of inflammation

5. Cultures and antibiotic sensitivity of suspected infectious site

   a. Should be obtained before onset of antibiotic therapy

   b. Specimens must be carefully collected and identified

   c. Preliminary results in 24 hours; final results in 72 hours

6. Highly sensitive C-reactive protein (hsCRP)—marker of inflammation

B. Diagnose

1. Inflammation—immediate, short-term, nonspecific response to the adverse effects of injury, i.e., physical irritants (trauma/foreign body) or chemical irritants (strong acids/alkalies) or invasion by microorganisms

2. Communicable diseases—caused by pathogenic microorganisms and transmitted by direct contact, droplet spread, contaminated articles, or through carriers (see Table 1)

3. Hospital-Acquired Infections (HAI)—nearly 2 million (5%) hospital clients acquire an infection in the hospital; most often caused by *Staphylococcus aureus*

C. Plan/Implementation

1. Treatment of infection or infectious disease with appropriate antibiotic medication

2. Standard Precautions (barrier)—used with all clients

   a. Primary strategy for infection control in all settings

   b. Most important way to reduce transmission of pathogens

Table 1 COMMON COMMUNICABLE DISEASES OF CHILDHOOD		
NAME/INCUBATION	**TRANSMISSION/CLINICAL PICTURE**	**NURSING CONSIDERATIONS**
Chickenpox (Varicella) 13–17 days	Prodromal: slight fever, malaise, anorexia Rash is pruritic, begins as macule, then papule, and then vesicle with successive crops of all three stages present at any one time; lymphadenopathy; elevated temperature Transmission: spread by direct contact, airborne, contaminated object	Isolation until all vesicles are crusted; communicable from 1 day before rash Avoid use of aspirin due to association with Reye's syndrome; use Acetaminophen Topical application of calamine lotion or baking soda baths Airborne and contact precautions in hospital
Diphtheria 2–5 days	Prodromal: resembles common cold Low-grade fever, hoarseness, malaise, pharyngeal lymphadenitis; characteristic white/gray pharyngeal membrane Transmission: direct contact with a carrier, infected client contaminated articles	Contact and droplet precautions until two successive negative nose and throat cultures are obtained Complete bedrest; watch for signs of respiratory distress and obstruction; provide for humidification, suctioning, and tracheostomy as needed; severe cases can lead to sepsis and death Administer antitoxin therapy
Pertussis (Whooping Cough) 5–21 days, usually 10	Prodromal: upper respiratory infection for 1–2 weeks Severe cough with high-pitched "whooping" sound, especially at night, lasts 4–6 weeks; vomiting Transmission: direct contact, droplet, contaminated articles	Hospitalization for infants; bedrest and hydration Complications: pneumonia, weight loss, dehydration, hemorrhage, hernia, airway obstruction Maintain high humidity and restful environment; suction; oxygen Administer erthromycin and pertussis immune globulin
Rubella (German Measles) 14–21 days	Prodromal: none in children, low fever and sore throat in adolescent Maculopapular rash appears first on face and then on rest of the body Symptoms subside first day after rash Transmission: droplet spread and contaminated articles	Contact precautions Isolate child from potentially pregnant women Comfort measures; antipyretics and analgesics Rare complications include arthritis and encephalitis Droplet precautions Risk of fetal deformity
Rubeola 10–20 days	Prodromal: fever and malaise followed by cough and Koplik's spots on buccal mucosa Erythematous maculopapular rash with face first affected; turns brown after 3 days when symptoms subside Transmission: direct contact with droplets	Isolate until 5th day; maintain bedrest during first 3–4 days Institute airborne and seizure precautions Antipyretics, dim lights; humidifier for room Keep skin clean and maintain hydration
Scarlet fever 2–4 days	Prodromal: high fever with vomiting, chills, malaise, followed by enlarged tonsils covered with exudate, strawberry tongue Rash: red tiny lesions that become generalized and then desquamate; rash appears within 24 hours Transmission: droplet spread or contaminated articles Group A beta-hemolytic streptococci	Droplet precautions for 24 hours after start of antibiotics Ensure compliance with oral antibiotic therapy Bedrest during febrile phase Analgesics for sore throat Encourage fluids, soft diet Administer penicillin or erythromycin

Table 1 COMMON COMMUNICABLE DISEASES OF CHILDHOOD *(CONTINUED)*		
NAME/INCUBATION	**TRANSMISSION/CLINICAL PICTURE**	**NURSING CONSIDERATIONS**
Mononucleosis 4–6 weeks	Malaise, fever, enlarged lymph nodes, sore throat, flulike aches, low-grade temperature Highest incidence 15–30 years old Transmission: direct contact with oral secretions, unknown	Advise family members to avoid contact with saliva (cups, silverware) for about 3 months Treatment is rest and good nutrition; strenuous exercise is to be avoided to prevent spleen rupture Complications include encephalitis and spleen rupture
Tonsillitis (streptococcal)	Fever, white exudate on tonsils Positive culture GpA strep	Antibiotics Teach parents serious potential complications: rheumatic fever, glomerulonephritis
Mumps 14–21 days	Malaise, headache, fever, parotid gland swelling Transmission: direct contact with saliva, droplet	Isolation before and after appearance of swelling Soft, bland diet Complications: deafness, meningitis, encephalitis, sterility

c. Standard precautions apply to contact with blood, body fluids, non intact skin, and mucous membranes from all clients

d. Handwashing

  1) Done immediately on contact with blood or bodily fluids

  2) Wash hands before putting on or taking off gloves, between client contacts, between procedures or tasks with same client, immediately after exposure to blood or bodily fluids

e. Gloves

  1) Use clean, non-sterile when touching blood, body fluids, secretions, excretions, contaminated articles

  2) Put on clean gloves just before touching mucous membranes or non intact skin, for touching blood, body fluids, secretions, contaminated items or if gloves torn or heavily soiled

  3) Change gloves between tasks/procedures

  4) Remove gloves promptly after use, before touching items and environmental surfaces

f. Masks, eye protection, face shield (Personal Protective Equipment)

  1) Used to protect mucous membranes of eyes, nose, mouth during procedures and client care activities likely to generate splashes or sprays of blood, bodily fluids, or excretions

g. Gowns (Personal Protective Equipment)

  1) Use clean, non-sterile gowns to protect skin and prevent soiling of clothing during procedures and client care activities likely to generate splashes and sprays of blood, bodily fluids, or excretions

  2) Should remove promptly, and wash hands after leaving client's environment

    h. Environmental control

        1) Do not need to use special dishes, glasses, eating utensils; can use either reusable or disposable

        2) Don't recap used sharps, or bend, break, or remove used needles

        3) Don't manipulate used needle with two hands; use a one-handed scoop technique. Place used sharps in a puncture-resistant container

        4) Use mouthpieces, resuscitation bags, or other devices for mouth-to-mouth resuscitation

    i. Client placement

        1) Private room if client has poor hygiene habits, contaminates the environment, or can't assist in maintaining infection control precautions (e.g., infants, children, altered mental status client)

        2) When cohorting (sharing room) consider the epidemiology and mode of transmission of the infecting organism

    j. Transport

        1) Use barriers (e.g., mask, impervious dressings)

        2) Notify personnel of impending arrival and precautions needed

        3) Inform client of ways to assist in prevention of transmission

3. Transmission-based precautions apply to clients with documented or suspected infections with highly transmissible or epidemiologically important pathogens; prevent spread of pathogenic microorganisms

    a. Airborne precautions

        1) Used with pathogens smaller than 5 microns that are transmitted by airborne route; droplets or dust particles that remain suspended in the air

        2) Private room with monitored negative air pressure with 6–12 air changes per hour (airborne infection isolation room)

        3) Keep door closed and client in room; susceptible persons should not enter room or wear N-95 HEPA filter

        4) Can cohort or place client with another client with the same organism, but no other organism

        5) Private room is the best situation

        6) Place mask on client if being transported

        7) Tuberculosis—wear fit-test respirator mask

        8) Example of disease in category: measles (rubeola), *M. tuberculosis*, varicella (chicken pox), disseminated zoster (shingles)

    b. Droplet precautions

        1) Used with pathogens transmitted by infectious droplets; droplets larger than 5 microns

        2) Involves contact of conjunctiva or mucous membranes of nose or mouth; happens during coughing, sneezing, talking, or during procedures such as suctioning or bronchoscopy

        3) Private room or with client with same infection but no other infection; wear mask if in close contact

      4) Maintain spatial separation of three feet between infected client and visitors or other clients; visitors wear mask if less than three feet

      5) Door may remain open

      6) Place mask on client if being transported

      7) Examples of disease in category: diphtheria, Group A streptococcus pneumonia, pneumonia or meningitis caused by *N. meningitidis* or H. influenzae Type B, Rubella, mumps, pertussis

   c. Contact precautions

      1) Needed with client care activities that require physical skin-to-skin contact (e.g., turn clients, bathe clients), or occurs between two clients (e.g., hand contact), or occurs by contact with contaminated inanimate objects in client's environment

      2) Private room or with client with same infection but no other infection

      3) Clean, non-sterile gloves for client contact or contact with potentially contaminated areas

      4) Change gloves after client contact with fecal material or wound drainage

      5) Remove gloves before leaving client's environment and wash hands with antimicrobial agent

      6) Wear gown when entering room if clothing will have contact with client, environment surfaces, or if client is incontinent, has diarrhea, an ileostomy, colostomy, or wound drainage

      7) Remove PPE (gown) before leaving room

      8) Use dedicated equipment or clean and disinfect between clients

      9) Example of diseases in category: infection caused by multidrug-resistant organisms (e.g., MRSA and vancomycin-resistant organisms), herpes simplex, herpes zoster, *clostridium difficile,* respiratory syncytial virus, pediculosis, scabies, rotavirus, hepatitis type A

▶ TUBERCULOSIS

A. Assessment

   1. Progressive fatigue, nausea, anorexia, weight loss

   2. Irregular menses

   3. Low-grade fevers over a period of time

   4. Night sweats

   5. Irritability

   6. Cough with mucopurulent sputum, occasionally streaked with blood; chest tightness and a dull aching chest; dyspnea

   7. Diagnostic procedures

     a. Skin testing (see Table 2)

     b. Sputum smear for acid-fast bacilli, induce by respiratory therapy in am and pm; not specific for TB

c. Chest x-ray routinely performed on all persons with positive PPD to detect old and new lesions; tubercles may be seen in lungs

d. QuantiFERON-TB Gold test;results within 24 hours

B. Diagnose

1. *Mycobacterium tuberculosis* (acid-fast gram-positive bacillus) transmitted by airborne droplets; bacillus multiplies in bronchi or alveoli, resulting in pneumonitis; may lie dormant for many years and be reactivated in periods of stress; may spread to other parts of body

2. Risk factors

   a. Close contact with someone who has active tuberculosis

   b. Immunocompromised

   c. IV drug abuser

   d. Persons who live in institutions

   e. Lower socioeconomic group

   f. Immigrants from countries with a high prevalence of tuberculosis (Latin American, Southeast Asia, Africa)

3. Incidence increasing in immigrant populations, poverty areas, elderly, alcoholics, drug abusers, and persons with AIDS

Table 2 TB SKIN TESTING	
TEST	**NURSING CONSIDERATIONS**
Mantoux Test Purified Protein Derivative (PPD)	Given intradermally in the forearm Read in 48–72 hours; measure induration across the forearm (palpable, hardened palpation, not the erythema) Results: 1. 15-mm or greater induration (hard area under the skin) = significant (positive) reaction for clients without certain risk factors. Does not mean that active disease is present, but indicates exposure to TB or the presence of inactive (dormant) disease 2. 10 mm–14.9 mm induration for clients at risk (ex: recent immigrants, injection drug users, children less than 4 years old) 3. 5 mm–9.9 mm for clients with AIDS, on immunosurpressant therapy, transplant clients.
Multiple Puncture Test (Tine)	Read test in 48–72 hours Vesicle formation = positive reaction Screening test only Questionable or positive reactions verified by Mantoux Test

C. Plan/Implementation

1. Notification of state health department; evaluation of contacts

2. Isoniazid prophylaxis—not recommended for those individuals greater than 35 years old who are at low risk because of increased risk of associated toxic hepatitis; persons less than 35 get 6–9 months therapy with isoniazid

   a. Household contacts

   b. Recent converters

   c. Persons under age 20 with positive reaction and inactive TB

   d. Susceptible health care workers

   e. Newly infected persons

   f. Significant skin test reactors with abnormal x-ray studies

   g. Significant skin test reactors up to age 35

3. Chemotherapy—to prevent development of resistant strains, two or three medications are usually administered concurrently; frequently a 6- or 9-month regimen of isoniazid and rifampin; ethambutol and streptomycin may be used initially

4. Isolation for 2–4 weeks (or three negative sputum cultures) after drug therapy is initiated; sent home before this (family already exposed)

5. Teaching

   a. Cover mouth and nose with tissue when coughing, sneezing, laughing; place tissues in plastic bag

   b. wear mask in crowds

   c. Avoid excessive exposure to dust and silicone

   d. Handwashing

   e. Must take full course of medications

   f. Encourage to return to clinic for sputum smears

   g. Good nutrition (increased iron, protein, vitamins B and C)

D. Evaluation

1. Has the spread of TB been prevented?

2. Is the client compliant with the medication regimen?

▶ HEPATITIS

A. Assessment

1. Fatigue

2. Jaundice (icterus), yellow sclera

3. Anorexia, RUQ pain and tenderness, malaise

4. Clay-colored stools, tea-colored urine

5. Pruritus: accumulation of bile salts under the skin

6. Liver function studies: elevated ALT, AST, alkaline phosphatase (ALP), bilirubin

7. Prolonged PT

8. Percutaneous liver biopsy

9. Antibodies to specific virus; e.g., anti-HAV

Table 3 CLASSIFICATIONS OF HEPATITIS				
TYPE	HIGH RISK GROUP	INCUBATION	TRANSMISSION	NURSING CONSIDERATIONS

Hepatitis A (HAV)	Young children
	
	Institutions for custodial care
	
	International travelers to developing countries
		15–50 days	Common in fall, early winter
			
			Fecal–oral
			
			Shellfish from contaminated water
			
			Poor sanitation
			
			Contaminated food handlers
			
			Oral–anal sexual activity
				Survives on hands
				
				Diagnostic tests—
				    Cultured in stool and detected in serum before onset of disease
				
				Prevention–improved sanitation; Hepatitis A vaccine
				
				Treated with gamma globulin early postexposure
				    No preparation of food

Hepatitis B (HBV)	Immigrants from areas of HBV endemicity
	
	Drug addicts
	
	Fetuses from infected mothers
	
	Homosexually active men
	
	Clients on dialysis
	
	Male prisoners
	
	Transfusion recipients
	
	Health care workers
		48–180 days	Blood and body fluids
			
			Parenteral drug abuse
			
			Sexual contact
			
			Hemodialysis
			
			Accidental contaminated needle exposure
			
			Maternal–fetal route
				Diagnostic tests—
				    Hepatitis B surface antigen, anti-HBc, anti-HBe
				    Treatment–Hepatitis B vaccine (Heptavax-B, Recombivax HB),
				    Hepatitis B immune globulin (HBIg) postexposure; interferon alpha-2b; lamivudir
				
				Chronic carriers—frequent; potential for chronicity 5-10%
				
				Complications: cirrhosis; liver cancer

Hepatitis C (HCV)	Persons receiving frequent blood transfusions International travelers Hemophilia clients	14–180 days	Contact with blood and body fluids IV drug users	May be asymptomatic Complications: cirrhosis; liver cancer Great potential for chronicity
Delta or Hepatitis D (HDV)	Drug addicts Concurrent HBV infection	14–56 days	Co-infects with Hepatitis B Close personal contact Parenteral transmission	Diagnostic test–HD Ag in serum

TYPE	HIGH RISK GROUP	INCUBATION	TRANSMISSION	NURSING CONSIDERATIONS
Hepatitis E	Persons living in under-developed countries	15–64 days	Oral-fecal Contaminated water	Resembles Hepatitis A Does not become chronic Usually seen in young adults Seen in travelers from Asia, Africa, Mexico
Toxic Hepatitis	Elderly Drug-induced (INH, diuretics, Tetracycline, carbon tetachloride, Tylenol, ETOH) Alcohol		Noninfectious inflammation of liver	Removal of causative substance Check level of consciousness Encourage fluids

Table 3 CLASSIFICATIONS OF HEPATITIS *(CONTINUED)*

B. Diagnose

1. Acute inflammatory disease of the liver resulting in cell damage from liver cell degeneration and necrosis

2. Potential nursing diagnoses

   a. Fatigue

   b. Physical mobility, impaired

   c. Impaired liver function

   d. Acute pain

   e. Deficient knowledge

3. Classifications (see Table 3)

C. Plan/Implementation

1. Frequent rest periods

2. If clients diagnosed with hepatitis A are diapered or incontinent, contact precautions in addition to standard precautions

3. Contact precautions in addition to standard precautions for clients diagnosed with hepatitis A

4. Diet low in fat, high in calories, carbohydrates and protein; no alcoholic beverages

5. For pruritus—calamine, short clean nails, antihistamines

6. Medications

   a. Vitamin K

   b. Antiviral drugs: interferon and lamivudine

   c. Post-exposure Hepatitis B vaccine

7. Teach client and family

   a. Avoid alcohol and potentially hepatotoxic prescription/OTC medications (particularly aspirin and sedatives)

   b. Balance rest and activity periods

   c. Techniques to prevent spread

    d. Cannot donate blood

    e. Note and report recurrence of signs and symptoms

D. Evaluation

  1. Has permanent liver damage been avoided?

  2. Has client comfort been maintained?

▶ LYME DISEASE

A. Assessment

  1. Stage 1

    a. Rash (erythematous papule that develops into lesion with a clear center) develops at site of tick bite within 2–30 days; concentric rings develop, suggesting a bull's-eye; lesion enlarges quickly

    b. Regional lymphadenopathy

    c. Development of flulike symptoms (malaise, fever, headache, myalgia, stiff neck, arthralgia, conjunctivitis) within one to several months, lasts 7–10 days and may reoccur

  2. Stage 2

    a. Develops within 1–6 months if untreated

    b. Cardiac conduction defects

    c. Neurologic disorders: facial paralysis; paralysis that is not permanent

  3. Stage 3

    a. Arthralgias, enlarged or inflamed joints occur within one to several months after the initial infection, chronic fatigue, cognitive disorders

    b. May persist for several years

B. Diagnose

  1. Multisystem infection transmitted to humans by tick bite

  2. Most common in summer months

C. Plan/Implementation

  1. Prevention

    a. Cover exposed areas when in wooded areas

    b. Check exposed areas for presence of ticks

  2. Nursing care

    a. Administer antibiotics for 3–4 weeks: doxycycline, ceftriaxone, azithromycin during stage 1

    b. Administer IV penicillin G during later stages

D. Evaluation

  1. Has infection been prevented by wearing proper clothing in wooded areas?

  2. If infected, has treatment been initiated early to prevent complications?

▶ **SEXUALLY TRANSMITTED INFECTIONS (STI)**

A. Assessment (see Table 4)

B. Diagnose—potential nursing diagnoses

   1. Health maintenance, altered

   2. Sexual patterns, altered

C. Plan/Implementation (see Table 4)

D. Evaluation

   1. Is client knowledgeable about treatment for STD?

   2. Have sexual contacts been notified and evaluated?

▶ **AIDS**

A. Assessment

   1. HIV positive—presence of HIV in the blood

   2. AIDS—syndrome with CD4/TC counts below 200

   3. Opportunistic infections

     a. *P. jiroveci(P. carinii)* pneumonia

       1) Gradually worsening chest tightness and shortness of breath

       2) Persistent, dry, nonproductive cough, rales

       3) Dyspnea and tachypnea

       4) Low-grade/high fever

       5) Progressive hypoxemia and cyanosis

     b. *C. albicans* stomatitis or esophagitis

       1) Changes in taste sensation

       2) Difficulty swallowing

       3) Retrosternal pain

       4) White exudate and inflammation of mouth and back of throat

Table 4 SEXUALLY TRANSMITTED INFECTIONS				
TYPE	SYMPTOMS	DIAGNOSTIC TESTS	TRANSMISSION AND INCUBATION	NURSING CONSIDERATIONS
Syphilis	Stage 1: painless chancre disappears within 4 weeks Stage 2: copper-colored rash on palms and soles; low-grade fever Stage 3: cardiac and CNS dysfunction	VDRL, RPR, FTA-ABS, MHA-TP (to confirm syphilis when VDRL and RPR are positive) Dark Field Microscopic examination	Mucous membrane or skin; congenital; kissing, sexual contact 10-90 days	Prevention—condoms Treat with penicillin G IM For PCN allergy—erythromycin for 10–15 days Ceftriaxone and tetracyclines (nonpregnant females) Retest for cure Abstinence from sexual activity until treatment complete Reportable disease
Gonorrhea	Thick discharge from vagina or urethra Frequently asymptomatic in females If female has symptoms, usually has purulent discharge, dysuria, and dyspareunia (painful intercourse) Symptoms in male include painful urination and a yellow-green discharge	Culture of discharge from cervix or urethra Positive results for other STD diagnostic tests	Mucous membrane or skin; congenital; vaginal, orogenital, anogenital sexual activity 2–7 days	IM ceftriaxone 1 time and PO doxycyline BID for 1 week; azithromycin IM aqueous penicillin with PO probenecid (to delay penicillin urinary excretion) PO azithromycin or doxycycline is used to treat chlamydia, which coexists in 45% of cases Spectinomycin if allergy to ceftriaxone Monitor for complications, pelvic inflammatory disease
Genital Herpes (HSV-2)	Painful vesicular genital lesions Difficulty voiding Recurrence in times of stress, infection, menses	Direct examination of cells HSV antibodies	Mucous membrane or skin; congenital Virus can survive on objects such as towels 3–14 days	Acyclovir (not cure) Emotional support Sitz baths Local medication Client must notify sexual contacts Monitor Pap smears on regular basis—increased incidence of cancer of cervix Precautions about vaginal delivery

Table 4 SEXUALLY TRANSMITTED INFECTIONS *(CONTINUED)*				
TYPE	SYMPTOMS	DIAGNOSTIC TESTS	TRANSMISSION AND INCUBATION	NURSING CONSIDERATIONS
Chlamydia	Men—dysuria, frequent urination, watery discharge Women—may be asymptomatic, thick discharge with acrid odor, pelvic pain, yellow-colored discharge; painful menses	Direct examination of cells Enzyme-linked ELISA	Mucous membrane; sexual contact 1–3 weeks	Notification of contacts May cause sterility Treat with azithromycin, doxycycline, erythromycin
Condylomata acuminata (genital warts)	Initially single, small papillary lesion spreads into large cauliflowerlike cluster on perineum and/or vagina or penis; may be itching/burning	Direct exam Biopsy HPV	Majority due to human papilloma virus (HPV) Mucous membrane; sexual contact; congenital 1–3 months	Curettage, cryotherapy with liquid nitrogen or podophyllin resin Kerotolytic medications Avoid intimate sexual contact until lesions are healed Strong association with incidence of genital dysplasia and cervical carcinoma Atypical, pigmented, or persistent warts should be biopsied Notify contacts

   c. *C. neoformans*—severe debilitating meningitis

     1) Fever, headache, blurred version

     2) Nausea and vomiting

     3) Stiff neck, mental status changes, seizures

   d. Cytomegalovirus (CMV)—significant factor in morbidity and mortality

     1) Fever, malaise

     2) Weight loss, fatigue

     3) Lymphadenopathy

     4) Retinochoroiditis characterized by inflammation and hemorrhage

     5) Visual impairment

     6) Colitis, encephalitis, pneumonitis

     7) Adrenalitis, hepatitis, disseminated infection

   e. Kaposi's sarcoma—most common malignancy

     1) Small purplish-brown, nonpainful, nonpruritic palpable lesions occurring on any part of the body

     2) Most commonly seen on the skin

     3) Diagnosed by biopsy

 4. Diagnostic tests

    a. Positive HIV antibody on enzyme-linked immunosorbent assay (ELISA) and confirmed by Western blot assay or indirect immunoflourescence assay (IFA)

    b. Viral load testing, CD4 to CD8 ratio, antigen assays

    c. Radioimmunoprecipitation assay (RIPA)

    d. CBC reveals leukopenia with serious lymphopenia, anemia, thrombocytopenia

B. Diagnose

  1. AIDS (acquired immunodeficiency syndrome)—a syndrome distinguished by serious deficits in cellular immune function associated with positive human immunodeficiency virus (HIV); evidenced clinically by development of opportunistic infections (e.g. *Pneumocystis jiroveci pneumonia*, Candida albicans, cytomegalovirus), enteric pathogens, and malignancies (most commonly Kaposi's sarcoma)

    a. High-risk groups

      1) Homosexual/bisexual men, especially with multiple partners

      2) Intravenous drug abusers

      3) Hemophiliacs via contaminated blood products

      4) Blood transfusion recipients prior to 1985

      5) Heterosexual partners of infected persons

      6) Children of infected women/in utero or at birth

    b. Transmission—contaminated blood or body fluids, sharing IV drug needles, sexual contact, transplacental and possibly through breast milk

    c. Time from exposure to symptom manifestation may be prolonged (10–12 years)

Table 5 NURSING CARE OF A CLIENT WITH ACQUIRED IMMUNE DEFICIENCY SYNDROME	
PROBLEM	**NURSING CONSIDERATIONS**
Fatigue	Provide restful environment Assist with personal care Monitor tolerance for visitors
Pain	Give meds as appropriate Assess level of pain
Disease susceptibility	Implement infection control precautions Handwashing on entering and leaving room Monitor for oral infections and meningitis Give antibiotics as ordered
Respiratory distress	Monitor vital signs, breath sounds Give bronchodilators and antibiotics as ordered Suction and maintain O_2 as ordered Monitor for symptoms of secondary infections

Table 5 NURSING CARE OF A CLIENT WITH ACQUIRED IMMUNE DEFICIENCY SYNDROME *(CONTINUED)*	
PROBLEM	**NURSING CONSIDERATIONS**
Anxiety, depression	Use tact, sensitivity in gathering personal data
	Encourage expression of feelings
	Respect client's own limits in ability to discuss problems
Anorexia, diarrhea	Monitor weight
	Encourage nutritional supplements
	Assess hydration

C. Plan/Implementation

   1. Preventive measures

      a. Avoidance of IV drug use (needle-sharing)

      b. Precautions regarding sexual patterns—sex education, condoms, avoid multiple partners

      c. Use standard precautions

   2. Nursing care (see Table 5)

      a. No effective cure; antiviral medications (e.g., Zidovudine, Aciclovir) are being used to slow progression of symptoms

      b. Treatment specific to the presenting condition

         1) Kaposi's sarcoma—local radiation (palliative), single agent/combination chemotherapy

         2) Fungal infections—nystatin swish and swallow, clotrimazole oral solution, amphotericin B with/without flucytosine

         3) Viral infections—Acyclovir, Ganciclovir

      c. Contact precautions in addition to standard precautions

      d. Nutrition—high protein and calories

      e. Symptomatic relief—comfort measures

      f. Maintain confidentiality

      g. Provide support

         1) Client and family coping—identify support systems

         2) Minimize social isolation—no isolation precautions are needed to enter room to talk to client, take VS, administer PO medications

         3) Encourage verbalization of feelings

      h. Client client/family discharge teaching

         1) Behaviors to prevent transmission—safe sex, not sharing toothbrushes, razors, and other potentially blood- contaminated objects

         2) Measures to prevent infections—good nutrition, hygiene, rest, skin and mouth care, avoid crowds

D. Evaluation

   1. Has client comfort been maintained?

   2. Is client knowledgeable about medication regimen?

▶ **POISON CONTROL**

A. Assessment

1. Airway, breathing, circulation (ABC)—treat the client first, then the poison

2. Identify poison—amount ingested, time of ingestion; save vomitus

3. Diagnostics

   a. Urine and serum analysis

   b. Long-bone x-rays if lead deposits suspected

   c. CAT scan, EEG

Table 6 TEACHING PREVENTION OF ACCIDENTAL POISONING IN CHILDREN	
ACTION	**RATIONALE**
Proper storage—locked cabinets	Once child can crawl, can investigate cabinets and ingest contents of bottles
Never take medicine in front of children	Children are interested in anything their parents take and will mimic taking medicine
Never leave medication in purse, on table, or on kitchen counter	Children will investigate area and ingest bottle contents
Never refer to medicine as candy	Increases interest in taking medicine when unsupervised
Leave medicines, cleaning supplies in original containers	Pill boxes, soda bottles increase attractiveness and inhibit identification of substance should poisoning occur
Provide activities and play materials for children	Encourages child's interest without endangering him/her
Teach need for supervision of small children	Small children cannot foresee potential harm and need protection

B. Diagnose—potential nursing diagnoses

1. Injury, risk for

2. Health maintenance, altered

C. Plan/Implementation

1. Prevention—most toxic ingestions are acute (see Table 6)

   a. Child-proofing—store all potentially poisonous substances in locked out-of-reach area

   b. Increased awareness of precipitating factors

      1) Growth and development characteristics—under/overestimating the capabilities of the child

      2) Changes in household routine

      3) Conditions that increase emotional tension of family members

2. Instructions for caretaker in case of suspected poison ingestion

   a. Recognize signs and symptoms of accidental poisoning—change in child's appearance/behavior; presence of unusual substances in child's mouth, hands, play area; burns, blisters and/or suspicious odor around child's mouth; open/empty containers in child's possession

   b. Initiate steps to stop exposure

   c. Call Poison Control Center—be prepared to provide information

     1) Substance—name, time, amount, route

     2) Child—condition, age, weight

   d. Poison Control Center (PCC) will advise to begin treatment at home or to bring child to an emergency facility

   e. Syrup of Ipecac is no longer recommended for treatment at home; Any Ipecac in the home should be disposed of safely

   f. No emetic or other substance should be given at home without consultation with the PCC or health care provider

   g. Save any substance, vomitus, stool, urine

   h. Induce vomiting only if indicated by Poison Control Center or health care provider

   i. Contraindications to inducing vomiting

     1) When child is in danger of aspiration—decreased level of consciousness, severe shock, seizure(s), diminished gag reflex

     2) When substance is petroleum distillate (lighter fluid, kerosene, paint remover) because of increased risk of aspiration pneumonia, or strong corrosive (acid/alkali drain cleaner), which may redamage esophagus and pharynx

   j. General considerations

     1) Water may be used to dilute the toxin; avoid giving large amounts of fluids when medication has been ingested because this may accelerate gastric emptying and speed drug absorption

     2) Milk may delay vomiting

     3) Do not attempt to neutralize a strong acid/alkali because this may cause a heat-producing reaction that can burn tissue

     4) There are only a few specific antidotes (physiologic antagonist reversing effect); there is no universal antidote

3. Emergency care in a health care facility

   a. Basic life support

     1) Respiratory—intubate if comatose, seizing, or no gag reflex; frequent blood gases

     2) Circulation

       a) IV fluids; maintain fluid and electrolyte balance

       b) Cardiac monitor—essential for comatose child and with tricyclic antidepressant or phenothiazine ingestion

   b. Gastric lavage and aspiration—client is intubated and positioned head down and on left side; large oro/nasogastrictube inserted and repeated irrigations of normal saline instilleduntil clear; not more than 10 ml/kg; must be done within 60 minutes

   c. Activated charcoal—absorbs compounds, forming a non-absorbable complex; 5–10 g for each g of toxin

     1) Give within 30 minutes of ingestion and after emetic

     2) Mix with water to make a syrup; given PO or via gastric tube

4. Hasten elimination
   a. Diuretics—for substances eliminated by kidneys
   b. Chelation—heavy metals (e.g., mercury, lead, and arsenic) are not readily eliminated from body; progressive buildup leads to toxicity; a chelating agent binds with the heavy metal, forming a complex that can be eliminated by kidneys, peritoneal hemodialysis (e.g. deferoxamine, dimercaprol, calcium EDTA)

5. Prevent recurrence—crisis intervention with nonjudgmental approach; acknowledge difficulty in maintaining constant supervision; explore contributory factors; discuss and educate about growth and development influences as well as passive (child restraint closures) and active safety measures

D. Evaluation

1. Has child's safety been maintained?

2. Are parents knowledgeable about ways to prevent accidental poisoning?

▶ ASPIRIN (SALICYLATE) POISONING

A. Assessment

1. Tinnitus, nausea, sweating, dizziness, headache

2. Change in mental status

3. Increased temperature, hyperventilation (respiratory alkalosis)

4. Later, metabolic acidosis, and respiratory acidosis, bleeding, and hypovolemia

B. Diagnose

1. Toxicity begins at doses of 150–200 mg/kg; 4 grams may be fatal to child
   a. Altered acid–base balance (respiratory alkalosis) due to increased respiratory rate
   b. Increased metabolism causes greater O_2 consumption, CO_2 and heat production
   c. Metabolic acidosis results in hypokalemia, dehydration, and kidney failure
   d. May result in decreased prothrombin formation and decreased platelet aggregation, causing bleeding

C. Plan/Implementation

1. Induce vomiting; initiate gastric lavage with activated charcoal

2. Monitor vital signs and laboratory values

3. Maintain IV hydration and electrolyte replacement; monitor I and O, skin turgor, fontanels, urinary specific gravity

4. Reduce temperature—tepid water baths or hypothermia blankets; prone to seizures

5. Vitamin K, if needed, for bleeding disorder; guaiac of vomitus/stools

6. IV sodium bicarbonate enhances excretion

D. Evaluation

1. Are the client's vital signs stable?

2. Is the client's acid–base balance restored?

► ACETAMINOPHEN POISONING

A. Assessment

1. First 2 hours, nausea and vomiting, sweating, pallor, hypothermia, slow-weak pulse

2. Followed by latent period (1–1.5 days) when symptoms abate

3. If no treatment, hepatic involvement occurs (may last up to 1 week) with RUQ pain, jaundice, confusion, stupor, coagulation abnormalities

4. Diagnostic tests—serum acetaminophen levels at least 4 hours after ingestion; liver function tests AST, ALT, and kidney function tests (creatinine, BUN)—change in renal and liver function is a late sign

B. Diagnose

1. Toxicity begins at 150 mg/kg

2. Major risk is hepatic necrosis

C. Plan/Implementation

1. Induce vomiting

2. *N*-Acetylcysteine–specific antidote; most effective in 8–10 hours; must be given within 24 hours; given PO every 4 hours × 72 hours or IV × 3 doses

3. Maintain hydration; monitor output

4. Monitor liver and kidney function

D. Evaluation

1. Have liver and kidney damage been prevented?

2. Has the client's hydration been maintained?

► LEAD TOXICITY (PLUMBISM)

A. Assessment

1. Physical symptoms

   a. Irritability

   b. Sleepiness

   c. Nausea, vomiting, abdominal pain, poor appetite

   d. Constipation

   e. Decreased activity

   f. Increased intracranial pressure (e.g., seizures and motor dysfunction)

2. Environmental sources

   a. Flaking, lead-based paint (primary source)

   b. Crumbling plaster

   c. Odor of lead-based gasoline

   d. Pottery with lead glaze

   e. Lead solder in pipes

3. Diagnostic tests

   a. Blood lead level less than or equal to 9 micrograms per deciliter is normal

   b. Erythrocyte protoporphyrin (EP) level

   c. CBC—anemia

    d. X-rays (long bone/GI)—may show radiopaque material, "lead lines"

B. Diagnose

1. Child—practice of pica (habitual and compulsive ingestion of nonfood substances); children absorb more lead than adults; paint chips taste sweet

2. Pathology—lead is slowly excreted by kidneys and GI tract; stored in inert form in long bones; chronic ingestion affects many body systems

    a. Hematological—blocks formation of hemoglobin, leading to microcytic anemia (initial sign) and increased erythrocyte protoporphyrin (EP)

    b. Renal—toxic to kidney tubules, allowing an abnormal excretion of protein, glucose, amino acids, phosphates

    c. CNS—increases membrane permeability, resulting in fluid shifts into brain tissue, cell ischemia, and destruction causing neurological and intellectual deficiencies with low-dose exposure; with high-dose exposure, intellectual delay, convulsions, and death (lead encephalopathy)

C. Plan/Implementation

1. Chelating agent—promotes lead excretion in urine and stool (dimercaprol, calcium disodium, EDTA); succimer, deferoxamine

    a. Maintain hydration

    b. Identify sources of lead and institute deleading procedures; involve local housing authorities as needed

    c. Instruct parents about supervision for pica and ways to encourage other activities for the child

D. Evaluation

1. Is a referral to social service/public health agency needed?

2. Is assistance with obtaining child care necessary?

▶ HAZARDS AND HAZARDOUS WASTE

A. Types of hazards

1. Chemical hazards—dusts, gases, fumes, mists

2. Psychophysiologic hazards—stress associated with job demands (e.g., rotating shifts, overtime, violence in the workplace)

3. Biologic hazards—exposure to infectious agents (e.g., TB, hepatitis B)

4. Ergonomic hazards—imbalance between individual and equipment, such as repetitive actions leading to carpal tunnel syndrome (ergonomics: study of interaction of human body with use of mechanical and electrical machines)

5. Safety hazards—precautions with equipment, fire safety, electrical systems

6. Hazardous materials (e.g., explosion from stored chlorine used for private swimming pool, radioisotope accident in nuclear medicine)

    a. Exposure—presence of hazardous waste in environment

    b. OSHA (Federal Occupational Safety and Health Administration) mandates acceptable levels of exposure to chemicals

    c. Dose—amount of substance inhaled, ingested, absorbed through skin or eyes

d. When there is a problem during transportation of chemical materials, information is provided from a central source; advises rescue and health care workers about the substance, its effect, and how to treat exposure

B. Hazardous materials causing immediate threat to life; client treated and then decontaminated

1. Chlorine
2. Cyanide
3. Ammonia
4. Phosgene
5. Hydrogen sulfide
6. Organophosphate insecticides
7. Nitrogen dioxide

C. Hazardous materials with cancer-causing potential; client decontaminated and then treated

1. Polychlorinated biphenyls

D. Ethical issues

1. Autonomy

   a. Workers have right to know about hazardous chemicals and materials in the workplace and community so that they can take appropriate action to protect themselves

   b. Workers have right to know critical health and safety information

   c. Information must be presented so that it is tailored to meet the needs of the work force, taking into account language and literacy

2. Beneficence (doing good)

   a. Involvement of worker groups in planning hazard communication training and designing written hazardous awareness materials;should integrate adult learning theory principles

E. Nursing care

1. Before treatment, determine

   a. Does chemical pose threat to caregivers?

   b. If yes, has client been decontaminated?

   c. If chemical poses no threat or decontamination has been completed,client can be treated

   d. If chemical poses threat and client has not been decontaminated but has immediate life-threatening condition, health care workers put on protective garments and provide care to stabilize client; environment is sealed to prevent spread of chemical

2. Goals

   a. Decontaminate individual
   b. Prevent spread of contamination
   c. Clean and remove contaminated water and waste
   d. Monitor personnel exposed

3. Preparation

   a. Cover floor from entrance to treatment room

  b. Seal off air vents

  c. Rope off designated area

  d. Security keeps nonessential personnel away from area

  e. Place needed equipment in treatment room

  f. Place equipment that may be needed outside treatment room

  g. Remove extraneous supplies from treatment room

4. Decontamination procedure

  a. Client walks, is wheeled, or is placed on a clean stretcher covered in plastic

  b. Client is transported over protected floor to treatment room

  c. Client is taken to decontamination shower accompanied by health care worker wearing protective clothing and a respirator (if needed)

  d. Client's clothing removed and placed in hazard bag (clothing contains 95% of contamination)

  e. Valuables placed in separate bag for later decontamination

  f. Client washes with soap and water, paying particular attention to body orifices (especially nostrils) and hairy areas

  g. Client shampoos hair

  h. Client's wounds are irrigated

  i. Waste water collected in container if there is no containment unit for shower

  j. If client was exposed to radiation, is then scanned with radiation detector meter with special attention to body orifices and hairy areas

  k. Floor covering is removed and placed in hazard bag

  l. Health care workers remove and bag protective clothing

  m. After shower, client puts on clean clothes, and steps onto clean floor

  n. Medical evaluation is then started

5. Decontamination procedure for client requiring care before decontamination

  a. Treatment room is considered to be contaminated

  b. Designated health care worker stands at door to transcribe documentation (medical records not taken into room) and get necessary equipment

  c. Health care workers may not enter or leave room without performing special procedures

▶ ACCIDENT PREVENTION

A. Newborn infant

1. Don't smoke around infants, increases risk of upper respiratory tract infections

2. Don't leave infant unattended in a high place or unstrapped in a safety seat

3. Use rear-facing car safety seat

4. Make sure furniture is free of lead-based paint

5. Crib slats should be no further apart than 2 3/8"; the mattress should be tight-fitting

6. Place infant flat on back after eating and for sleeping

B. 2 months old

1. Don't hold infant while smoking or drinking hot liquid

2. Set water heater at 120–130°F; test bath water temperature with inner aspect of the wrist before immersing infant

C. 4 months old

1. Keep small objects and small pieces of food out of infant's reach

2. Don't use teething biscuits—they become small and can obstruct airway

3. Teach older siblings/children not to give infant small things

D. 6 months old

1. Child-proof the home, especially the kitchen and bathroom; remove all dangerous items or place out of reach

2. Use safety gates at bottom/top of stairs; use drawer safety latches, plug fillers

3. Keep poison control number on phone; use as needed

E. 9 months old

1. Use nonskid rugs, socks with nonskid strips, nonskid strips in bathtub

2. Keep wastebaskets covered or out of reach

3. Pad sharp edges of furniture

4. Never leave child unattended near water or in bathtub

5. Don't use electrical appliances near water

F. 1 to 3 years old

1. Don't use toys with small pieces or give food with small pieces (peanuts, hard candy and a responsible adult present when near water

2. Hold child's hand when walking near the street

3. Encourage the child to sit down while eating

4. Secure all medications in locked area; have Poison Control number available

5. Turn pot handles toward the back of the stove and cover all electrical outlets

6. Use rear-facing car seat until child reaches height and weight allowed by car safety seat manufacturers; after age 2 years or has outgrown a rear-facing car seat, use forward-facing car seat with harness as long as possible

G. 3 to 6 years old

1. Use bicycle helmet; ride bicycle on right-hand side of the road or on sidewalk; make sure the bicycle is the correct size, feet should touch the ground when sitting on the bicycle seat

2. Teach child not to eat things from outside (e.g., mushrooms) until checked by parents

3. Look both ways before crossing street

4. If weight or height above forward-facing limit, use belt-positioning booster seat until seat belt fits properly

H. 6 to 11 years old

1. Obey traffic signals while on bike; use reflectors on bike; wear light clothing

2. When playing group sports look for teams divided by size and maturation, not by age; use protective equipment; helmet while bike riding, skateboarding or rollerblading

I. Adolescent

1. Teach appropriate ways to deal with anger and threats

2. Teach safety for swimming and diving

3. Use car safety restraint; lap and seat belts

4. Teach hazards of drinking and driving

J. Adult

1. Use car safety restraint

2. Teach responsible behavior to reduce sexually transmitted diseases and alcohol-related accidents

3. Suicide prevention

4. Handgun control and safety

5. Motorcycle helmet use

6. Smoke and carbon monoxide detector use; fire extinguisher use

K. Elderly

1. At risk for injuries

   a. Muscle weakness

   b. Changes in balance

   c. Gait abnormalities

   d. Slowed reaction time

   e. Use of medications

   f. Chronic medical conditions (e.g., Parkinson's disease)

   g. Changes in vision, hearing, smell

2. Remove throws rugs, door thresholds; make sure floors are smooth and nonslip

3. Clear pathways of furniture

4. Use solid chairs with arm rests

5. Provide good lighting with accessible switches; use night light

6. Adapt kitchen and bathroom; use raised toilet seat, grab bars

7. Use cordless phone

8. Teach correct way to go up and down stairs; use hand rail, don't limit vision by carrying large load

9. Don't wear long gowns or robes or pants with flowing material

10. Wear sturdy, comfortable, nonskid shoes; don't wear flimsy slippers

11. Keep pet feeding dishes out of main walkway

12. Maintain mobility through exercise and assistive devices

▶ DISASTER PLANNING

A. Assessment—greatest good for the greatest number of people

1. Resources used for clients with strongest probability of survival

2. Nurses make tough decisions about which order clients will be seen

3. Decisions are based on assessment of injuries and knowledge of probable outcomes

4. Use Airway, Breathing, Circulation, neurologic Dysfunction (ABCDs) to prioritize

B. Planning

1. Triage under usual conditions

   a. Emergent—immediate threat to life

   b. Urgent—major injuries requiring immediate treatment

   c. Nonurgent—minor injuries that do not require immediate treatment

2. Triage with mass casualties

   a. Red—unstable clients who require immediate care to save life (e.g., occluded airway, active hemorrhaging); first category seen

   b. Yellow—stable clients who can wait 30–60 minutes for treatment (e.g., moderate burn, eye injury); second category to be seen

   c. Green—stable clients who can wait longer to be treated (e.g., "walking wounded"); third category to be seen

   d. Black—unstable clients having massive injuries that will probably prove fatal (e.g., massive body trauma); last category to be treated; supportive and comfort measures provided (e.g., pain control)

   e. DOA (dead on arrival)

C. Implementation

1. Care standardized according to standing orders

   a. IV fluids

   b. Lab tests

   c. Diagnostic procedures

   d. Medications (e.g., analgesics, tetanus prophylaxis, antibiotics)

2. Specialists become "generalists"

3. Nurses may have expanded responsibilities (e.g., suturing, surgical airway)

4. Use of diagnostic procedures may be limited (e.g., CT scans) with multiple trauma

5. Use of hospital resources determined by designated disaster medical officer

6. Areas of hospital are used as needed for treatment

7. Resources are obtained to provide emotional and spiritual care to clients and families

8. Person is designated to deal with media and traffic control

9. Measures are implemented to track unidentified clients

10. Procedures for handling evidence from disaster may be implemented

11. Hospitals practice disaster drills several times a year

D. Evaluation

1. Have the clients been cared for in an orderly fashion?

2. Have clients' physical needs been met?

▶ **BIOTERRORISM**

Table 7 BIOTERRORISM			
TYPE	SYMPTOMS	TRANSMISSION AND INCUBATION	NURSING CONSIDERATIONS
Anthrax Cutaneous	1–7 days after exposure: itching with small papule or vesicle 2 days after lesion formation: enlarged painless lesion with necrotic center 7–10 days after lesion formation: black eschar forms; sloughs after 12th day	Skin contact 1–7 days No person-to-person transmission High risk: exposure to contaminated animal hides, veterinarians, personnel who handle contaminated materials, military	Standard precautions Decontamination • Bag clothes in labeled, plastic bags • Do not agitate clothes • Instruct client to shower thoroughly with soap and water and shampoo hair • Wear gloves, gown, and respiratory protection • Decontaminate surfaces with bleach solution (one-part household bleach to nine-parts water) • Administer oral fluoroquinolones for post-exposure prophylaxis • Administer doxycycline, erythromycin, ciprofloxacin
Anthrax Inhalation	Initial: sore throat, mild fever, muscles aches, malaise followed by possible brief improvement 2–3 days later: abrupt onset of respiratory failure and shock, fever, hemorrhagic meningitis	Aerosolized spores 1–7 days up to 60 days No person-to-person transmission	Standard precautions Ventilator support for respiratory therapy IV and PO ciprofloxacin and doxycycline
Botulism	Drooping eyelids, weakened jaw clench, dysphasia, blurred vision, symmetric descending weakness, 12–72 hours after exposure respiratory dysfunction; may cause death	Contaminated food 12–36 hours Aerosol inhalation 24–72 hours No person-to-person transmission	Standard precautions Contact health department and Centers for Disease Control and Prevention (CDC) if suspicion of single case Supportive care
Plague Bubonic	Fever, headache, general illness, painful, swollen regional lymph nodes (bubo); develops into septicemia and plague pneumonia	Infected rodent to man by infected fleas 2–8 days	Standard precautions for treatment of bubo; Droplet precautions for plague pneumonia Administer antibiotics Apply insecticides to kill fleas, control rat population

Table 7 BIOTERRORISM *(CONTINUED)*			
TYPE	**SYMPTOMS**	**TRANSMISSION AND INCUBATION**	**NURSING CONSIDERATIONS**
Pneumonic Plague	2–4 days after exposure, fever, productive cough containing infectious particles, chest pain, hemoptysis, bronchopneumonia, rapid shock, and death	Aerosolized inhalation 1–3 days Person-to-person transmission occurs through large aerosol droplets	Droplet precautions until 72 hours of antibiotic therapy Place in private room or cohort with clients with same diagnosis Administer antibiotics: Streptomycin, ciprofloxacin, doxycycline Decontamination • Bag clothes in labeled, plastic bags • Do not agitate clothes • Instruct client to shower thoroughly with soap and water and shampoo hair • Wear gloves, gown, and respiratory protection • Decontaminate surfaces with bleach solution (one-part household bleach to nine-parts water)
Smallpox	Occur in 10–17 days; fever, myalgia synchronous onset of rash that is most prominent on face and extremities (palms and soles included), rash scabs over in 1–2 weeks	Airborne and droplet exposure, contact with skin lesions Client infectious until scabs separate (about 3 weeks)	Airborne, contact, and standard precautions place in private room with door closed, monitored negative air pressure, 6–12 air exchanges per hour Decontaminate items contaminated by infectious lesions using contact precautions; single case is considered a public health emergency If exposed, administer vaccination within 3 days of contact; vaccination does not give lifelong immunity

Note: The plagues (bubonic and pneumonic) are included together.

Chapter 8

HEALTH PROMOTION AND MAINTENANCE

Units

1. **Growth and Development**

2. **Childbearing—Normal**

3. **Childbearing—Maternal Complications**

4. **Childbearing—Neonatal Normal**

5. **Neonatal Complications**

6. **Reproduction**

7. **Prevention and Early Detection of Disease**

GROWTH AND DEVELOPMENT Unit 1

▶ HEALTH MAINTENANCE

A. Assessment

1. Factors influencing growth and development
   a. Genetic, hereditary, prenatal
   b. Environmental
      1) Family, cultural
      2) Socioeconomic and culture
      3) Living environment
   c. Gender
   d. Parental
   e. Stress
   f. Relationships and attachments
   g. Physical, nutrition and emotional health (see Table 1)

2. Expected stages of play development
   a. Age characteristics
      1) Exploratory—(holding toys: age 0–1 yr)
      2) Toys as adult tools—(imitation: age 1–7 yr)
      3) Games and hobbies (age 8–12 yr)
   b. Social characteristics
      1) Solitary play—alone, but enjoys presence of others, interest centered on own activity (infancy)
      2) Parallel play—plays alongside, not with, another; characteristic of toddlers, but can occur in other age groups (toddler)
      3) Associative play—no group goal; often follows a leader (preschool)
      4) Cooperative play—organized, rules, leader/follower relationship established (school-age)

3. Physical measurements compared with expected norms
   a. Height
   b. Weight
   c. Head circumference
   d. Chest circumference

4. Screening tests
   a. Denver II—evaluates children from birth to 6 years in 4 skill areas: personal–social, fine motor, language, gross motor
      1) Age adjusted for prematurity by subtracting the number of months preterm
      2) Questionable value in testing children of minority/ethnic groups
   b. Stanford-Binet
   c. I.Q. related to genetic potentialities and environment; intelligence tests used to determine I.Q.; mental age × 100 = I.Q./chronological age

KAPLAN) NURSING   453

Table 1 OVERVIEW OF ERIKSON'S DEVELOPMENTAL TASKS THROUGHOUT THE LIFE SPAN				
AGE	STAGE	ERIKSON'S TASK	POSITIVE OUTCOME	NEGATIVE OUTCOME
Birth to 1 year	Infancy	Trust vs. mistrust	Trusts self and others	Demonstrates an inability to trust; withdrawal, isolation
1 year to 3 yrs	Toddler	Autonomy vs. shame and doubt	Exercises self-control and influences the environment directly	Demonstrates defiance and negativism
3 to 6 yrs	Preschool	Initiative vs. guilt	Begins to evaluate own behavior; learns limits on influence in the environment	Demonstrates fearful, pessimistic behaviors; lacks self-confidence
6 to 12 yrs	School-age	Industry vs. inferiority	Develops a sense of confidence; uses creative energies to influence the environment	Demonstrates feelings of inadequacy, mediocrity, and self-doubt
12 to 20 yrs	Adolescence	Identity vs. role diffusion	Develops a coherent sense of self; plans for a future of work/education	Demonstrates inability to develop personal and vocational identity
20 to 40 yrs	Young adulthood	Intimacy vs. isolation	Develops connections to work and intimate relationships	Demonstrates an avoidance of intimacy and vocational career commitments
40 to 65 yrs	Middle adulthood	Generativity vs. stagnation	Involved with established family; expands personal creativity and produc-tivity	Demonstrates lack of interests, commitments Preoccupation with self-centered concerns
65+ yrs	Late adulthood	Integrity vs. despair	Identification of life as meaningful	Demonstrates fear of death; life lacks meaning

B. Diagnose
1. Potential nursing diagnoses
   a. Knowledge deficit
   b. Decreased growth
   c. Decreased development
   d. Changes in growth and development pattern
2. Process—sequence is orderly and predictable; rate tends to be variable within (more quickly/slowly) and between (earlier/later) individuals
3. Growth—increase in size (height and weight); tends to be cyclical, more rapid *in utero*, during infancy, and adolescence

4. Development—maturation of physiological and psychosocial systems to more complex state
   a. Developmental tasks—skills and competencies associated with each developmental stage that have an effect on subsequent stages of development
   b. Developmental milestone—standard of reference to compare the child's behavior at specific ages
   c. Developmental delay(s)—variable of development that lags behind the range at a given age
5. Muscular coordination and control—proceeds in head-to-toe (cephalocaudal), trunk-to-periphery (proximodistal), gross-to-fine developmental pattern

C. Plan/Implementation
1. Establish a therapeutic relationship
2. Identify age-appropriate behavioral milestones
3. Educate caregivers on proper health care for children
   a. Health care provider visits, immunization schedules, childhood diseases
   b. Review diet and exercise patterns
4. Observe for alterations of parenting
   a. Behavior patterns of parents and child
   b. Identify healthy relationships and unhealthy relationships, e.g., failure to thrive, indications of child abuse
5. Observe and document screening
6. Promote socialization, activity, play
   a. Promote improved social skills and decreased social isolation
   b. Provide simple activities or tasks to promote self-esteem
7. Meet basic health and safety needs (hygienic, nutritional, rest and exercise)
8. Recognize spans and ranges of normalcy

D. Evaluation
1. Are all aspects of child's growth and development within normal limits for individual child?
2. Do parents have an understanding of child's developmental needs?
3. Have factors negatively impacting child's growth and development been eliminated or lessened?

▶ INFANCY—BIRTH TO 12 MONTHS

A. Assessment (see Table 2)

1. Physical growth and development (see Table 2)

2. Developmental milestones (see Table 2)

3. Attachment established during first year

B. Diagnose

1. Potential nursing diagnoses

   a. Injury, risk for

   b. Parenting, risk for altered

2. Potential problems in infancy

   a. Injury

   b. Failure to thrive

   c. Development delay

C. Plan/Implementation

1. Screen infants routinely for growth and development

2. Evaluate infant/parent relationships during feeding activities

3. Begin anticipatory guidance activities with parents

4. Select age-appropriate toys (see Table 2)

5. Introduce complementary foods

   a. Introduce only one food at a time for each two-week period

   b. Least allergenic foods are usually given in first half of the first year (iron-fortified rice cereal); more allergenic foods, (e.g., egg, orange juice) are offered in last half of first year; usual order: cereal, fruits, vegetables, potatoes, meat, egg, orange juice

6. Document age-appropriate social skills, social attachments, reaction to separation

   a. Phases of separation anxiety

      1) Protest—cries/screams for parents; inconsolable by others

      2) Despair—crying ends; less active; disinterested in food/play; clutches "security" object if available

      3) Denial—appears adjusted; evidences interest in environment; ignores parent when he/she returns; resigned, not contented

Table 2 INFANT GROWTH AND DEVELOPMENT	
1 MONTH	**7 MONTH**
Head sags Early crawling movements	Sits for short periods using hands for support Grasps toy with hand (partially successful) Fear of strangers begins to appear Lability of mood (abrupt mood shifts)
2 MONTH	**8 MONTH**
Closing of posterior fontanelle Diminished tonic neck and Moro reflexes Able to turn from side to back Eyes begin to follow a moving object Social smile first appears	Anxiety with strangers
3 MONTH	**9 MONTH**
Can bring objects to mouth at will Head held erect, steady Binocular vision Smiles in mother's presence Laughs audibly	Elevates self to sitting position Rudimentary imitative expression Responds to parental anger Expressions like "dada" may be heard
4 MONTH	**10 MONTH**
Appearance of thumb apposition Absent tonic neck reflex Evidence of pleasure in social contact Drooling Moro reflex absent after 3–4 mo	Crawls well Pulls self to standing position with support Brings hands together Vocalizes one or two words
5 MONTH	**11 MONTH**
Birth weight usually doubled Takes objects presented to him/her	Erect standing posture with support
6 MONTH	**12 MONTH**
Average weight gain of 4 oz per week during second 6 mo Teething may begin (lower central incisors) Can turn from back to stomach Early ability to distinguish and recognize strangers	Birth weight usually tripled Needs help while walking Sits from standing position without assistance Eats with fingers Usually says two words in addition to "mama" and "dada"
AGE-APPROPRIATE TOYS	
Birth to 2 months	Mobiles 8–10 inches from face
2–4 mo	Rattles, cradle gym
4–6 mo	Brightly colored toys (small enough to grasp, large enough for safety)
6–9 mo	Large toys with bright colors, movable parts, and noisemakers
9–12 mo	Books with large pictures, large push-pull toys, teddy bears

D. Evaluation

1. Has infant's growth and development progressed within normal limits?
2. Is parent/infant relationship secure?
3. Do parents demonstrate increased knowledge about injury prevention?

▶ TODDLER—12 TO 36 MONTHS

A. Assessment (see Table 3)

1. Growth and development (see Table 3)
2. Begins to establish independence

B. Diagnose

1. Potential nursing diagnoses
   a. Injury, risk for
   b. Poisoning, risk for
   c. Nutrition: less than body requirements, altered
2. Potential problems in toddlerhood
   a. Negativism
   b. Safety, abuse

C. Plan/Implementation

1. Routine screening of toddler growth and development
2. Evaluate toddler, parent reactions to separation
3. Continue anticipatory guidance activities with parents
4. Reinforce the desirability of stable daily routines for play, feeding and rest
5. Select age-appropriate toys (see Table 3)

D. Evaluation

1. Has growth and development progressed within normal limits?
2. Do parents demonstrate knowledge of household hazards?
3. Have parents learned to cope with temperament?

Table 3 TODDLER GROWTH AND DEVELOPMENT	
15 MONTH	**24 MONTH**
Walks alone	Early efforts at jumping
Builds 2-block tower	Builds 5- to 6-block tower
Throws objects	300-word vocabulary
Grasps spoon	Obeys easy commands
Names commonplace objects	
18 MONTH	**30 MONTH**
Anterior fontanelle usually closed	Walks on tiptoe
Walks backward	Builds 7- to 8-block tower
Climbs stairs	Stands on one foot
Scribbles	Has sphincter control for toilet training
Builds 3-block tower	
Oral vocabulary—10 words	
Thumb sucking	
AGE-APPROPRIATE TOYS	
Push-pull toys	Dolls
Low rocking horses	Stuffed animals

PRESCHOOL—36 MONTHS TO 6 YEARS

A. Assessment (see Table 4)
   1. Growth and development (see Table 4)
   2. Psychosexual development begins
B. Diagnose
   1. Potential nursing diagnoses
      a. Injury, risk for
      b. Grieving, dysfunctional
      c. Difficulty in group situations
   2. Potential problems in preschool years
      a. Fear of injury, mutilation, and punishment
      b. Safety
C. Plan/Implementation
   1. Screen school-aged children routinely for growth and development
   2. Evaluate parent/child relationships
   3. Continue anticipatory guidance activities with parents
   4. Reinforce the desirability of stable daily routines for play, feeding, and rest
   5. Reinforce the idea of parents as role models who allow their children to make age-appropriate decisions
   6. Select age-appropriate toys (see Table 4)

Table 4 PRESCHOOL GROWTH AND DEVELOPMENT	
3 YEARS	**5 YEARS**
Copies a circle	Runs well
Builds bridge with 3 cubes	Jumps rope
Less negativistic than toddler, decreased tantrums	Dresses without help
Learns from experience	2,100-word vocabulary
Rides tricycle	Tolerates increasing periods of separation from parents
Walks backward and downstairs without assistance	Beginnings of cooperative play
Undresses without help	Gender-specific behavior
900-word vocabulary, uses sentences	Skips on alternate feet
May invent "imaginary" friend	Ties shoes
4 YEARS	
Climbs and jumps well	
Laces shoes	
Brushes teeth	
1,500-word vocabulary	
Skips and hops on one foot	
Throws overhead	
AGE-APPROPRIATE TOYS AND ACTIVITIES	
Child imitative of adult patterns and roles. Offer playground materials, housekeeping toys, coloring books, tricycles with helmet.	

D. Evaluation

1. Have parents established the child's routines of play, feeding, and sleep?

2. Has child demonstrated coping skills regarding separations from parents?

3. Has child demonstrated day and night continence?

4. Does child have firm basis for development of positive body image?

▶ SCHOOL AGE—6 TO 12 YEARS

A. Assessment (see Table 5)

1. Growth and development (see Table 5)

2. Intense period of industry and productivity

3. Begins logical patterns of thought

4. Peer relationships important

5. Likes and dislikes established

Table 5 SCHOOL-AGE GROWTH AND DEVELOPMENT	
6 YEARS	**9 YEARS**
Self-centered, show-off, rude	Skillful manual work possible
Extreme sensitivity to criticism	Conflicts between adult authorities and peer group
Begins losing temporary teeth	Better behaved
Appearance of first permanent teeth	Conflict between needs for independence and dependence
Ties knots	Likes school
7 YEARS	**10–12 YEARS**
Temporal perception improving	Remainder of teeth (except wisdom) erupt
Increased self-reliance for basic activities	Uses telephone
Team games/sports/organizations	Capable of helping
Develops concept of time	Increasingly responsible
Boys prefer playing with boys and girls with girls	More selective when choosing friends
8 YEARS	Develops beginning of interest in opposite sex
Friends sought out actively	Loves conversation
Eye development generally complete	Raises pets
Movements more graceful	
Writing replaces printing	
AGE-APPROPRIATE TOYS, GAMES, AND ACTIVITIES	
Construction toys	Participation in repair, building, and mechanical activities, household chores
Use of tools, household and sewing tools, table games, sports	

B. Diagnose

1. Potential nursing diagnoses

   a. Injury, risk for

   b. Grieving, dysfunctional

   c. Difficulty with social relationships, school

   d. Difficulty with body image, self-esteem, self-concept

2. Potential problems in school-age years

   a. Enuresis: bed-wetting

   b. Encopresis: incontinence of feces

   c. Safety: injuries, head lice are common

C. Plan/Implementation

1. Screen school-aged children routinely for growth and development

2. Evaluate parent/child relationships

3. Continue anticipatory guidance activities with parents

4. Reinforce the desirability of stable daily routines for play, feeding, and rest

5. Reinforce the idea of parents as role models who allow their children to make age-appropriate decisions

6. Select age-appropriate toys (see Table 5)

7. Encourage physical activity

D. Evaluation

1. Have parents and child coped with problems with urinary or bowel elimination?

2. Has child adjusted to challenges of school?

3. Have parents been educated regarding pubescent changes?

4. Has child successfully avoided injury?

▶ ADOLESCENCE—12 TO 20 YEARS

A. Assessment (see Table 6)

1. Growth and development (see Table 6)

2. Body image very important

3. Peer and social relationships very important

4. Identity/autonomy important

B. Diagnose

1. Potential nursing diagnoses

   a. Injury, risk for

   b. Self-esteem disturbance

   c. Health maintenance, altered

2. Potential problems in adolescence

   a. Adolescent pregnancy

   b. Poor self-image

   c. Safety

   d. Drug and alcohol misuse/abuse

   e. AIDS

   f. High school dropout

   g. Violence

Table 6 ADOLESCENT GROWTH AND DEVELOPMENT	
PHYSICAL DEVELOPMENT—PUBERTY	**FEMALE CHANGES**
Attainment of sexual maturity	Increase in pelvic diameter
Rapid alterations in height and weight	Breast development
Girls develop more rapidly than boys	Altered nature of vaginal secretions
Onset may be related to hypothalmic activity, which influences pituitary gland to secrete hormones affecting testes and ovaries	Appearance of axillary and pubic hair
	Menarche—first menstrual period
Testes and ovaries produce hormones (androgens and estrogens) that determine development of secondary sexual characteristics	**PHYSICAL DEVELOPMENT—ADOLESCENT**
	More complete development of secondary sexual characteristics
Pimples or acne related to increased sebaceous gland activity	Improved motor coordination
	Wisdom teeth appear (ages 17–21)
Increased sweat production	**PSYCHOSEXUAL DEVELOPMENT**
Weight gain proportionally greater than height gain during early stages	Masturbation as expression of sexual tension
	Sexual fantasies
Initial problems in coordination—appearance of clumsiness related to rapid, unsynchronized growth of many systems	Experimental sexual intercourse
	PSYCHOSOCIAL DEVELOPMENT
Rapid growth may cause easy fatigue	Preoccupied with rapid body changes, what is "normal"
Preoccupation with physical appearance	Conformity to peer pressure
MALE CHANGES	Moody
Increase in genital size	Increased daydreaming
Breast swelling	Increased independence
Appearance of pubic, facial, axillary, and chest hair	Moving toward a mature sexual identity
Deepening voice	
Production of functional sperm	
Nocturnal emissions	

C. Plan/Implementation

1. Screen the adolescent routinely for growth and development

2. Evaluate parent/child/peer relationships

3. Continue anticipatory guidance activities with parents and adolescents

4. Reinforce the desirability of stable daily routines for work and rest

5. Continue to reinforce the idea of parents and significant others as role models who allow their children to make age-appropriate decisions

6. Counsel adolescent to delay impulsive actions with long-term consequences (e.g., adolescent pregnancy, drug and alcohol misuse, AIDS, high school dropout), and the use of problem-solving skills

7. Encourage the development of educational/vocational options

8. Promote appropriate, safe approaches to resolve conflicts with peers and adults

D. Evaluation

1. Has parents' understanding/perception of adolescent's developmental needs increased?

2. Does adolescent have a larger repertoire of adaptive coping mechanisms?

3. Does adolescent/parent identify and use coping mechanisms?

4. Is adolescent comfortable with body image?

5. Do adolescent and parents recognize risks involved with motor vehicles, alcohol, etc.?

6. Does adolescent have social peer groups?

▶ 20 TO 40 YEARS

A. Assessment (see Table 7)

1. Growth and development (see Table 7)

2. Work, career important

3. Establishes intimacy

B. Diagnose—potential nursing diagnoses

1. Altered health maintenance

2. Altered self-esteem

3. Difficulty with relationships

4. Potential for increased stress

C. Plan/Implementation

1. Meet physical and mental health needs

2. Evaluate relationships, especially with chosen partner

3. Observe responses to stress

4. Anticipatory guidance

D. Evaluation

1. Have client's physical and emotional needs been met?

2. Has client coped, adapted to stressors?

3. Is client committed to relationships and career?

4. Is client knowledgeable about aging process?

5. Is client satisfied with life at this point?

Table 7 ADULTHOOD GROWTH AND DEVELOPMENT		
20 TO 33 YEARS	**33 TO 40 YEARS**	**35 TO 40 YEARS**
Decreased hero worship	Period of discovery, rediscovery of interests and goals	(There in some overlap in years)
Increased reality	Increased sense of urgency	Self-questioning
Independent from parents	Life more serious	Fear of middle age and aging
Possible marriage, partnership	Major goals to accomplish	Reappraises the past
Realization that everything is not black or white, some "gray" areas	Plateaus at work and marriage, partnership	Discards unrealistic goals
Looks towards future, hopes for success	Sense of satisfaction	Potential changes of work, marriage, partnership "Sandwich" generation—concerned with children and aging parents
Peak intelligence, memory		Increased awareness of mortality
Maximum problem-solving ability		Potential loss of significant others

▶ 40 TO 65 YEARS

A. Assessment (see Table 8)

1. Physical functioning (see Table 8)

2. Cognitive functioning (see Table 8)

3. Relationships change

4. Work, career important

B. Diagnose—potential nursing diagnoses

1. Decreased cognitive and physical functioning

2. Altered family

3. Self-care deficit

4. Altered body image

C. Plan/Implementation

1. Help client adjust to changes of aging

2. Help client adjust to changing roles

3. Anticipatory guidance

D. Evaluation

1. Does client have realistic self-expectations?

2. Is client adapting and accepting limits?

3. Have the client's physical and psychosocial needs been met?

Table 8 MIDDLE ADULTHOOD GROWTH AND DEVELOPMENT		
40 TO 55 YEARS	**48 TO 60 YEARS**	**50 TO 65 YEARS**
Graying hair, wrinkling skin	Evaluates past	Increasing physical decline
Pains and muscle aches	Sets new goals	Increasingly forgetful
Realization—future shorter time span than past	Defines value of life, self	Accepts limitations
Menopause	Assesss legacies—professional, personal	Modification of lifestyle
Decreased sensory acuity	Serenity and fulfillment	Decreased power Retirement
Powerful, policy makers, leaders	Balance between old and young	Less restricted time, able to choose different activities
Relates to older and younger generations	Accepts changes of aging	

▶ 65 AND ABOVE

A. Assessment (see Table 9)

1. Physical and cognitive functioning (see Table 9)

2. Significant relationships change

3. Activities may be limited

4. Decreased sense of taste and smell

5. Financial constraints

B. Diagnose

1. Self-care deficit

2. Isolation

3. Altered relationships

4. Decreased independence

5. Family processes, altered

C. Plan/Implementation

1. Assist clients with adjusting to lifestyle changes

2. Allow client to verbalize concerns

3. Prevent isolation

4. Provide assistance as required

D. Evaluation

1. Has client successfully adjusted to decreased abilities and increased dependence?

2. Is client involved in activities for physical and mental stimulation?

3. Is the client in a safe environment?

4. Does client see life as meaningful?

Table 9 ADULTHOOD GROWTH AND DEVELOPMENT	
65 TO 80 YEARS	**GREATER THAN 80 YEARS**
Physical decline	Signs of aging very evident
Loss of significant others	Few significant relationships
Appraisal of life	Withdrawal, risk of isolation
Appearance of chronic diseases	Self-concern
Reconciliation of goals and achievements	Accepting of death, face mortality
Changing social roles	Increased losses
	Decreased abilities

▶ INTELLECTUAL DELAY

A. Assessment

1. Sensory deficits (see Table 10)

2. Physical anomalies

3. Delayed growth and development

B. Diagnose: Sub-average intellectual function (I.Q. less than 70) with concurrent impairment in adaptive functioning; onset under the age of 18

1. Characteristics

a. Lack of, or destruction of, brain cells

2. Causes

a. Heredity

b. Infection

c. Fetal anoxia

d. Cranial or chromosomal abnormalities

e. Intracranial hemorrhage

C. Plan/Implementation

1. Assist parents with adjustment

2. Provide sensory stimulation

		Table 10 INTELLECTUAL DELAY		
CLASSIFICATION	I.Q. RANGE	PRESCHOOL GROWTH AND DEVELOPMENT	SCHOOL TRAINING AND EDUCATION	ADULT SOCIAL/ VOCATIONAL LEVEL
I. Mild	55–70	Slow to walk, feed self, and talk compared with other children	With special education, can learn reading and math skills for third-to-sixth grade level	Can achieve social/ vocational self-maintenance May need occasional psychosocial support
II. Moderate	40–55	Delays in motor development Can do some self-help activities	Responds to training Does not progress with reading or math skills Poor communication skills	Sheltered, usually incapable of self-maintenance
III. Severe	25–40	Marked delay in development May be able to help self minimally	Can profit from habit training Has some understanding of speech	Dependent on others for care Can conform to routine
IV. Profound	Under 25	Significant delay, minimal-capacity functioning	May respond to skill training Shows basic emotional responses	Incapable of self-maintenance, needs nursing care

3. Encourage socially acceptable behavior

4. Provide emotional support

D. Evaluation

1. Have parents adjusted to disabilities of child?

2. Has child obtained optimal functioning?

▶ FETAL ALCOHOL SYNDROME

A. Assessment

1. Thin upper lip, epicanthal folds, maxillary hypoplasia

2. Intellectual deficiencies, motor deficiencies, microcephaly, and hearing disorders

3. Irritability during infancy and hyperactivity during childhood

4. Small for gestational age

B. Diagnose

1. Leading cause of intellectual delay

2. Caused by excessive alcohol ingestion during pregnancy

3. Preventable if mother avoids alcohol during pregnancy

C. Plan/Implementation

1. Prevention

   a. Instruct women to stop consuming alcohol 3 months before conception

   b. There is no safe level of alcohol consumption during pregnancy

2. At birth

   a. Swaddle infant and decrease environmental stimuli

   b. Administer sedatives to decrease symptoms of withdrawal

3. Monitor infant's weight gain

4. Promote nutritional intake

D. Evaluation

1. Has the mother stopped drinking?

2. Has child achieved optimal functioning?

▶ DOWN SYNDROME

A. Assessment

1. Intellectual delay—I.Q. range from 20 to 70

2. Marked hypotonia; short stature

3. Altered physical development—epicanthal folds, low-set ears, protruding tongue, low nasal bridge

B. Diagnose

1. Characteristics

   a. Chromosomal abnormality involving an extra chromosome (number 21)

2. Causes

   a. Unknown

   b. Associated with maternal age greater than 35

C. Plan/Implementation

1. Provide stimulation—OT, PT, special education

2. Observe for signs of common physical problems: 30–40% have heart diseases; 80% have hearing loss; respiratory infections are common

3. Establish and maintain adequate nutrition, parental education, and support

D. Evaluation

1. Has child achieved optimal functioning?

2. Have parents adjusted to child's disability?

▶ LEARNING DISABILITIES

A. Assessment

1. Hyperkinesis (sometimes absent)

2. Decreased attention span, i.e., attention deficit disorder (ADD)

3. Perceptual deficits

4. Aggression/depression

B. Diagnose

    1. Characteristics

        a. Learning and behavioral disorders that occur because of CNS malfunctioning

        b. Neuropsychological testing—reveals individual differences

        c. Average to high I.Q.

C. Plan/Implementation

    1. Reduce frustration

    2. Special educational intervention; small class size

    3. Provide safety and security

    4. Administer medications, e.g., Ritalin, Dexedrine

    5. Refer to appropriate resources—special education, parent support groups

D. Evaluation

    1. Is child developing to his/her greatest potential?

    2. Have referrals been made to appropriate resources?

▶ **HUMAN SEXUALITY**

A. Assessment

1. Physical appearance
2. Physical limitations
3. Sexual role performance problems
   a. Infertility
   b. Frigidity
   c. Impotence
   d. Premature ejaculation
   e. Inability to achieve orgasm
   f. Dyspareunia (pain with intercourse)
4. Sexual role functioning
   a. Homosexuality
   b. Bisexuality
   c. Sexual ambiguity
   d. Transsexual surgery
   e. Transvestism

B. Diagnose

1. Expression of person's sexual identity
2. Involves sexual relationships and self-concept

C. Plan/Implementation

1. Don't allow your personal beliefs to interfere with your ability to help client express concerns
2. Remain nonjudgmental
3. Acknowledge feelings may be uncomfortable
4. Provide information as needed

D. Evaluation

1. Has client been able to verbalize concerns about sexuality?
2. Have client's needs regarding sexuality been met?

▶ **PREGNANCY**

A. Assessment

1. Estimated date of birth (EDB)
   a. Naegele's rule—count back three months from first day of last menstrual period and add seven days and one year
   b. Ultrasonography—estimates fetal age from head measurements

    c. Fundal height—measurement of fundal height from the top of symphysis pubis to the top of the fundus with a flexible, nonstretchable tape measure, used as a gross estimate of dates

      1) Above the level of symphysis—between 12 and 14 weeks

      2) At the umbilicus or 20 cm—about 20 weeks

      3) Rises about 1 cm/week until 36 weeks, after which it varies

2. Obstetric classification

    a. Gravida—the total number of pregnancies regardless of duration (includes present pregnancy); nulligravida—woman who has never been pregnant

    b. Para—number of past pregnancies that have gone beyond the period of viability (capability of the fetus to survive outside of the uterus-after 20 weeks gestation or greater than 500 g) regardless of the number of fetuses (eg twins) or whether the infant was born alive or dead

    c. Term—born from beginning of 38 to end of 42 week

    d. Abortion—any pregnancy that terminates before the period of viability

3. Characteristic findings

    a. Uterus—increases in size, at 12–14 weeks, above symphysis pubis

    b. Cervix—softens, mucus plug in canal, bluish color (Chadwick's sign)

    c. Abdomen—stretches, striae

    d. Breasts—enlarged, tender

    e. Blood volume—increases 30% and peaks at 28 weeks

    f. Cardiac output—increased by 750 ml/min

    g. Ventilation—decreased tidal volume in third trimester

    h. Digestion—decreased peristalsis and increased pressure

    i. Skin

      1) Pink or reddish streaks (striae gravidarum) on breasts, abdomen, buttocks, and/or thighs; result of fat deposits causing stretching of the skin

      2) Increased pigmentation on the face; blotchy brown areas on the forehead and cheeks (chloasma or "mask of pregnancy"); on the abdomen, dark line from the umbilicus to the symphysis pubis (linea nigra)

      3) Minute vascular spiders

      4) Umbilicus is pushed outward and by the seventh month, depression disappears, becomes a darkened area on the abdominal wall

      5) Sweat and sebaceous glands more active

    j. Urinary—frequency and stasis result from pressure

    k. Endocrine

      1) Placenta—produces estrogen, progesterone, human chorionic gonadotrophin (hCG), human placental lactogen (hPL)

      2) Pituitary—elevated estrogen and progesterone, suppressed LH, FSH, and oxytocin

          3) Weight gain—steady, consistent is ideal; based on pre-pregnancy BMI

            a) BMI less than 18.5; total weight gain range 28–40 lb

            b) BMI 18.5–24.9; total weight gain range 25–35 lb

            c) BMI 25–29.9; total weight gain 15–25 lb

            d) BMI greater than 30; weight gain total 11–20 lb

4. Diagnostic test—hCG is measured by radioimmunoassay in blood and urine; serum more sensitive, so results are more accurate and available earlier

5. Verifying pregnancy

    a. Presumptive—changes felt by woman: amenorrhea, nausea/vomiting ("morning sickness"), breast sensitivity, fatigue, quickening (maternal perception of fetal movement occurring between 16 and 20 weeks of gestation), urinary frequency

    b. Probable—changes observed by examiner: uterine enlargement, soufflé and contractions, positive urine pregnancy tests, Hegar's sign (softening and compressibility of isthmus of uterus), Chadwick's sign (bluish color of cervix)

    c. Positive—definite signs of pregnancy: fetal heartbeat (8–12 weeks by Doptone and by 18–20 weeks auscultation), palpation of fetal movement, visualization of fetus by ultrasound

6. Fetal assessment

    a. Fetal heart rate (FHR)—a significant predictor of fetal well-being; at term 120–160 beats/min

    b. Fetal movement (FM)—a regular pattern of 10 movements in one hour twice a day is a good indicator of fetal well-being; fewer than three movements in a one-hour period should be reported

B. Diagnose

1. Potential nursing diagnoses

    a. Deficient knowledge

    b. Risk for ineffective role performance

    c. Risk for imbalanced nutrition: less than body requirements

    d. Risk for fetal injury

2. Fertilization—union of ovum and spermatozoa, occurs about 24 hours after ovulation; usually outer third of fallopian tube

3. Implantation

    a. Upper part of uterus

    b. About one week after fertilization

4. Early placental development

    a. Combination of endometrium and fetal chorionic layer (maternal and embryonic parts)

    b. Chorion produces human chorionic gonadotrophin (hCG)

    c. Transmits nutrients from maternal bloodstream by a number of mechanisms

      d. Transfer of oxygen from mother to fetus by diffusion

      e. Removes waste products of fetal metabolism into mother's bloodstream from which they will be excreted

C. Plan/Implementation

    1. Encourage prenatal care

    2. Manage discomforts of pregnancy (see Table 1)

D. Evaluation

    1. Have woman's physical needs been met?

    2. Is client knowledgeable about her pregnancy?

Table 1 DISCOMFORTS OF PREGNANCY	
ASSESSMENT	**NURSING CONSIDERATIONS**
Nausea and vomiting (morning sickness)	May occur any time of day Dry crackers on arising Eat small, frequent meals Avoid strong odors and greasy foods
Constipation, hemorrhoids	Bulk foods, fiber, stool softeners Generous fluid intake Encourage regularity, routine
Leg cramps	Increase calcium intake Dorsiflex feet, local heat
Breast soreness	Well-fitting bra Bra may be worn at night
Backache	Emphasize posture and good body mechanics Careful lifting Good shoes Pelvic tilt exercises
Heartburn	Small frequent meals Antacids—avoid those containing phosphorus Decrease fatty and fried foods Avoid supine position after meals
Dizziness	Slow, deliberate movements Support stockings Monitor intake
Vertigo, lightheadedness	Vena cava or maternal hypotensive syndrome Turn on left side
Urinary frequency	Kegel exercises Decrease fluids before bed Report signs of infection

▶ FETAL DEVELOPMENT

A. Assessment

1. Maternal considerations

   a. High-risk group

   b. Environment

   c. Medications, drugs, alcohol

   d. Nutrition–should be no attempt at weight reduction

   e. Age

2. Genetic considerations

   a. African Americans for sickle-cell disease, Northern European descendants of Ashkenazi Jews for Tay-Sachs disease,Mediterranean ancestry for thalassemia; couples with a history of a child with a defect; family history of a structural abnormality orsystemic disease that may be hereditary; closely related parents; women over 40

   b. Chromosomal alteration–may be numeric or structural

      1) Down's syndrome (trisomy 21)–increased in women over 35 years; characterized by a small, round head with flattened occiput, low-set ears, large fat pads at the nape of a short neck, protruding tongue, small mouth and high palate, epicanthal folds with slanted eyes, hypotonic muscles with hypermobility of joints, short, broad hands with inward curved little finger, transverse simian palmar crease, mental deficiencies

      2) Turner's syndrome (female with only one X)–characterized by stunted growth, fibrous streaks in ovaries, usually infertile, no intellectual impairment, occasionally perceptual problems

      3) Klinefelter's syndrome (male with extra X)–normal intelligence to mild intellectual delay, usually infertile

   c. Autosomal defects–defects occurring in any chromosome pair other than the sex chromosomes

      1) Autosomal dominant–union of normal parent with affected parent gene; the affected parent has a 50% chance of passing on the abnormal gene in each pregnancy; BRCA-1 and BRCA-2 breast cancer, Type 2 diabetes, Marfan syndrome, polycystic kidney disease

      2) Autosomal recessive–requires transmission of abnormal gene from both parents for expression of condition; cystic fibrosis, sickle cell disease

      3) Sex-linked transmission traits–trait carried on a sex chromosome (usually the X chromosome); may be dominant or recessive, but recessive is more prevalent; e.g., hemophilia, color blindness

    d. Inborn errors of metabolism—disorders of protein, fat, or carbohydrate metabolism due to absent or defective enzymes that generally follow a recessive pattern of inheritance

        1) Phenylketonuria (PKU)—disorder due to autosomal recessive gene creating a deficiency in the liver enzyme phenylalanine hydroxylase, which metabolizes the amino acid phenylalanine; results in metabolites accumulation in the blood; toxic to brain cells

        2) Tay-Sachs disease—autosomal recessive trait resulting from a deficiency of hexosaminidase A, resulting in apathy and regression in motor and social development and decreased vision

        3) Cystic fibrosis (mucoviscidosis or fibrocystic disease of the pancreas)—an autosomal recessive trait characterized by generalized involvement of exocrine glands, resulting in altered viscosity of mucus-secreting glands throughout the body

3. Diagnostic tests

    a. Alpha-fetal protein (AFP) test—fetal serum protein to predict neural tube defects, threatened abortion, fetal distress; decreased AFP levels suggest possible Down syndrome

        1) Done between 16 and 18 weeks

        2) High incidence of false-positive results (delivered normal neonates)

        3) Usual concurrent test for presence of acetylcholinesterase

    b. Chorionic villus sampling (CVS)—early antepartal test to diagnose fetal karyotype, sickle-cell anemia, PKU, Down syndrome, Duchenne muscular dystrophy

        1) Done between 8 and 12 weeks

        2) Complications include bleeding, spontaneous abortion, rupture of membranes

        3) Rh-negative mother should receive Rho(D) immune globulin (IGIM) after test to prevent Rh isoimmunization

        4) Ultrasound used to guide; sample of fetal placental tissue

        5) Full bladder required

    c. Amniocentesis—amniotic fluid is aspirated by a needle inserted through the abdominal and uterine walls

        1) Done at 16 weeks to detect genetic disorder; possible after 14 weeks gestation

        2) Done at 30 weeks to assess L/S ratio (lecithin/sphingomyelin) to determine lung maturity

        3) Prior to the procedure, the client's bladder should be emptied if greater than 20 weeks gestation; ultrasonography (x-ray only if necessary) is used to avoid trauma from the needle to the placenta, fetus

        4) Test results take 2 to 4 weeks

       5) Complications include premature labor, infection, Rh isoimmunization, abruptio placentae, amniotic embolism; Rh-negative mother should receive Rho(D) immune globulin (IGIM) after procedure

       6) Monitor fetus electronically after procedure, monitor for uterine contractions

       7) Teach client to report decreased fetal movement, contractions, abdominal discomfort, fluid loss, or fever after procedure

    d. Ultrasound—transducer on abdomen transmits sound waves that show fetal image on screen

       1) As early as five weeks to confirm pregnancy, gestational age

       2) Multiple purposes—to determine position, number, measurement of fetus(es) and other structures (placenta)

       3) Client must drink fluid prior to test to have full bladder to assist in clarity of image

       4) No known harmful effects for fetus or mother

       5) Noninvasive

    e. Non-stress test (NST)—ultrasound transducer records fetal movements, and Doppler ultrasound measures fetal heart rate to assess fetal well-being after 28 weeks

       1) Client should eat snacks

       2) A reactive non-stress test (good finding) is two or more FHR accelerations of 15 bpm lasting 15 seconds over a 20-minute interval, and return of FHR to normal baseline

    f. Contraction stress test (CST), either nipple stimulation or oxytocin stimulation—evaluates fetal response to stress of labor

       1) Performed after 28 weeks

       2) Woman in semi-Fowler's or side-lying position

       3) Positive contraction-stress; decelerations with at least 50% of contractions; potential risk to fetus, cesarean may be necessary

       4) Negative contraction stress test—no late decelerations with a minimum of three contractions lasting 40–60 seconds in 10-minute period

       5) Monitor for post-test labor onset

    g. Estriol levels—serial 24-hour maternal urine samples or serum specimens to determine fetoplacental status; decreasing levels usually indicate deterioration

B. Diagnose—potential nursing diagnoses

  1. Knowledge deficits

  2. Lack of prenatal care

C. Plan/Implementation

1. Teach optimal nutrition and exercise

2. Advise avoidance of hazards

   a. Urinary tract infections (UTI)—lower tract characterized by urinary frequency and urgency, dysuria, and sometimes hematuria; manifested in upper tract by fever, malaise, anorexia, nausea, abdominal/back pain; confirmed by greater than 100,000/ml bacterial colony count by clean catch urine; sometimes asymptomatic; treated with sulfa-based medications and ampicillin

   b. TORCH test series—group of maternal systemic infections that can be transmitted across the placenta or by ascending infection (after rupture of membranes [ROM]) to the fetus; infection early in pregnancy may produce significant and devastating fetal deformities, whereas later infection may result in overwhelming active systemic disease and/or CNS involvement causing severe neurological impairment or death of newborn

      1) Toxoplasmosis (protozoa; transplacental to fetus)—discourage eating undercooked meat and handling cat litter box

      2) Other

         a) Syphilis

         b) Varicella/shingles (transplacental to fetus or droplet to newborn)—caution susceptible woman about contact with the disease and zoster immune globulin for exposure

         c) Group B beta-hemolytic streptococcus (direct or indirect to fetus during labor and delivery)—treated with penicillin

         d) Hepatitis B (transplacental and contact with secretions during delivery)—screen and immunize maternal carriers; treat newborn with HBIg

         e) Hepatitis A—need to encourage good handwashing techniques

         f) AIDS (as with hepatitis)—titers in newborn may be passive transfer of maternal antibodies or active antibody formation

      3) Rubella (transplacental)—prenatal testing required by law; caution susceptible woman about contact; vaccine is not given during pregnancy

      4) Cytomegalovirus (CMV)—transmitted in body fluids; detected by antibody/serological testing

      5) Herpes 2 (transplacental, ascending infection within 4–6 hours after ROM or contact during delivery if active lesions)—cesarean delivery if active lesions

3. Teach/prepare for procedures

4. Teach danger signs of pregnancy

   a. Gush of fluid or bleeding from vagina

   b. Regular uterine contractions

   c. Severe headaches, visual disturbances, abdominal pain, or persistent vomiting

   d. Fever or chills

e. Swelling in face and fingers

f. Decrease in fetal movement

5. Teach client to report decrease in fetal movement

D. Evaluation

1. Has client remained free of complications and is fetus in stable condition?

2. Does client have sufficient knowledge of pregnancy and childbirth?

▶ LABOR AND DELIVERY

A. Assessment

1. Characteristic findings

a. Onset

1) Lightening—subjective sensation as fetus descends into pelvic inlet

a) Primipara (occurs up to two weeks prior to delivery)

b) Multipara (may not occur until labor begins)

2) Softening of cervix

3) Expulsion of mucus plug (show)

4) Uterine contractions that are progressive and regular

b. Cervical changes

1) Effacement—progressive thinning and shortening of cervix (0–100%)

2) Dilation—opening of cervix os during labor (0–10 cm)

c. Rupture of membranes—rupture of amniotic sac (ROM)

1) Check fetal heart tones to assess for fetal distress

2) Prolapsed cord

a) Symptoms—premature rupture of membranes, presenting part not engaged, fetal distress, protruding cord

b) Nursing care—call for help, push against presenting part to relieve pressure on cord, place in Trendelenburg or knee- chest position

c) Treatment successful—fetal heart tones remain unchanged

2. Fetal monitoring

a. Intermittent auscultation

b. Electronic monitoring

1) External—ultrasound over fetal back monitors, FHR and a pressure transducer monitors uterine tone

a) Transabdominal, noninvasive

b) Client needs to decrease extra-abdominal movements

2) Internal—fetal scalp probe provides FHR, and an internal transducer provides intra-uterine pressure readings

a) Membranes must be ruptured, cervix sufficiently dilated, and presenting part low

b) Invasive procedure

    c. Results of monitoring

       1) Normal FHR 120–160; must obtain a baseline

3. Tachycardia (greater than 160 bpm lasting longer than 10 minutes)—early sign of fetal hypoxia, associated with maternal fever, fetal anemia, fetal or maternal infection, drugs (atropine, vistaril), maternal hyperthyroidism, fetal heart failure; nonreassuring sign when associated with late decelerations, severe variable decelerations, or absence of variability

4. Bradycardia (less than 110 bpm lasting longer than 10 minutes) —late sign of fetal hypoxia, associated with maternal drugs (anesthetics), prolonged cord compression, fetal congenital heart block, maternal supine hypotensive syndrome; nonreassuring sign when associated with loss of variability and late decelerations

5. Variability—beat to beat fluctuation; measured by EFM only

    a. Normal (6–25 bpm)–indicator of fetal well-being

    b. Absent (0–2 bpm) or decreased (3–5 bpm) may be associated with fetal sleep state, fetal prematurity, reaction to drugs (narcotics, barbiturates, tranquilizers, anesthetics), congenital anomalies, hypoxia, acidosis; if persists for more than 30 minutes, may indicate fetal distress

    c. Increased (greater than 25 bpm)–significance unknown

6. Accelerations—15 bpm rise above baseline followed by a return; usually in response to fetal movement or contractions; indicates fetal well-being

7. Decelerations—fall below baseline lasting 15 seconds or more, followed by a return to baseline

    a. Early: onset close to the beginning or before peak of contraction; most often uniform mirror image of contraction on tracing; associated with head compression, in second stage with pushing; reassuring pattern

    b. Late: onset after contraction is established; usually begins at the peak of the contraction, with slow return to baseline after the contraction is complete; indicative of fetal hypoxia because of deficient placental perfusion; caused by PIH, maternal diabetes, placenta previa, abruption placentae; nonreasurring sign

    c. Variable decelerations—transient U/V-shaped reduction occurring at any time during uterine contracting phase; decrease usually more than 15 bpm, lasting 15 seconds, return to baseline in less than 2 minutes from onset, indicative of cord compression, which may be relieved by change in mother's position; ominous if repetitive, prolonged, severe, or slow return to baseline, administer O_2, discontinue oxytocin

    d. Nursing interventions for abnormal results

       1) None for early decelerations

       2) For late decelerations (at the first sign of abnormal tracing)—position mother left side-lying (if no change, move to other side, Trendelenburg or knee-chest position); administer oxygen by mask, start IV or increase flow rate, stop oxytocin if appropriate, prepare for C-section

       3) For variable decelerations—reposition mother to relieve pressure on the umbilical cord

8. Factors affecting labor and delivery

    a. Lie—relationship of spine of fetus to spine of mother; longitudinal (parallel), transverse (right angles), oblique (slight angle off a true transverse lie)

    b. Presentation—part of fetus that presents to (enters) maternal pelvic inlet

       1) Cephalic/vertex—head (95% of labors)

       2) Breech/buttocks (3–4%)

          a) Frank (most common)—flexion of hips and extension of knees

          b) Complete—flexion of hips and knees

          c) Footing/incomplete—extension of hips and knees

       3) Shoulder (transverse lie)—rare

    c. Attitude—relationship of fetal parts to each other; usually flexion of head and extremities on chest and abdomen to accommodate to shape of uterine cavity

    d. Position—relationship of fetal reference point to maternal pelvis (see Figure 1); to find best location for FHR assessment, determine the location of the fetal back; weeks of gestation may alter the location, as well

       1) Fetal reference point

          a) Vertex presentation—dependent upon degree of flexion of fetal head on chest; full flexion—occiput (O); full extension—chin (M); moderate extension (military)—brow (B)

          b) Breech presentation—sacrum (S)

          c) Shoulder presentation—scapula (SC)

       2) Maternal pelvis is designated per her right/left and anterior/posterior

       3) Expressed as standard three-letter abbreviation; e.g., LOA = left occiput anterior, indicating vertex presentation with fetal occiput on mother's left side toward the front of her pelvis (see Figure 1). To find best location for FHR assessment, determine the location of the fetal back. Weeks of gestation may alter the location, as well

          a) LOA—left occiput anterior, most common; FHR best heard below umbilicus on mother's left side

          b) LOP—left occiput posterior

          c) ROA—right occiput anterior

          d) ROP—right occiput posterior

          e) LSA—left sacrum anterior

          f) RSA—right sacrum anterior

       4) Configuration and diameter of pelvis

       5) Distensibility of uterus

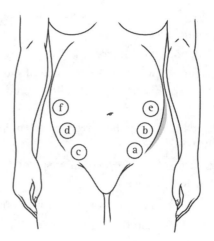

Figure 1 Determining Position

e. Station—level of presenting part of fetus in relation to imaginary line between ischial spines (zero station) in midpelvis of mother (see Figure 2)

1) −5 to −1 indicates a presenting part above zero station (floating); +1 to +5, a presenting part below zero station

2) Engagement—when the presenting part is at station zero or below

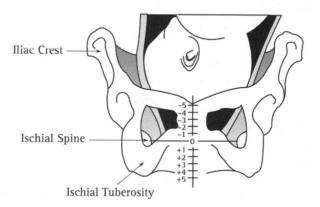

Figure 2 Station of Presenting Part

f. Contractions

1) Three phases

a) Increment—steep crescent slope from beginning of the contraction until its peak

b) Acme/peak—strongest intensity

c) Decrement—diminishing intensity

2) Characteristics of contractions

a) Frequency: time frame in minutes from the beginning of one contraction to the beginning of the next one or the peak of one contraction to the peak of the next; frequency less than every two minutes should be reported

b) Duration: time frame in seconds from the beginning of a contraction to its completion; more than 90 seconds should be reported because of potential risk of uterine rupture or fetal distress

c) Intensity: the strength of a contraction at acme; may be assessed by subjective description from the woman, palpation (mild contraction—slightly tense uterus easy to indent with fingertips; moderate—firm fundus difficult to indent with fingertips; strong—rigid, board-like fundus)

g. True vs. false labor (see Table 2)

Table 2 TRUE VS. FALSE LABOR	
TRUE	**FALSE**
Cervix progressively effaced and dilated	Cervical changes do not occur
Contractions—regular with increasing frequency (shortened intervals), duration, and intensity	Contractions—irregular with usually no change in frequency, duration, or intensity
Discomfort radiates from back around the abdomen	Discomfort is usually abdominal
Contractions do not decrease with rest	Contractions may lessen with activity or rest

h. Stages of labor

1) Stage 1—beginning to complete cervical dilation (0–10 cm)

2) Stage 2—complete dilation to birth of baby

3) Stage 3—birth to delivery of placenta

4) Stage 4—first 4 hours after delivery of placenta

i. Cultural influences

j. *Not all members of a culture will choose actions below.*

1) Japan—natural childbirth, may labor silently

2) China—stoic response to pain, side-lying position for labor and birth

3) India—female relatives present

4) Laos—may use squatting position for birth

k. Participation in childbirth preparation classes

B. Diagnose—potential nursing diagnoses

1. Potential knowledge deficits

2. Difficulty adapting and coping with stress

3. Risk of complications

4. Need for pain management

5. Labor may not progress

C. Plan/Implementation

1. Monitor progress—maternal

   a. First stage of labor: beginning of labor to complete cervical dilation

      1) Phase one (latent): 0–3 cm; contractions 10–30 sec long, 5–30 min apart; mild to moderate

      2) Phase two (active): 4–7 cm; contractions 40–60 sec long, 3–5 min apart; moderate to strong

      3) Phase three (transition): 8–10 cm; contractions 45–90 sec long, 1½–2 min apart; strong

   b. Second stage of labor: complete cervical dilation to delivery of fetus

      1) Phase 1: 0 to +2 station; contractions 2–3 min apart

      2) Phase 2: +2 to +4 station; contractions 2–2.5 min apart; increase in dark red bloody show; increased urgency to bear down

      3) Phase 3: +4 to birth; contractions 1–2 min apart; fetal head visible; increased urgency to bear down

   c. Third stage of labor: birth and delivery of placenta

      1) Placental delivery—slight gush of blood and lengthening of umbilical cord; check for remaining fragments

   d. Fourth stage of labor: first 4 hours after delivery

2. Monitor progress—fetal

   a. During labor check FHR

   b. Manage fetal distress (see Table 3)

| Table 3 MANAGEMENT OF FETAL DISTRESS ||
ASSESSMENT	NURSING CONSIDERATIONS
Irregular fetal heartbeat	Turn client onto left side Give supplemental oxygen Check for cord prolapse Start intravenous line
Umbilical cord prolapse	Elevate presenting part off the cord Call for help Place client in Trendelenburg or knee-chest position Give supplemental oxygen Start intravenous line

3. Monitor discomfort/exhaustion/pain control—support client in choice of pain control

   a. Relaxation techniques taught during pregnancy where breathing is taught as a relaxed response to contraction

   b. Low back pain—advise massage of sacral area

   c. Use different breathing techniques during different phases of labor

   d. Encourage rest between contractions

4. Keep couple informed of progress

5. Administer analgesic (consider: orders, client request, stage of labor, and fetal well-being)
   a. May prolong labor
   b. Local/block/general
6. Educate client about anesthetics
   a. Systemic analgesics
      1) Opioid agonists—morphine; risk of maternal and fetal respiratory depression and sedation
      2) Opioid agonist-antagonist analgesics—butophanol, nalbuphine—less risk of respiratory depression
   b. Nerve block analgesia and anesthesia
      1) Local—for episiotomy; lidocaine, chloroprocaine; may be given with epinephrine
      2) Pudendal nerve block—for episiotomy or when forceps or vacuum extractor used
   c. Spinal anesthesia (block)—used for Cesarean birth; local anesthetic with fentanyl injected into subarachnoid space at level or 3rd to 5th lumbar vertebrae; risk of maternal hypotension and respiratory depression, fetal distress; postdural puncture headache
   d. Epidural anesthesia or analgesia (block)—most popular
      1) Lumbar—injected into epidural space between 4th and 5th lumbar vertebrae; bupivacaine, ropivacaine, fentanyl, sufentanil; may be client-controlled epidural analgesia
   e. Combined spinal-epidural analgesia—opioid injected into epidural space followed by local anesthetic
7. Prepare for delivery
   a. Normal spontaneous
   b. Vaginal birth after cesarean (VBAC)
8. Newborn care at delivery—immediate actions
   a. Establish airway
   b. Observe for Apgar score at 1 and 5 minutes
   c. Clamp umbilical cord
   d. Maintain warmth
   e. Place identification band on baby and mother

D. Evaluation
   1. Can mother participate effectively in delivery process?
   2. Is mother able to rest between contractions?
   3. Has mother established eye contact with neonate after birth?
   4. Have complications with mother been avoided?

▶ **POSTPARTUM**

A. Assessment (see Table 4)

1. Physical

2. Cultural influences

Table 4 FOURTH STAGE OF LABOR		
FIRST 1–2 HOURS		**NURSING CONSIDERATIONS**
Vital signs (BP, pulse)	q 15 min	Follow protocol until stable
Fundus	q 15 min	Position—at the level of the umbilicus for the first 12 hours, then descends by one finger breadth each succeeding day, pelvic organ usually by day 10
Lochia (color, volume)	q 15 min	Lochia (endometrial sloughing)—day 1–3 rubra (bloody with fleshy odor; may be clots); day 4–9 serosa (pink/brown with fleshy odor); day 10+ alba (yellow–white); at no time should there be a foul odor (indicates infection)
Urinary	Measure first void	May have urethral edema, urine retention
Bonding	Encourage interaction	Emphasize touch, eye contact

B. Diagnose—potential nursing diagnoses

1. Physical mobility, impaired

2. Parenting, risk for altered

3. Self-care deficit

C. Plan/Implementation

1. If ordered, Rho(D) immune globulin (IGIM) to mother—Rho(D) immune globulin (IGIM) promotes lysis of fetal Rh-positive RBCs circulating in maternal bloodstream before Rh-negative mother develops her own antibodies to them

2. Assess lochia color and volume

3. Check episiotomy and perineum for signs and symptoms of infection

4. Assess for attachment/bonding—influenced by maternal psychosocial-cultural factors, infant health status, temperament, and behaviors, circumstances of the prenatal, intrapartal, postpartal, and neonatal course; evidenced initially by touching and cuddling, naming, "en face" positioning for direct eye contact, later by reciprocity and rhythmicity in maternal–infant interaction

5. Promote successful feeding

6. Nonnursing woman—suppress lactation

   a. Mechanical methods—tight-fitting bra for 72 hours, ice packs,minimize breast stimulation

7. Nursing woman—successful lactation is dependent on infant sucking and maternal production and delivery of milk (letdown/milk ejection reflex); monitor and teach preventive measures for potential problems (see Table 5)

  a. Nipple irritation/cracking

    1) Nipple care—clean with warm water, no soap, and dry thoroughly; absorbent breast pads if leaking occurs; apply breast milk to nipples and areola after each feeding and air dry; apply warm compresses after each feeding and air dry

    2) Position nipple so that infant's mouth covers a large portion of the areola and release infant's mouth from nipple by inserting finger to break suction

    3) Rotate breastfeeding positions

Table 5 LACTATION PRINCIPLES	
BREAST CARE—ANTEPARTUM AND POSTPARTUM	**INITIATING BREAST FEEDING**
Soap on nipples should be avoided during bathing to prevent dryness	Relaxed position of mother is essential—support dependent arm with pillow
Redness or swelling can indicate infection and should always be investigated	Alternate which breast is offered first
	Five minutes on each breast is sufficient at first—teach proper way to break suction
	Most of the areola should be in infant's mouth to ensure proper sucking

  b. Engorgement—nurse frequently (every 30 minutes to 3 hours) and long enough to empty breasts completely (evidenced by sucking without swallowing); warm shower or compresses to stimulate letdown; alternate starting breast at each feeding; mild analgesic 20 minutes before feeding and ice packs between feedings for pronounced discomfort

  c. Plugged ducts—area of tenderness and lumpiness often associated with engorgement; may be relieved by heat and massage before feeding

  d. Expression of breast milk—to collect milk for supplemental feedings, to relieve breast fullness or to build milk supply; may be manually expressed or pumped by a device and refrigerated for no more than 48 hours or frozen in plastic bottles (to maintain stability of all elements) in refrigerator freezer for 2 weeks and deep freezer for 2 months (do not thaw in microwave or on stove)

  e. Medications—most drugs cross into breast milk; check with health care provider before taking any medication

8. "Postpartum blues" (day 3–7)—normal occurrence of "roller coaster" emotions, weeping, "letdown feeling"; usually relieved with emotional support and rest/sleep; report if prolonged or later onset

9. Urinary incontinence

    a. Kegel exercises–tighten pubococcygeal muscles, hold for count of 3, then relax; do 10 times tid

    b. Avoid diuretics such as caffeine

10. Sexual activities–abstain from intercourse until episiotomy is healed and lochia has ceased (usually 3–4 weeks); may be affected by fatigue, fear of discomfort, leakage of breast milk, concern about another pregnancy; assess and discuss couple's desire for and understanding about contraceptive methods; breastfeeding does not give adequate protection; oral contraceptives should not be used during breastfeeding

D. Evaluation

1. Has bonding been initiated?

2. Are feeding techniques established?

3. Is uterine involution progressing normally?

4. Has client received anticipatory guidance?

▶ PARENTING

A. Assessment

1. Knowledge of growth and development

2. Family composition

3. Family dynamics

4. Cultural influences

5. Resources available to parents

6. Support mechanisms

7. Previous experiences, age of parents

8. Attachments, interpersonal relationships

9. Communication between parents and with child

10. Expectations of parents

11. Motivation and commitment of parents

B. Diagnose–potential nursing diagnoses

1. Risk for impaired parenting

2. Readiness for enhanced knowledge

3. Readiness for enhanced family processes

4. Readiness for enhanced parenting

C. Plan/Implementation

1. Promote realistic age-appropriate expectations (social, motor, language)

2. Provide anticipatory guidance

3. Educate regarding routine health care

4. Observe response to stress

5. Encourage active participation

6. Support as needed

D. Evaluation

1. Is there an understanding of development needs? Are age-appropriate decisions made?

2. Are there signs of adaptive coping?

3. Is there participation in screening?

4. Has normal bonding occurred?

5. Does the child respond appropriately to the parent and to others?

6. Can the parent interpret the needs of the child?

7. Has acceptable behavior been defined and are limits being set? Is there an acceptable means of discipline?

8. Has successful teaching occurred?

9. Do the parents experience a sense of satisfaction?

10. Are there sufficient data or is there a need for further assessment?

▶ SPONTANEOUS ABORTION (UNPLANNED TERMINATION OF A PREGNANCY)

A. Assessment

1. Persistent uterine bleeding and cramp-like pain

2. Laboratory finding—negative or weakly positive urine pregnancy test

3. Obtain history, including last menstrual period

4. Types (see Table 1)

Table 1 CLINICAL CLASSIFICATION OF SPONTANEOUS ABORTION		
TYPE	ASSESSMENT	NURSING CONSIDERATIONS
Threatened	Vaginal bleeding and cramping Soft uterus, cervix closed	Ultrasound for intrauterine sac, quantitative hCG Decrease activity for 24–48 hours, avoid stress, no sexual intercourse for 2 weeks after bleeding stops Monitor amount and character of bleeding; report clots, tissue, foul odor
Inevitable, if cervical dilation cannot be prevented	Persistent symptoms, hemorrhage, moderate to severe cramping Cervical dilation and effacement	Monitor for hemorrhage (save and count pads) and infection; if persistent or increased symptoms, D and C Emotional support for grief and loss
Incomplete	Persistent symptoms, expulsion of part of products of conception	Administer IV/blood, oxytocin D and C or suction evacuation
Complete	As above, except no retained tissue	Possible methylergonovine; no other treatment if no evidence of hemorrhage or infection
Missed—fetus dies *in utero* but is not expelled	May be none/some abating of above symptoms Cervix is closed If retained greater than 6 weeks, increased risk of infection, DIC, and emotional distress	D and C evacuation within 4–6 weeks After 12 weeks, dilate cervix with several applications of prostaglandin gel or suppositories of laminaria (dried sterilized seaweed that expands with cervical secretions)
Habitual—3 or more	May be incompetent cervix, infertility	Cerclage (encircling cervix with suture)

B. Diagnose

1. Causes

   a. Chromosomal abnormalities

   b. Teratogenic drugs

   c. Abnormalities of female reproductive tract

2. Potential nursing diagnosis

   a. Anxiety, fear

   b. Deficient knowledge

   c. Deficient fluid volume

   d. Grieving

3. Termination of pregnancy spontaneously at any time before the fetus has attained viability

C. Plan/Implementation

1. Monitor vital signs

2. Monitor for bleeding, cramping, pain

3. Monitor hydration status and electrolyte balance

4. Administer Rho(D) immune globulin (IGIM) as needed

5. Save all tissues

6. Teach purpose of bedrest

7. Prepare client for surgical procedure if indicated (D and C, therapeutic abortion)

8. Provide emotional support for grief and loss

D. Evaluation

1. Has the woman adjusted to the loss of the pregnancy?

2. Have complications been prevented?

▶ ECTOPIC PREGNANCY

A. Assessment

1. Missed period

2. Unilateral lower quadrant pain after 4–6 weeks of normal pregnancy

3. Rigid, tender abdomen

4. Referred shoulder pain can occur

5. Low hematocrit, low hCG levels in urine and blood

6. Bleeding—gradual oozing to frank bleeding

B. Diagnose

1. Pain due to implantation of egg outside of uterus

2. Potential for anxiety and grieving

3. Potentially life-threatening to mother due to hemorrhage

4. Causes

   a. Pelvic inflammatory disease (PID)

   b. Previous tubal surgery

   c. Congenital anomalies of the fallopian tubes

C. Plan/Implementation
   1. Prepare for surgery
   2. Monitor for shock preoperatively and postoperatively
   3. Provide emotional support and expression of grief
   4. Administer Rho(D) immune globulin (IGIM) to Rh-negative women
   5. Discharge teaching

D. Evaluation
   1. Has the woman adjusted to the loss of the pregnancy?
   2. Have complications been prevented?

▶ HYPERTENSION/PREECLAMPSIA/ECLAMPSIA

A. Preexisting hypertension (HTN)—diagnosed and treated before the 20th week of pregnancy; requires strict medical and obstetrical management

B. Gestational Hypertension—characterized by hypertension (systolic pressure greater than 140 mm Hg and/or diastolic pressure greater than 90 mm Hg) without proteinuria after 20 weeks gestation and resolving by 12 weeks postpartum; treated with frequent evaluation of BP and protein in urine

C. Preeclampsia and Eclampsia
   1. Assessment—increased risk in African Americans, primigravida older than 35 years or younger than 17 years, multiple fetuses or history of and renal disease, family history of hypertension in previous pregnancy; prenatal screening at each visit for symptomatology

Table 2 CHARACTERISTICS OF PREECLAMPSIA AND ECLAMPSIA					
CONDITION	BP	PROTEINURIA	SEIZURES	HYPERREFLEXIA	OTHER
Mild preeclampsia	Greater than 140/90 mm Hg after 20 weeks gestation	300 mg/L per 24 h Greater than 1+ random sample	No	No	Mild facial edema Weight gain (greater than 4.5 lb/wk)
Severe preeclampsia	Greater than 160/110 mm Hg	Greater than 500 mg/ L per 24 h Greater than 3+ random sample	No	Yes	Headache Oliguria Blurred vision RUQ pain Thrombocytopenia HELLP (hemolysis, elevated liver enzymes, low platelet count)
Eclampsia	Greater than 160/110 mm Hg	Marked proteinuria	Yes	No	Same as severe preeclampsia Severe headache Renal failure Cerebral hemorrhage

Table 3 PREECLAMPSIA AND ECLAMPSIA TREATMENT	
CONDITION	**TREATMENT**
Mild preeclampsia	Bed rest in left lateral position Monitor BP daily 6–8 8 oz drinks/day Frequent follow up
Severe preeclampsia	Depends on fetal age Only cure is delivery of fetus (induction of labor) Control BP (hydralyzine), prevent seizures (magnesium sulfate) Prevent long term morbidity and maternal mortality Emotional support if delivery prior to age of viability
Eclampsia (Medical Emergency)	Support through seizures and potential coma Ensure patent airway, O_2 support DIC management Delivery of fetus Emotional support if delivery prior to age of viability In cases of severe hypertension, seizures may still occur 24–48 h postpartum; monitor magnesium sulfate or hydralazine if continued postpartum

D. Evaluation

1. Has the infant been delivered safely?

2. Have complications been prevented?

3. Is the family coping effectively?

▶ PLACENTA PREVIA

A. Assessment

1. First- and second-trimester spotting

2. Third trimester bleeding that is sudden, bright-red, potentially profuse, *painless*

3. Ultrasonography—classified by degree of obstruction

B. Diagnose

1. The placenta is implanted in the lower uterine segment, usually near or over the cervical opening; placenta may partially or totally cover cervical os

2. Potential nursing diagnoses

   a. Impaired fetal gas exchange

   b. Risk for deficient fluid volume

   c. Deficient knowledge

   d. Risk for maternal injury

   e. Anxiety and fear

C. Plan/Implementation

1. Hospitalization initially

   a. Bedrest side-lying or Trendelenburg position for at least 72 hours

  b. Ultrasound to locate placenta

  c. No vaginal, rectal exam (if becomes necessary, must be done in OR under sterile conditions)

  d. Amniocentesis for lung maturity; monitor for changes in bleeding and fetal status

  e. Assess Daily Hgb and Hct

  f. Weigh peripads (1 gram = 1 mL blood loss)

  g. Two units of cross-matched blood available

  h. Assess amount of blood loss

2. Send home if bleeding ceases and pregnancy to be maintained

  a. Limit activity

  b. No douching, enemas, coitus

  c. Assess fetal movement

  d. Non stress test at least every 1–2 weeks

  e. Assess complications

3. Delivery by cesarean if evidence of fetal maturity, excessive bleeding, active labor, other complications

D. Evaluation

1. Was the infant delivered safely?

2. Were complications prevented?

▶ ABRUPTIO PLACENTAE—(PREMATURE SEPARATION OF PLACENTA)

A. Assessment

1. *Painful,* dark red vaginal bleeding; bleeding may be scant to profuse

2. Abdomen (uterus) is tender, painful, tense

3. Possible fetal distress, maternal shock

4. Contractions

B. Diagnose

1. Premature separation of the placenta

2. Occurrence increased with maternal hypertension and cocaine abuse

3. Potential nursing diagnoses

  a. Deficient fluid volume

  b. Impaired fetal gas exchange

  c. Acute pain

  d. Anxiety and fear

C. Plan/Implementation

1. Monitor for maternal shock and fetal distress

  a. Blood loss seen may not match symptoms

  b. Could have rapid fetal distress

2. Prepare for immediate delivery

3. Monitor for postpartal complications

   a. Disseminated intravascular coagulation (DIC)—bleeding gums, bleeding around IV insertion sites

   b. Pulmonary emboli

   c. Infection

   d. Renal failure

D. Evaluation

1. Has the woman's fluid and electrolyte balance been maintained?

2. Have complications been prevented?

▶ DIABETES

A. Assessment

1. Urine screening for ketones

2. Blood sugar levels; oral glucose tolerance test

3. Glucose tolerance test (1-h test at 24–28 weeks) for women at average risk

   a. Age 25 or older

   b. Obesity

   c. Family history of diabetes in first-degree relative

   d. Hispanic, African American, Native American, or Asian American

   e. History of abnormal glucose tolerance

4. Glycosylated hemoglobin (HbA_{1C})—(indicates past serum glucose levels over previous 3 months); normal is 3.5–6%

B. Diagnose

1. Potential nursing diagnoses

   a. Deficient knowledge

   b. Risk for risk-prone health behaviors

   c. Risk for unstable blood glucose

   d. Imbalanced nutrition: less than body requirements

2. Classification

   a. Type 1—complications more common

   b. Type 2

   c. Gestational diabetes (GDM)—increased demand for insulin during pregnancy

   d. Impaired fasting glucose tolerance

3. Diabetes increases risk for

   a. Maternal infections—UTIs and vaginal yeast infections

   b. Hypertensive states of pregnancy

   c. Hydramnios (greater than 2,000 ml amniotic fluid) and consequent preterm labor

   d. Macrosomia (large for gestational age but may have immature organ systems)

   e. Congenital anomalies (neural tube defects)

   f. Prematurity and stillbirth

      g. Respiratory distress syndrome (RDS)

      h. Untreated ketoacidosis can cause coma and death of mother and fetus

  4. Gestational diabetes

      a. Hyperglycemia after 20 weeks when insulin need accelerates

      b. Usually controlled by diet

      c. Oral hypoglycemics not used—teratogenic and increase risk of neonatal hypoglycemia

      d. Risk factors

         1) Obesity

         2) Family history of diabetes

         3) History of gestational diabetes

         4) Hypertension, preeclampsia/eclampsia, recurrent UTIs, monilial vaginitis, polyhydramnios; previously large infant (9-lb, 4,000 g or more)

         5) Previously unexplained death/anomaly or stillbirths

         6) Glycosuria, proteinuria on two or more occasions

  5. Testing for diabetes—at 24–28 weeks for all gravidas

      a. Screen blood glucose level 1 hour after 50 g concentrated glucose solution

      b. Three-hour glucose tolerance test; normal findings:
         FBS—less than 92 mg/dL (5.1 mmol/L)

         1 hour—less than 180 mg/dL (10 mmol/L)

         2 hours—less than 153 mg/dL (8.5 mmol/L)

         3 hours—less than 140 mg/dL (7.8 mmol/L)

      c. If two or more abnormal findings, significant for diabetes

      d. Glycosylated hemoglobin (HbA1c)—measures control past three months; elevations (greater than 6%) in first trimester associated with increased risk of congenital anomalies and spontaneous abortion; in the last trimester, elevations with macrosomia

C. Plan/Implementation

  1. Reinforce need for careful monitoring throughout pregnancy, including frequent medical/nursing evaluations

  2. Evaluate understanding of modifications in diet/insulin coverage

  3. Teach client and at least one significant other

      a. Diet—eat prescribed amount of food daily at same times; daily exercise

      b. Home glucose monitoring

      c. Insulin—purpose, dosage, administration, action, adverse effects, potential change in amount needed during pregnancy as fetus grows and immediately after delivery, no oral hypoglycemics (teratogenic)

  4. Assist with stress reduction

  5. Fetal surveillance

D. Evaluation

1. Does client remain free of hypoglycemia and hyperglycemia?

2. Are the mother and infant free from complications?

3. Does the client demonstrate compliance?

4. Do the woman and family show effective coping?

▶ CARDIAC DISEASE

A. Assessment

1. Chest pain

2. Dyspnea on exertion; dyspnea at rest; edema

3. Monitor vital signs and do EKG as heart lesion (especially with mitral valve involvement) may become aggravated by pregnancy

B. Diagnose

1. Potential nursing diagnoses

   a. Acute pain

   b. Decreased cardiac output

   c. Impaired fetal gas exchange

   d. Anxiety/fear

   e. Deficient knowledge

   f. Activity intolerance

   g. Maternal injury

2. Treatment of heart disease in pregnancy is determined by the functional capacity of the heart, and type of delivery will be influenced by the mother's status and the condition of fetus

C. Plan/Implementation

1. Encourage rest and adequate nutrition during pregnancy

2. Assess maternal vital signs and fetal heart rate

3. Encourage moderation in physical activity

4. Teach importance of avoidance and early treatment of upper respiratory infections

5. Be alert for signs of heart failure: increase of dyspnea; tachycardia; weight gain

6. Assess activity level during labor

   a. Assess vital signs frequently

   b. Place client on cardiac monitor and on external fetal monitor.

   c. Maintain bedrest with mother in side-lying or semi-recumbent position

   d. Administer oxygen as prescribed

   e. Assess for signs of pulmonary edema and heart failure

   f. Provide emotional support

D. Evaluation

1. Was the infant delivered safely?

2. Were cardiac complications in the mother prevented?

▶ SYPHILIS

A. Assessment

1. Blood tests (VDRL)

2. Primary lesion (chancre) located on internal or external genitalia

   a. Secondary stage may be unnoticeable

3. Previous obstetrical history of spontaneous abortion, premature births, or full-term stillbirth

4. Method of infection

   a. Congenital

   b. Acquired—sexually

B. Diagnose—potential nursing diagnoses

1. Delayed growth and development

2. Deficient knowledge

C. Plan/Implementation

1. Administer penicillin, which crosses placenta, thereby additionally treating fetus

D. Evaluation

1. Has the infection been successfully treated?

2. Have complications in the infant been prevented?

▶ GONORRHEA

A. Assessment

1. Positive culture of vaginal secretions

2. Purulent discharge or asymptomatic

B. Diagnose

1. Potential nursing diagnoses

   a. Risk for infection

   b. Deficient knowledge

2. May complicate pregnancy and cause sterility

C. Plan/Implementation

1. Teach about antibiotic as ordered

2. Instill prophylactic medication into baby's eyes after delivery

D. Evaluation

1. Have complications in the infant been avoided?

▶ PRE-EXISTING INFECTIONS

A. Assessment

1. History

2. Exposure—especially rubella, syphilis, herpes, HIV, CMV

3. Screening

   B. Diagnose

      1. Risk for infection

      2. Deficient knowledge

   C. Plan/Implementation

      1. Assist with cultures; antibody levels

      2. Teach administration of medications as ordered

      3. Prepare for possible cesarean section, surgical procedure

   D. Evaluation

      1. Have complications in the infant been avoided?

      2. Does mother have knowledge about pre-existing infection?

▶ GESTATIONAL TROPHOBLASTIC DISEASE (HYDATIDIFORM MOLE)

   A. Assessment

      1. Elevated hCG levels

      2. Uterine size greater than expected for dates

      3. No FHR

      4. Minimal dark red/brown vaginal bleeding with passage of grapelike clusters

      5. No fetus by ultrasound

      6. Increased nausea and vomiting and associated gestational hypertension

   B. Diagnose

      1. Degenerative anomaly of chorionic villi

   C. Plan/Implementation

      1. Curettage to completely remove all molar tissue that can become malignant

      2. Pregnancy is discouraged for 1 year

      3. hCG levels are monitored for 1 year (if continue to be elevated, may require hysterectomy and chemotherapy)

      4. Contraception discussed; IUD not used

      5. Administer Rho(D) immune globulin (IGIM) to Rh-negative women

   D. Evaluation

      1. Has the woman adjusted to the lack of a viable pregnancy?

      2. Has the Rh-negative woman received Rho(D) immune globulin (IGIM)?

▶ PRETERM LABOR

   A. Assessment

      1. Occurs between 20 and 37 weeks gestation, uterine contractions and cervical changes

      2. Risk factors

         a. African American

         b. Older than 35 or younger than 17

         c. Low socioeconomic status

     d. Previous preterm labor or birth

     e. Medical disease

     f. Smoking or substance abuse

     g. Problems with pregnancy

B. Diagnose—potential nursing diagnoses

   1. Acute pain

   2. Risk for fetal injury

   3. Deficient knowledge

C. Plan/Implementation

   1. Bedrest, side-lying

   2. Uterine monitoring, daily weights

   3. Maintain good nutrition

   4. Relaxation techniques

   5. Administration of medication (e.g., terbutaline)

D. Evaluation

   1. Has client complied with treatment?

   2. Has client given birth at or near term to a healthy mature infant?

▶ INDUCTION OF LABOR

A. Assessment

   1. Mother cannot have CPD

   2. Fetus must have mature vertex presentation

   3. Fetus must have engaged head

   4. Mother has "ripened" cervix, or it is induced to "ripen"

   5. Indications

     a. Diabetes

     b. Postmaturity

     c. Gestational hypertension

     d. Fetal jeopardy

     e. Logistical factors—(rate of rapid birth, distance from hospital)

B. Diagnose—potential nursing diagnoses

   1. Risk for maternal and fetal injury

   2. Deficient knowledge

C. Plan/Implementation

   1. Assess fetus continuously by external monitor

   2. Monitor BP, pulse, progress of labor of mother

   3. Prepare for amniotomy (rupture of membranes)

   4. Begin oxytocin administration

     a. Begin at 0.5–1 milliunits/min; increase dose 1–2 milliunits/min at intervals of 30–60 minutes until desired contractions; can administer up to 20 mU/min (follow unit/health care provider policy/order)

     b. Piggyback to principal intravenous line

     c. Administer via infusion pump

       d. Usual contraction pattern: q 2–3 minutes, lasting for 90 seconds or less

       e. Stop infusion if fetal distress or hypertonic contractions begin (contractions that last more than 90 seconds or occur more frequently than every 2 minutes)

D. Evaluation

    1. Has the woman delivered safely?

    2. Have complications been prevented?

▶ CESAREAN DELIVERY

A. Assessment

    1. Dystocia (abnormal or difficult labor)

    2. Previous Cesarean birth

    3. Breech presentation or CPD

    4. Fetal distress

    5. Active maternal gonorrhea or herpes type 2 infections

    6. Prolapsed umbilical cord

    7. Hypertensive states of pregnancy

    8. Placenta previa, abruptio placentae

    9. Fetal anomalies (e.g., hydrocephaly)

B. Diagnose

    1. Potential nursing diagnoses

       a. Anxiety

       b. Powerlessness

       c. Deficient knowledge

    2. Classification

       a. Vertical incision

          1) More blood loss

          2) Rapid delivery

       b. Low-segment transverse incision

          1) Less blood loss

          2) Vaginal birth after cesarean (VBAC) a possibility

C. Plan/Implementation

    1. Obtain lab tests—type and crossmatch, urinalysis, CBC

    2. Provide routine preop care; IV fluid

    3. Insert indwelling bladder catheter

    4. Provide emotional support; as a new mother first, surgical client second

    5. Administer preop medication—usually lower narcotic dose than routine preop medication

    6. Monitor for hemorrhage

       a. Assess fundus for firmness and location; massage if boggy

       b. Assess skin incision and dressing for signs of for excessive bleeding

       c. Assess vital signs for evidence of shock

    7. Routine postop care

8. Provide comfort measures and medications to control pain

9. Splint the incision site while the client does deep breathing exercises

10. Give the mother her infant as soon as possible to promote parent/child bonding

11. Encourage ambulation

D. Evaluation

1. Has the infant been delivered safely?

2. Have complications been prevented?

▶ PRECIPITOUS DELIVERY OUTSIDE HOSPITAL SETTING

A. Assessment

1. Determine that transport to hospital/birthing center is not possible

2. Evaluate mother's cognitive status and explain actions

B. Diagnose—potential nursing diagnoses

1. Risk for maternal and fetal injury

2. Deficient knowledge

C. Plan/Implementation

1. Remain with client

2. Prepare sterile or clean environment

3. Support infant's head; apply slight pressure to control delivery

4. Slip a nuchal cord, if present, over head

5. Rotate infant externally as head emerges

6. Deliver shoulders, trunk

7. Dry baby and place on mother's abdomen

8. Hold placenta as delivered

9. Wrap baby in blanket and put to breast

10. Check for bleeding and fundal tone

11. Arrange transport to hospital

12. Support mother and family

D. Evaluation

1. Has the infant been delivered safely?

2. Have complications been prevented?

▶ POSTPARTUM HEMORRHAGE

Definition: blood loss greater than 500 mL after a vaginal birth or 1000mL after a Cesarean birth

A. Assessment

1. Uterine tone and location

2. Blood loss amount:

   a. Accurate measurement of blood loss is accomplished by weighing peri pads.

   b. Large: Blood loss greater than 6 inches (15 cm) to saturated on a peri pad in 1 hour (50–80 mL)

   c. Moderate amount: Blood loss greater than 4 inches (10 cm) but less than 6 inches (15 cm) on peri pad in 1 hour (25–50 mL)

3. Lochia regressing to a previous stage

4. History

   a. Multiparity

   b. Retained placental fragments

   c. Overdistended uterus

   d. Prolonged labor or delivery of large infant

B. Diagnose—potential nursing diagnoses

   1. Deficient fluid volume

   2. Risk for infection

   3. Risk for maternal injury

   4. Impaired parenting

C. Plan/Implementation

   1. Massage uterus post delivery if not firm

   2. Assess involution for early identification of problems

   3. Administer oxytocin, ergonovine or methylcryonovine maleate, prostaglandin as ordered

      a. Produces contractions of uterus

      b. Controls postpartum hemorrhage

      c. Potential adverse effects are hypertension, nausea, and vomiting

   4. Monitor for signs of shock

D. Evaluation

   1. Has the woman's fluid balance been maintained?

   2. Have complications been prevented?

▶ POSTPARTUM INFECTION

A. Assessment

   1. Temperature 100.4°F or higher on any two consecutive postpartum days exclusive of the first 24 hours; chills, tachycardia

   2. Abdominal pain or severe afterpains, perineal discomfort

   3. Lochia—foul odor, prolonged rubra phase, decreased or increased amount

   4. Localized tenderness

   5. Diagnostic tests

      a. Blood cultures, culture of lochia, urine cultures, increased erythrocyte sedimentation rate (ESR)

      b. White blood cell count—significant increase over a 6-hour time period

   B. Diagnose—potential nursing diagnoses

      1. Risk for infection

      2. Deficient knowledge

   C. Plan/Implementation

      1. Encourage early ambulation

      2. Change peripads frequently

      3. Provide adequate nutrition, fluid intake, and sleep

      4. Monitor for signs of infection

      5. Administer antibiotics if ordered

   D. Evaluation

      1. Have complications been prevented?

      2. Does client have adequate understanding of good hygiene techniques?

▶ POSTPARTUM DEPRESSION

A. Assessment

      1. Decrease in estrogen and progesterone may precipitate "baby blues"

      2. Occurs during first year, often by fourth week

      3. Possibly associated with changing hormone levels

      4. Sadness and crying

      5. Difficulty concentrating

      6. Fatigue

      7. Appetite and sleep disturbances

B. Diagnose—potential nursing diagnoses

      1. Insomnia

      2. Risk for self-directed violence

      3. Interrupted family processes

      4. Anxietydisturbed thought processes

C. Plan/Implementation

      1. Encourage verbalization of feelings and identification of concerns

      2. Assess potential for suicide

      3. Consult with medical and psychiatric staff

      4. Support groups

      5. Administer medication

      6. Assist with care of baby

D. Evaluation

      1. Is the woman able to cope with the stress of a newborn?

      2. Is the woman able to verbalize her feelings?

▶ **NORMAL NEWBORN**

Table 1 NEWBORN ASSESSMENT		
SYSTEM	**ASSESSMENT**	**NURSING CONSIDERATIONS**
Respiration/perfusion	Rate—quiet vs. active Labored—retractions, grunting Color, heart rate, heart murmurs Nose breather	Keep airway patent Limit activities—decreases O_2 consumption Monitor blood gases/blood pressure Keep supplemental O_2 use limited to that required Monitor for respiratory distress (increased respiratory rate, grunting, nasal flaring, intercostals retractions) Prepare for possible intubation

Nutrition	Weight and length
	Head circumference
	Bottle feeding
	Chest circumference
	Situations that increase demand:
	  Sepsis
	    Ventilatory distress
	    Stress
		Monitor volume of fluid intake
		Dipstick and specific gravity on urine
		Caloric value of intake
		Monitor output volume in first 24 hours

Heat regulation	Ability to maintain normal body temperature
	Acidosis may develop if poor temperature regulation
		Provide regular monitoring
		Adjust environmental temperature appropriately:
		  Body covering
		    Warmer or isolette

Table 1 NEWBORN ASSESSMENT *(CONTINUED)*		
SYSTEM	**ASSESSMENT**	**NURSING CONSIDERATIONS**

CNS	Reflexes:
	  Tonic neck
	  Babinski
	  Moro
	  Autonomics—sucking, rooting, swallowing
	Fontanelles—bulging or flat
	Severe hypo- or hyperactivity
	Activity/sleep/cry:
	  Hyperirritable
	  Depressed
	Anatomical anomalies:
	  Cranial—hydrocephalus, microcephaly
	  Spinal
	Paralysis/paresis:
	  Erb's palsy
	  Bell's palsy
	  Lower extremities
		Respond to life-threatening problems immediately:
		  Absence of swallow reflex
		  Bulging fontanelle
		  Cranial nerve injuries

Parenting	Infant—behavior, individual differences
	Mother/father:
	  Pattern of touching
	  Reciprocity of interaction
	  Age and development level
	  Guilt, anxiety, grief reactions
	  Ability to interact
		Report any deviations

Circumcision	Observe for infection, bleeding	Record first voiding after procedure Apply dressing

A. Assessment (see Table 1)

  1. Airway—bulb suctioning—mouth first, then nose

  2. Apgar score (performed at 1 and 5 minutes of age)

    a. Scoring (see Table 2)

    b. Interpretations

      1) 0–3: poor

      2) 4–6: fair

      3) 7–10: excellent

Table 2 APGAR SCORE			
	0	1	2
Heart rate	Absent	Slow (less than 100 bpm)	Normal (greater than 100 bpm)
Respiratory effort	Absent	Slow, irregular	Good cry
Muscle tone	Flaccid	Some flexion	Active
Reflexes	No response	Weak cry	Vigorous cry
Color	Blue, pale	Body pink, extremities blue	Completely pink
TOTAL _____			

3. Measurements at term
   a. Weight—6–9 lb (2,700–4,000 g); normal five to ten percent weight loss in first few days should be regained in 1–2 weeks
   b. Length—19–21 inches (48–53 cm)
   c. Head circumference—13–14 inches (33–35 cm); 1/4 body length
   d. Chest—1 inch less than head circumference, 12–13 inches (30.5–33 cm)

4. Vital signs
   a. Temperature
      1) Rectal—not recommended as routine because of potential for rectal mucosa irritation and increased risk of perforation
      2) Axillary—97.7–99.7°F (36.5–37.6°C); thermometer should remain in place at least 3 minutes unless an electronic thermometer is used
   b. Apical rate—100 bpm (sleep); 120–140 bpm (awake); up to 180 bpm (crying); assessed by auscultation for 1 full minute when infant not crying
   c. Respirations—30–60 breaths/min; primarily diaphragmatic and abdominal, synchronous with chest movements; may be short (less than 15 sec) periods of apnea; since neonate is an obligatory nose breather, it is important to keep nose and mouth clear
   d. Blood pressure—65/41 mm Hg in arm and calf

5. Posture
   a. Maintains fetal position for several days
   b. Resistance to extension of extremities

6. Skin—sensitive to drying
   a. Erythematous (beefy red) color for a few hours after birth; then pink or as expected for racial background; acrocyanosis (bluish discoloration of hands and feet) is normal for 24 hours
   b. Vernix caseosa—protective gray-white fatty substance of cheesy consistency covering the fetal/newborn skin; do not attempt vigorous removal

c. Lanugo—light distribution of downy, fine hair may be over the shoulder, forehead, and cheeks; extensive amount is indicative of prematurity

d. Milia—distended sebaceous glands appearing as tiny, white, pinpoint papules on forehead, nose, cheeks, and chin of neonate that disappear spontaneously in a few days or weeks

e. Pigmentation

1) Mongolian spots—bluish gray or dark nonelevated pigmentation area over the lower back and buttocks present at birth in some infants (African American, Hispanic, Asian)

2) Birthmarks

a) Telangiectatic nevi ("stork bites")—cluster of small, flat, red localized areas of capillary dilatation usually on eyelids, nose, nape of neck; can be blanched by the pressure of the finger; usually fade during infancy

b) Nevus vasculosus (strawberry mark)—raised, demarcated, dark red, rough-surfaced capillary hemangioma in dermal and subdural layers; grow rapidly for several months and then begin to fade; usually disappear by 7 years of age

c) Nevus flammeus (port wine stain)—reddish, usually flat, discoloration commonly on the face or neck; does not grow and does not fade

7. Head—may appear asymmetrical because of overriding of cranial bones during labor and delivery (molding)

a. Fontanelles—"soft spots" at junction of cranial bones

1) Anterior fontanel—diamond shaped 2.5–4 cm, easily felt, usually open and flat (may be moderate bulging with crying/stooling); sustained bulging occurs with increased intracranial pressure, depression with dehydration; may be slight pulsation; closes by 18 months of age

2) Posterior—triangular 0.5–1 cm, not easily palpated; closes between 8 and 12 weeks of life

b. Cephalhematoma—collection of blood under the periosteum of a cranial bone appearing on first and second day; does not cross suture line; disappears in weeks to months

c. Caput succedaneum—localized soft swelling of the scalp often associated with a long and difficult birth; present at birth; overrides the suture line; fluid is reabsorbed within hours to days after delivery

d. Face—symmetrical distribution and movement of all features; asymmetry may signify paralysis of facial cranial nerve (Bell's palsy)

e. Eyes—eyelids may be edematous; pupils equal and react to light; absence of tears, corneal reflex, blink reflex, areas of subconjunctival hemorrhage

f. Mouth—sucks well when stimulated; hard and soft palate intact when examined with clean-gloved finger, gag reflex, rooting reflex

g. Ears—tops (pinnae) should be parallel with the inner and outer canthus of eyes; low-set ears are associated with chromosomal abnormalities, intellectual delay and/or internal organ abnormalities; hearing is evaluated by an arousal response to loud or moderately loud noise unaccompanied by vibration, startle reflex

8. Chest—breast enlargement lasting up to 2 weeks may occur in both males and females

9. Abdomen

   a. Cylindrical and slightly protuberant

   b. Umbilical cord—initially white and gelatinous with 2 arteries and 1 vein, shriveled and black by 2–3 days, falls off within 1–2 weeks; foul-smelling discharge is indicative of infection requiring immediate treatment to prevent septicemia

   c. First stool is black and tarry (meconium) passed within 12–24 hours; followed by thin green-brown transitional stools the third day; then 1–2 formed pale yellow to light brown stools/day with formula feeding or loose golden yellow stools with sour milk odor with every breast feeding

10. Genitourinary—urine is present in bladder at birth, but neonate may not void for 12–24 hours (may be brick-red spots on diaper from passage of uric acid crystals); thereafter usually voids pale yellow urine 6–10 times/day

    a. Female—labia relatively large and approximated; may have normal thick white discharge; a white cheese-like substance (smegma) and/or blood tinge (pseudomenstruation)

    b. Male—testes can be felt in scrotum

11. Trunk and extremities

    a. Arms and legs symmetric in shape and function

    b. Hips abduct to > 60°; symmetric inguinal and buttocks creases indicating no hip dislocation

    c. Foot in straight line

12. Reflexes

    a. Rooting and sucking—turns toward any object touching/stroking cheek/mouth, opens mouth, and sucks rhythmically when finger/nipple is inserted into mouth (usually disappears by 4–7 months)

    b. Pupillary—constriction on exposure of light

    c. Palmar grasp—pressure on palm elicits grasp (fades by 3–4 months)

    d. Plantar grasp—pressure on sole behind toes elicits flexion (lessens by 8 months)

    e. Tonic neck—fencing position; lying on back with head turned to one side, arm and leg on that side of body will be in extension while extremities on opposite side will be flexed (disappears by 3–4 months)

    f. Moro—elicited by sudden disturbance in the infant's immediate environment, body will stiffen, arms in tense extension followed by embrace gesture with thumb and index finger in a "c" formation (disappears after 3–4 months)

g. Positive-supporting—infant will stiffen legs and appear to stand when held upright

h. Stepping reflex—when held upright with one foot touching a flat surface, will step alternatingly (fades 4–5 months)

i. Babinski's sign—stroking the sole of the foot from heel upward across ball of foot will cause all toes to fan (reverts to usual adult response by 12 months)

B. Diagnose—potential nursing diagnoses

1. Airway clearance, ineffective

2. Thermoregulation, ineffective

3. Growth and development, altered

C. Plan/Implementation

1. Establish airway and maintain

2. Observe for Apgar score at 1 and 5 minutes

3. Clamp umbilical cord

4. Maintain warmth and keep exposure to environment minimal

5. Place identification band on baby and mother

6. Administer prophylactic medications

   a. Eye prophylaxis

   b. Administer intramuscular vitamin K—for first 3–4 days of life (the neonate is unable to synthesize vitamin K)

7. Record first stool and urine

8. Weigh and measure baby

9. Observe and support mother–infant bond

10. Begin and monitor feeding schedule

    a. Before initiating first formula feeding, check for readiness (active bowel sounds, absence of abdominal distention, and lusty cry) and for absence of gagging, choking, regurgitating associated with tracheoesophageal fistula or esophageal atresia by giving a small amount of sterile water (glucose is irritating to lungs)

    b. Since colostrum is readily absorbed by the gastrointestinal and respiratory system, breastfeeding may be started immediately after birth

11. Umbilical cord care—clean cord and surrounding skin; no tub baths until cord falls off; fold diapers below to maintain dry area; report redness, drainage, foul odor

12. Care of penis

    a. Uncircumcised—do not force retraction of foreskin (complete separation of foreskin and glans penis takes from 3–5 years); parents should be told to gently test for retraction occasionally during the bath, and when it has occurred, gently clean glans with soap and water

b. Circumcised (surgical removal of prepuce/foreskin)

   1) Ensure signed permission before procedure; provide comfort measures during and after procedure

   2) Postprocedure monitor for bleeding and voiding, apply A and D ointment or petroleum jelly (except when Plastibell is used)

   3) Teach parents to clean area with warm water squeezed over penis and dry gently; a whitish yellow exudate is normal and should not be removed; if Plastibell is used, report to pediatrician if it has not fallen off in about 8 days

D. Evaluation

   1. Did the infant make an optimal transition to extrauterine life?

   2. Have complications been prevented?

▶ RESPIRATORY DISTRESS SYNDROME (RDS)

A. Assessment

1. Labored respiration after several minutes or hours of normal respiration initially

2. Cyanosis, expiratory grunting, nasal flaring, intercostal and subcostal retractions, tachypnea (greater than 60 breath/min)

3. Unresponsiveness, apneic episodes

4. Diagnostic tests

    a. Ultrasound—biparietal diameter

    b. Amniocentesis

    1) Lipid level

    2) Creatinine level

    3) L/S ratio

    c. PO_2 less than 50 mm Hg; CO_2 greater than 60 mm Hg

B. Diagnose

1. Causes

    a. Prematurity

    b. Surfactant deficiency disease

2. Potential nursing diagnosis

    a. Impaired gas exchange

    b. Impaired spontaneous ventilation

    c. Risk for infection

    d. Risk for impaired parent infant attachment

C. Plan/Implementation

1. Maintain body temperature

2. Maintain neutral thermal environment

3. Parenteral nutrition during acute phase (nipple and gavage feeding contraindicated)

4. IV fluids

5. Maintain patent airway

6. Positioning—side-lying with head supported by small folded blanket or on back with neck slightly extended

7. Suctioning as needed

8. PEEP or CPAP—keep nasal prongs in place; high frequency ventilation

9. Oxygen hood or mechanical ventilation

10. Medications—antibiotics, diuretics, vitamin E, surfactant

D. Evaluation

1. Is the newborn able to maintain respirations?

2. Is the newborn able to maintain a patent airway?

▶ PERINATAL ASPHYXIA

A. Assessment

1. Meconium staining (nonbreech)

2. Signs of intracranial damage, increased pressure, altered fontanelles, seizures, bradycardia

3. Abnormal respirations with cyanosis and decreased respiratory rate

B. Diagnose

1. Potential nursing diagnoses

   a. Impaired gas exchange

   b. Ineffective tissue perfusion

2. Predisposing conditions

   a. Small for gestational age

   b. Maternal history of heavy cigarette smoking; preeclampsia/eclampsia; multiple gestations

C. Plan/Implementation

1. Prepare for aggressive ventilatory assistance

2. Keep airway open

D. Evaluation

1. Is tissue perfusion adequate?

2. Is neurological status normal?

▶ HYPERBILIRUBINEMIA

A. Assessment

1. Physiologic jaundice—caused by immature hepatic function, resolving cephalohematoma; jaundice after 24 hours, peaks at 72 hours, lasts 5–7 days; no treatment necessary

2. Breast-feeding jaundice (early onset)—caused by poor milk intake; onset 2–3 days, 72 hours peak; treated by frequent breastfeeding, caloric supplements

3. Breastmilk jaundice (late onset)—caused by factor in breast milk; onset 4–5 days, peak 10–15 days; treated by discontinuing breast feeding for 24 hours

4. Pathologic jaundice (Hemolytic anemia)—caused by blood antigen incompatibility; onset first 24 hours; peak variable; treated by phototherapy, exchange transfusions

B. Diagnose—potential nursing diagnoses

1. Risk for injury (CNS involvement)

2. Risk for injury (effects of treatment)

C. Plan/Implementation

1. Assess serum bilirubin levels (term 2–5 d less than 12 mg/dL (less than 205 μ mol/L))

2. Observe depth and extent for jaundice

3. Observe behavior of infant

4. Phototherapy

    a. Increase fluid intake

    b. Observe for adverse effects

    c. Patch eyes; uncover eyes every 2 hours

    d. Expose as much skin as possible; cover genitals

    e. Provide sensory stimulation

    f. Provide opportunities for bonding

5. Exchange transfusion if necessary to remove excess bilirubin

D. Evaluation

1. Have complications been prevented?

2. Has bonding taken place?

▶ HEMOLYTIC DISEASE OF NEWBORN (PATHOLOGIC JAUNDICE)

A. Assessment

1. Jaundice within 24 hours of birth

2. Serum bilirubin level elevates rapidly

3. Hematocrit decreased, anemia due to hemolysis of large number of erythrocytes

4. Coombs Test—detects antibodies attached to circulating erythrocytes, performed on cord blood sample

B. Diagnose

1. Destruction of RBCs from antigen–antibody reaction

2. Baby's Rh antigens enter mother; mother produces antibody; antibodies re-enter baby and causes hemolysis and jaundice

3. Rare during first pregnancy

C. Plan/Implementation

1. Assist in early identification

2. Phototherapy with fluorescent lighting—alters nature of bilirubin to aid excretion; infant's eyes and genitals must be covered

3. Exchange transfusion, if indicated—removes bilirubin and maternal hemolytic antibodies

D. Evaluation

1. Has child been protected from eye irritation and dehydration during phototherapy?

2. Has parent/child relationship been maintained during treatments?

▶ NECROTIZING ENTEROCOLITIS

A. Assessment

1. Feeding intolerance, bile-colored vomiting, abdominal distension

2. Blood in stool

3. Temperature instability

4. Hypothermia

5. Lethargy

6. Onset 4–10 days after feeding started

7. Diagnostics

    a. Hematest–positive stools

    b. Abdominal radiograph shows air in bowel wall

B. Diagnose–potential nursing diagnoses

1. Nutrition; less than body requirements, imbalanced

2. Deficient fluid volume

C. Plan/Implementation

1. Stop oral feedings; NPO; insert nasogastric tube; observe for 24–48 hours

2. Administer antibiotics and intravenous fluids as ordered

3. Handle infant carefully; avoid tight diapering

4. Provide caloric needs via PN or small oral feedings

5. Careful handwashing

D. Evaluation

1. Have the infant's nutritional needs been met?

▶ HYPOGLYCEMIA

A. Assessment

1. Blood sugar less than 35 mg/dL(1.9 mmol/L)(normal 40–80 mg/dL)(2.2-4.4 mmol/L)

2. Jitteriness

3. Irregular respiratory effort

4. Cyanosis

5. Weak, high-pitched cry

6. Lethargy

7. Twitching

8. Eye-rolling

9. Seizures

B. Diagnose–potential nursing diagnoses

1. Deficient knowledge

2. Risk for unstable blood glucose

C. Plan/Implementation

1. Monitor glucose level soon after birth and repeat in 4 hours

2. Administer glucose carefully to avoid rebound hypoglycemia

3. Initiate feedings if infant not lethargic; reassess glucose levels immediately before feeding

D. Evaluation

1. Have the infant's glucose levels returned to normal?

▶ NARCOTIC-ADDICTED INFANTS/NEONATAL ABSTINENCE SYNDROME (NAS)

A. Assessment

1. High-pitched cry, hyperreflexivity, decreased sleep

2. Diaphoresis, tachypnea (greater than 60/min), restlessness

3. Tremors, uncoordinated sucking, frequent sneezing and yawning, nonnutritive sucking

4. Drug withdrawal from narcotics, barbiturates, or cocaine; may manifest as early as 12–24 hours after birth, up to 7–10 days after delivery

B. Diagnose—potential nursing diagnoses

1. Risk for injury

2. Nutrition, less than body requirements, imbalanced

3. Risk for impaired parent/child attachment

C. Plan/Implementation

1. Assess muscle tone, irritability, vital signs

2. Administer phenobarbital, chlorpromazine, diazepam, paregoric, methadone as ordered

3. Report symptoms of respiratory distress

4. Reduce environmental stimulation (e.g., dim lights, decrease noise level)

5. Provide adequate nutrition/fluids; provide pacifier for nonnutritive sucking

6. Monitor mother–child interactions

7. Wrap infant snugly, rock, and hold tightly

D. Evaluation

1. Are environmental stresses decreased?

2. Have further complications been prevented?

3. Has adequate hydration been maintained?

▶ COLD STRESS

A. Assessment

1. Mottling of skin or cyanosis

2. Abnormal blood gases (metabolic acidosis), hypoxia, hypoglycemia

B. Diagnose

1. Infant unable to increase activity and lacks a shivering response to cold

2. Heat is produced through metabolic process

3. Oxygen consumption and energy are diverted from maintaining normal brain cell, cardiac function, and growth to thermogenesis

4. Causes

   a. Hypoxemia (PO_2 less than 50 torr)

   b. Intracranial hemorrhage or any CNS abnormality

   c. Hypoglycemia (less than 40 mg/dL)(less than 2.2 mmol/L)

C. Plan/Implementation

1. Place in heated environment immediately after birth; dry infant immediately

2. Maintain neutral thermal environment

   a. Double-walled or servocontrolled incubator

   b. Radiant warming panel

   c. Open bassinet with cotton blankets and head covered

   d. Place infant on mother's abdomen

3. Monitor temperature

4. Fabric-insulated cap for head

D. Evaluation

1. Have complications been prevented?

▶ NEONATAL SEPSIS

A. Assessment

1. Temperature instability, especially hypothermia

2. Poor sucking, vomiting, diarrhea, feeding intolerances

3. Lethargy, convulsive activity

4. Episodes of apnea

5. Lack of weight gain, dehydration

B. Diagnose—predisposing factors

1. Prematurity

2. Maternal signs and symptoms of infection (beta-hemolytic streptococcal vaginosis)

3. Invasive procedures and resuscitation

4. Premature rupture of membranes; prolonged rupture of membranes

5. Prolonged labor or delivery by cesarean section or forceps

6. Aspiration of meconium fluid

C. Plan/Implementation

1. Administration of prophylactic antibiotics for 7–10 days

2. Administer oxygen

3. Temporarily discontinue oral feedings

4. Transfusion with fresh, irradiated granulocytes or polymorphonuclear leukocytes

5. IV gammaglobulin to prevent nosocomial infection

D. Evaluation

1. Have the infant's nutritional needs been met?

▶ CLEFT LIP AND PALATE

A. Assessment

1. Cleft lip—small or large fissure in facial process of upper lip or up to nasal septum, including anterior maxilla

2. Cleft palate—midline, bilateral, or unilateral fissures in hard and soft palate

B. Diagnose

1. Definition—congenital malformation

2. Lip is usually repaired during 1 to 3 months of age

3. Palate is usually repaired before child develops altered speech patterns; between 12–18 months

C. Plan/Implementation

1. Parents will have strong reaction to birth of defective infant—provide support and information

2. Assess infant's ability to suck

3. Surgical repair

   a. Preoperative

      1) Maintain adequate nutrition

      2) Feed with soft nipple, special lamb's nipple, Brechet feeder (syringe with rubber tubing), or cup; feed slowly and burp often

   b. Postoperative

      1) Maintain airway

         a) Observe for respiratory distress, aspiration, or blockage from edema, check ability to swallow

         b) Provide suction equipment and endotracheal tube at bedside

      2) Guard suture line

         a) Keep suture line clean and dry

         b) Use lip-protective devices, i.e., Logan bow or tape (see Figure 1)

         c) Maintain side-lying position on unaffected side

         d) Clean suture line with cotton-tipped swab dipped in saline, then apply thin coat of antibiotic ointment

         e) Minimize crying with comfort measures—rocking, cuddling

         f) Use elbow restraints as needed

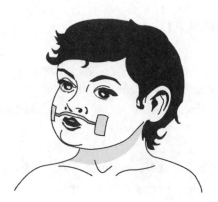

Figure 1 Logan Bow

3) Provide nutrition

  a) Use feeding techniques to minimize trauma—usually very slow to feed

  b) Burp baby frequently during feedings

4) Facilitate parents' positive response to child

5) Provide referrals to speech therapy and orthodontists as needed

D. Evaluation

1. Has defect been repaired?

2. Have infant's nutritional needs been met?

▶ NORMAL REPRODUCTION

A. Assessment

   1. Knowledge of normal sexual function

   2. Prevention of illness through self-care

   3. Promotion of health through control of fertility

   4. Cultural influences

B. Diagnose

   1. Potential nursing diagnoses

      a. Health-seeking behaviors (reproduction)

      b. Readiness for enhanced knowledge

      c. Anxiety related to reproductive health

   2. Diagnostic tests and procedures (e.g., culdoscopy, laparoscopy)

C. Plan/Implementation

   1. Provide privacy

   2. Assess knowledge

   3. Teach about breast self-exam (BSE), Pap test, mammogram, testicular self-exam

   4. Instruct client in breast self-examination

      a. Examine monthly

         1) Menstruating women—1 week after onset of menstrual period

         2) Nonmenstruating women—American Cancer Society suggests a routine, such as the first day of each month

      b. Procedure

         1) Inspect breasts in mirror

         2) Examine breasts first with arms at sides, second with arms above head, and third with hands on hips

         3) Use finger pads of 3 middle fingers to palpate breasts to detect unusual growths while lying down

         4) Look for dimpling or retractions

         5) Examine nipples for discharge, changes, swelling

   5. Provide information about mammography

      a. Assess knowledge of procedure

      b. Schedule after menstrual period (less breast sensitivity)

      c. Inform client that test may cause discomfort: compresses breast between 2 sheets of x-ray film

6. Provide health teaching about testicular self-exam
   a. Procedure
      1) Support testes in palm of one hand and palpate between thumb and forefinger
      2) Best performed in shower when cremaster muscles are relaxed and testes are pendulous
   b. Schedule once monthly
7. Assess knowledge of birth control
   a. Factors
      1) Impact of age, developmental level
      2) Desires of both partners
      3) Capability of use
      4) Permanent or temporary
   b. Plan—teach methods of contraception (see Table 1)
8. Assess knowledge of menopause, climacteric
   a. Menstruation ceases
   b. Symptoms related to hormone changes—vasomotor instability, emotional disturbances, atrophy of genitalia, uterine prolapse
   c. Estrogen replacement therapy (ERT)—contraindicated if family history of breast or uterine cancer, hypertension, or thrombophlebitis
   d. Kegel exercises—for strengthening pubococcygeal muscles
   e. Supplemental calcium—(1 gram HS) to slow osteoporosis
   f. Regular exercise and good nutrition

D. Evaluation
   1. Has the client developed a plan for control of fertility?
   2. Does the client understand self-care techniques?

▶ REPRODUCTIVE DISORDERS

A. Assessment (see Table 2)

B. Diagnose—potential nursing diagnoses
   1. Sexuality patterns, ineffective
   2. Sexual Dysfunction
   3. Readiness for enhanced knowledge

C. Plan/Implementation (see Table 2)

D. Evaluation
   1. Have complications been avoided?
   2. Is the client knowledgeable about prevention of infection?

Table 1 METHODS OF CONTRACEPTION	
METHOD	**NURSING CONSIDERATIONS**
Oral contraceptives—"the pill"	• Action—inhibits the release of FSH, resulting in anovulatory menstrual cycles; close to 100% effective • Adverse effects—nausea and vomiting (usually occurring the first 3 months), increased susceptibility to vaginal infections • Contraindications—hypertension, thromboembolic disease, and history of circulatory disease, varicosities, or diabetes mellitus • Teaching—swallow whole at the same time each day; one missed pill should be taken as soon as remembered that day or two taken the next day; more than one missed pill requires use of another method of birth control for the rest of the cycle; consume adequate amounts of vitamin B; report severe/persistent chest pain, cough and/or shortness of breath, severe abdominal pain, dizziness, weakness and/or numbness, eye or speech problems, severe leg pain
Hormone injections— methoxyprogesterone	• Injectable progestin that prevents ovulation for 12 weeks. • Convenient because it is unrelated to coitus (requires no action at the time of intercourse) and is 99.7% effective. • Injections must be given every 12 weeks. The site should not be massaged after the injection because this accelerates the absorption and decreases the effectiveness time. • Menstrual irregularity, spotting, and breakthrough bleeding are common. • Return to fertility is 6 to 12 months
MPA and estradiol	• A monthly injectable contraceptive. Similar to oral contraceptives in chemical formulation, but has the advantage of monthly rather than daily dosing. • Provides effective, immediate contraception within 5 days of the last normal menstrual period (LNMP). • Menstrual periods less painful and with less blood loss than medroxyprogesterone acetate • Return to fertility is 2 to 4 months
Intrauterine device (IUD)	• Action—presumed either to cause degeneration of the fertilized egg or render the uterine wall impervious to implantation; nearly 100% effective • Inserted by health care provider during the client's menstrual period, when the cervix is dilated • Adverse effects—cramping or excessive menstrual flow (for 2–3 months), infection • Teaching—check for presence of the IUD string routinely, especially after each menstrual period; report unusual cramping, late period, abnormal spotting/bleeding, abdominal pain or pain with intercourse, exposure to STI's, infection, missing/shorter/longer IUD string
Condom—rubber sheath applied over the penis	• Action—prevents the ejaculate and sperm from entering the vagina; helps prevent sexually transmitted disease; effective if properly used; OTC • Teaching—apply to erect penis with room at the tip every time before vaginal penetration; use water-based lubricant, e.g., K-Y jelly, never petroleum-based lubricant; hold rim when withdrawing the penis from the vagina; if condom breaks, partner should use contraceptive foam or cream immediately
Female (vaginal) condom	• Allows the woman some protection from disease without relying on the male condom. • The device is a polyurethane pouch inserted into the vagina, with flexible rings at both ends. The closed end with its ring functions as a diaphragm. The open end with its ring partially covers the perineum. • The female condom should not be used at the same time that the male partner is using a condom. • Failure rates are high with the female condom, at about 21%. • Increased risk of infections.

Table 1 METHODS OF CONTRACEPTION *(CONTINUED)*	
METHOD	NURSING CONSIDERATIONS
Diaphragm—flexible rubber ring with a latex-covered dome inserted into the vagina, tucked behind the pubic bone, and released to cover the cervix	• Action—prevents the sperm from entering the cervix; highly effective if used correctly • Must be fitted by health care provider and method of inserting practiced by the client before use • Risk—urinary tract infection (UTI) and toxic shock syndrome (TSS) • Teaching—diaphragm should not be inserted more than 6 hours prior to coitus; best used in conjunction with a spermicidal gel applied to rim and inside the dome before inserting; additional spermicide is necessary if coitus is repeated; remove at least once in 24 hours to decrease risk of toxic shock syndrome; report symptoms of UTI and TSS
Vaginal spermicides (vaginal cream, foam, jellies)	• Action—interferes with the viability of sperm and prevents their entry into the cervix; OTC • Teaching—must be inserted before each act of intercourse; report symptoms of allergic reaction to the chemical
Subdermal implant	• Action—effective for 5 years; requires surgical insertion and removal • Adverse effects—irregular bleeding, nausea, skin changes
Natural family planning (rhythm method, basal body temperature, cervical mucus method)	• Action—periodic abstinence from intercourse during fertile period; based on the regularity of ovulation; variable effectiveness • Teaching—fertile period may be determined by a drop in basal body temperature before and a slight rise after ovulation and/or by a change in cervical mucus from thick, cloudy, and sticky during nonfertile period to more abundant, clear, thin, stretchy, and slippery as ovulation occurs
Coitus interruptus	• Action—man withdraws his penis before ejaculation to avoid depositing sperm into vagina; variable effectiveness

Sterilization	• Vasectomy (male)—terminates the passage of sperm through the vas deferens
	  • Usually done in health care provider's office under local anesthesia; permanent and 100% effective
	  • Teaching—postprocedure discomfort and swelling may be relieved by mild analgesic, ice packs, and scrotal support; sterility not complete until the proximal vas deferens is free of sperm (about 3 months), another method of birth control must be used until two sperm-free semen analysis; success of reversal by vasovasostomy varies from 30 to 85%.
	• Tubal ligation (female)—fallopian tubes are tied and/or cauterized through an abdominal incision, laparoscopy, or minilaparotomy
	  • Teaching—usual postop care and instructions; intercourse may be resumed after bleeding ceases
	  • Success of reversal by reconstruction of the fallopian tubes is 40-75%

Table 2 PROBLEMS OF THE REPRODUCTIVE TRACT		
DISORDER	ASSESSMENT	NURSING CONSIDERATIONS
Infertility	Inability to conceive after a year of unprotected intercourse Tests include check of tubal patency, sperm analysis Affects approximately 10–15% of all couples	Support and assist clients through tests Allow expression of feelings and refer to support groups as needed Alternatives include artificial insemination, *in vitro* fertilization, adoption
Simple vaginitis	Yellow discharge, itching, burning	Douche, antibiotics, sitz baths
Atrophic vaginitis	Occurs after menopause Pale, thin, dry mucosa, itching, dyspareunia	Treated with topical estrogen cream, water-soluble vaginal lubricants, antibiotic vaginal suppositories and ointments
Candida albicans	Odorless, cheesy white discharge Itching, inflamed vagina and perineum	Topical clotrimazole Nystatin

Table 2 PROBLEMS OF THE REPRODUCTIVE TRACT *(CONTINUED)*		
DISORDER	**ASSESSMENT**	**NURSING CONSIDERATIONS**
Toxic shock syndrome (TSS)	Sudden-onset fever, vomiting, diarrhea, drop in systolic blood pressure, and erythematous rash on palms and soles	Early diagnosis critical to avoid involvement with other organ systems Managed with antibiotics, fluid and electrolyte replacement Educate about use of tampons
Pelvic inflammatory disease (PID)	Local infection spreads to the fallopian tubes, ovaries, and other organs Malaise, fever, abdominal pain, leukocytosis, and vaginal discharge Risk factors—20 years old or younger, multiple sex partners, IUD, vaginal douching, smoking, history of STIs, history of PID	Managed with antibiotics, fluid and electrolyte replacement, warm douches to increase circulation, rest Can cause adhesions that produce sterility
Mastitis	Reddened, inflamed breast Exudate from nipple Fever, fatigue, leukocytosis, pain	Systemic antibiotics, warm packs to promote drainage, rest, breast support
Fibrocystic changes	Multiple cyst development Free-moving, tender, enlarged during menstrual period and about 1 week before	Review importance and technique of breast self-exam Provide frequent monitoring for changes Prepare for possibility of aspiration, biopsy, or surgery Diet changes and vitamin supplements Benign, but associated with increased risk of breast cancer
Cancer of the cervix	Early—asymptomatic Later—abnormal bleeding, especially postcoital Risk factors—low socioeconomic status, began sexual activity or had pregnancy at a young age, multiple sexual partners	Preparation for tests, biopsy Internal radiation therapy Pap smear
Breast cancer	Small, fixed, painless lump Rash, or in more advanced cases, change in color, puckering or dimpling of skin, pain and/or tenderness, nipple retraction or discharge Axillary adenopathy Risk factors—family history of mother, sister, or daughter developing premenopausal breast cancer, age greater than 50, menses begins before age 12, no children or first pregnancy occurs after age 30, menopause after age 55	Mammography screening Prepare for surgery and/or radiation, chemotherapy
Uterine fibroids (myomas)	Low back pain, fertility problems, Menorrhagia	Benign tumors of myometrium Size and symptoms determine action Prepare for possible hysterectomy (removal of uterus) or myomectomy (partial resection of uterus)

Table 2 PROBLEMS OF THE REPRODUCTIVE TRACT (CONTINUED)		
DISORDER	**ASSESSMENT**	**NURSING CONSIDERATIONS**
Uterine displacement/prolapse	Weak pelvic support, sometimes after menopause Pain, menstrual interruption, fertility problems Urinary incontinence	Kegel exercises—isometric exercises of the muscle that controls urine flow (pubococcygeus, or PC muscle) can improve pelvic musculature support Pessary—device inserted into vagina that gives support to uterus in cases of retroversion or prolapse; must be inserted and rechecked by health professional Hormone replacement therapy—improves pelvic muscle tone Surgical intervention—colporrhaphy (suturing fascia and musculature to support prolapsed structures)
Endometriosis	Found in colon, ovaries, supporting ligaments, causes inflammation and pain Causes dysmenorrhea and infertility, backache Most common in young nulliparous women	Advise client that oral contraceptives suppress endometrial buildup or that surgical removal of tissue is possible Inform client that symptoms abate after childbirth and lactation

Endometrial cancer	Watery discharge, irregular menstrual bleeding, menorrhagia
	
	Diagnosed by endometrial biopsy or curettage
	
	Risk factors—age greater than 55, postmenopausal bleeding, obesity, diabetes mellitus, hypertension, unopposed estrogen replacement therapy
		Internal radiation implants:
		  Must restrict movements; bedrest with air mattress
		  Enema, douche, low-residue diet, ample fluids
		  Indwelling catheter and fracture pan for elimination
		  Visitors and professionals wear protective garments and limit exposure time
		  Dislodged implant must be handled with special tongs and placed in lead-lined container for removal; call hospital radiation therapy specialist first
		Hysterectomy:
		  Subtotal—removal of fundus only
		  Total—removal of the uterus (vagina remains intact)
		  Total abdominal hysterectomy with bilateral salpingooophorectomy (TAH-BSO)—removal of uterus, fallopian tubes, and ovaries
		  Radical—removal of lymph nodes as well as TAH-BSO
		  Assess for hemorrhage, infection, thrombophlebitis
		  If ovaries removed, estrogen replacement therapy (ERT) may be needed

Ovarian cyst	Pelvic discomfort Palpable during routine exam	May do biopsy or removal to prevent necrosis Monitor by sonography
Ovarian cancer	Family history of ovarian cancer, client history of breast, bowel, endometrial cancer, nulliparity, infertility, heavy menses, palpation of abdominal mass (late sign), diagnosis by ultrasound, CT, x-ray, IVP	Surgical removal, chemotherapy, staging of tumor after removal Foster verbalization of feelings, ensure continuity of care, encourage support systems

Table 2 PROBLEMS OF THE REPRODUCTIVE TRACT *(CONTINUED)*		
DISORDER	ASSESSMENT	NURSING CONSIDERATIONS
Orchitis	Complication of mumps, virus, STI may cause sterility, pain, and swelling	Prophylactic gammaglobulin if exposed to mumps virus Administration of drugs specific for organism Ice packs to reduce swelling, bedrest, scrotal support
Prostatitis	May be complication of lower UTIs Acute—fever, chills, dysuria, purulent penile discharge; elevated WBC and bacteria in urine Chronic—backache, urinary frequency, enlarged, firm, slightly tender prostate	Antibiotics, sitz baths Increased fluid intake Activities to drain the prostate

Benign prostatic hypertrophy (BPH)	Enlargement of the glandular and cellular tissue of the prostate, resulting in compression on the urethra and urinary retention; most often in men over 50 years old
	
	Dysuria, frequency, urgency, decreased urinary stream, hesitancy, and nocturia; later symptoms may be cystitis, hydronephrosis, or urinary calculi
	
	KUB, x-ray, IVP, and cystoscopy demonstrate prostate enlargement and urinary tract change
		Preoperative
		  Promote urinary drainage
		  Assure nutrition
		  Correct fluid and electrolyte balance
		  Antibiotics
		  Acid-ash diet to treat infection
		Postoperative
		  Assure patency of three-way Foley catheter; may have continuous irrigation with normal saline to remove clots (CBI)
		  If traction on catheter (pulled taut and taped to abdomen or leg to prevent bleeding), keep client's leg straight
		  Monitor drainage (reddish-pink and progress to clear)
		  Discourage attempts to void around catheter; control/treat bladder spasms
		  Teach bladder retraining by contracting and relaxing sphincter; instruct to avoid heavy lifting, straining at bowel movement, prolonged travel; inform about potential for impotence and discuss alternative ways of expressing sexuality

Prostate cancer	Urinary urgency, frequency, retention Back pain or pain radiating down leg Risk factors—increasing age	Hormonal and chemotherapy; surgical removal

PREVENTION AND EARLY DETECTION OF DISEASE

▶ HEALTH AND WELLNESS

A. Wellness—person functions at highest potential for well-being

B. Health promotion

   1. Activities that assist person to develop resources that improve quality of life

   2. Alteration of personal habits, lifestyle, environment to reduce risks and enhance health and well-being

C. Concepts

   1. Self-responsibility

      a. Individual has control over life

      b. Individual can make choices that promote health

   2. Nutritional awareness—properly balanced diet

   3. Stress reduction and management—manages stress appropriately

   4. Physical fitness—regular exercise promotes health

      a. Improves cardiovascular functioning

      b. Decreases cholesterol and LDLs

      c. Reduces weight

      d. Prevents body degeneration and osteoporosis

      e. Improves flexibility, muscle strength, endurance

D. Programs

   1. General wellness

   2. Smoking cessation

   3. Exercise/physical conditioning

   4. Weight control

   5. Stress management

   6. Nutritional awareness

   7. Work safety

▶ HEALTH SCREENING

A. Newborn

   1. PKU (phenylketonuria)—absence of enzyme needed to metabolize essential amino acid phenylalanine; Guthrie blood test

   2. Hypothyroidism—deficiency of thyroid hormones; heel-stick blood sample

   3. Galactosemia—error of carbohydrate metabolism

   4. Sickle-cell disease—abnormally shaped hemoglobin

   5. HIV (human immunodeficiency virus)

B. Infant/child

1. Developmental screening—Denver-II

2. Carrier screening for siblings and family members of a child with cystic fibrosis

3. Cholesterol screening for children with family history of hyperlipidemia, xanthomas, sudden death, early angina, or MI (less than 50 yr men, less than 60 yr women) in siblings, parents, uncles, aunts, grandparents

4. Lead poisoning—children (6–72 months) at highest risk

   a. Live in deteriorated housing

   b. Siblings or close peer with lead poisoning

   c. Household member with hobbies (e.g., stained glass) or lead-related occupations

5. Neuroblastoma—measure VMA and HVA (catecholamine metabolities)

C. School-age

1. Hearing and vision tests at 4 yr, 5 yr, then yearly during school

2. Height, weight

3. Dental exam

4. Medical assessment

5. Psychological exams

D. Adolescent

1. Developmental screening

2. PD

3. Sexuality

   a. Menstrual history

   b. Extent of sexual activity

   c. Contraceptive knowledge

4. Affect—symptoms of depression

5. Breast self-exam or testicular exam

6. Pelvic with pap smear—if sexually active or 18 years old, performed annually

E. Adult/elderly

1. Breast self-exam or testicular exam (see Table 1)

2. Cancer screenings

   a. Sigmoidoscopy—greater than 50 years old, performed every 10 years

   b. Fecal occult blood test—greater than 50 years old, performed yearly

   c. Digital rectal exam—greater than 40 years old, performed yearly

   d. Colonoscopy—beginning at age 50, every 10 years

   e. Pelvic exam for women—18–40 years old, performed every 3 years with Pap test

   f. Endometrial tissue sample for women who are at risk at menopause

   g. Mammography for women 35–39 years old once as baseline, after 40 yearly

   h. Health counseling and cancer check-ups—greater than 40 years old, performed yearly

3. Hypertension screening (see Tables 2 and 3)

4. Diabetes screening

5. Hearing and vision screening

Table 1 SELF-CARE: REPRODUCTIVE SYSTEM		
TEST	**AGE TO BEGIN (YRS)**	**REPEAT**
Breast self-exam	18–20	Monthly
Papanicolaou test (Pap smear)	18, or at least start of sexual activity	Yearly
Mammogram	35–39 40 and older	Once as baseline Annually
Testicular self-exam	onset of puberty	Monthly

Table 2 BLOOD PRESSURE SCREENING (MM HG)*		
SYSTOLIC	**DIASTOLIC**	**FOLLOW-UP RECOMMENDED**
less than 120	less than 80	Recheck in 2 years
120–139	80–89	Recheck in 1 year
140–159	90–99	Confirm within 2 months
160–179	100–109	Evaluate or refer to source of care within 1 month
180–209	110–119	Evaluate or refer to source of care within 1 week
≥210	≥120	Evaluate or refer to source of care immediately

Recommendations are for adults age 18 and older.

Table 3 ERRORS IN BLOOD PRESSURE MEASUREMENT	
Inaccurately high	Cuff is too short or too narrow (e.g., using a regular blood pressure cuff on an obese arm), or the brachial artery may be positioned below the heart
High diastolic	Unrecognized auscultatory gap (a silent interval between systolic and diastolic pressures that may occur in hypertensive clients or because you deflated the blood pressure cuff too rapidly); immediate reinflation of the blood pressure cuff for multiple blood pressure readings (resultant venous congestion makes the Korotkoff sounds less audible); if the client supports his or her own arm, then sustained muscular contraction can raise the diastolic blood pressure by 10%
Inaccurately low	Cuff is too long or too wide; the brachial artery is above the heart
Low systolic	Unrecognized auscultatory gap (a rapid deflation of the cuff or immediate reinflation of the cuff for multiple readings can result in venous congestion, thus making the Korotkoff sounds less audible and the pressure appear lower)

▶ **IMMUNITY**

A. Assessment

1. Antigen/antibody response

    a. Antigen—a foreign protein that stimulates antibody formation response

    b. Antibody—protective protein that acts as a defense mechanism

2. Active immunity

    a. Permanent

    b. Antigenic substance stimulates the individual's own antibody formations (e.g., tetanus)

3. Passive immunity

    a. Temporary

    b. Resistance acquired by introduction of antibodies from a source other than the individual (e.g., gamma globulin, breast feeding)

B. Diagnose

1. Antigen/antibody response—functions to neutralize, eliminate, or destroy substances recognized as foreign (nonself) by the body before the occurrence of potential harm to body tissues

C. Plan/Implementation

1. Recommended immunization schedule for infants and children (see Table 4) and adults (see Tables 5 and 6)

2. Contraindications to immunization

    a. Severe febrile illness

    b. Live viruses should not be given to anyone with altered immune system, e.g., undergoing chemotherapy, radiation, or with immunological deficiency

    c. Previous allergic response to a vaccine

    d. Recently acquired passive immunity, e.g., blood transfusion, immunoglobulin

3. Interrupted schedule or uncertain immunity status

    a. Not necessary to repeat immunizations when the schedule is interrupted; continue schedule at next visit or when immunization is again appropriate

    b. If there is no evidence of immunizations and the child is less than 7 years old give: DTaP, IPV, Tine; 4–6 weeks later MMR; 1 month after second immunization give DTaP and IPV; repeated in another month and again in 10–16 months

    c. Can give DTaP, IPV, MMR

4. Nursing care (see Table 6)

D. Evaluation

1. Do the parents know what adverse effects of the immunization their child may experience?

2. Did the child receive the immunizations as scheduled?

Table 4 CHILDHOOD IMMUNIZATION

Figure 1. Recommended immunization schedule for persons aged 0 through 18 years – United States, 2016.
(FOR THOSE WHO FALL BEHIND OR START LATE, SEE THE CATCH-UP SCHEDULE [FIGURE 2]).

These recommendations must be read with the footnotes that follow. For those who fall behind or start late, provide catch-up vaccination at the earliest opportunity as indicated by the green bars in Figure 1. To determine minimum intervals between doses, see the catch-up schedule (Figure 2). School entry and adolescent vaccine age groups are shaded.

Vaccine	Birth	1 mo	2 mos	4 mos	6 mos	9 mos	12 mos	15 mos	18 mos	19–23 mos	2-3 yrs	4-6 yrs	7-10 yrs	11-12 yrs	13–15 yrs	16–18 yrs
Hepatitis B[1] (HepB)	1st dose	←------ 2nd dose ------→			←---------------------------------- 3rd dose ----------------------------------→											
Rotavirus[2] (RV) RV1 (2-dose series); RV5 (3-dose series)			1st dose	2nd dose	See footnote 2											
Diphtheria, tetanus, & acellular pertussis[3] (DTaP: <7 yrs)			1st dose	2nd dose	3rd dose			←------ 4th dose ------→				5th dose				
Haemophilus influenzae type b[4] (Hib)			1st dose	2nd dose	See footnote 4		3rd or 4th dose, See footnote 4									
Pneumococcal conjugate[5] (PCV13)			1st dose	2nd dose	3rd dose		←------ 4th dose ------→									
Inactivated poliovirus[6] (IPV: <18 yrs)			1st dose	2nd dose	←---------------------------------- 3rd dose ----------------------------------→							4th dose				
Influenza[7] (IIV; LAIV)					Annual vaccination (IIV only) 1 or 2 doses							Annual vaccination (LAIV or IIV) 1 or 2 doses		Annual vaccination (LAIV or IIV) 1 dose only		
Measles, mumps, rubella[8] (MMR)					See footnote 8		←------ 1st dose ------→					2nd dose				
Varicella[9] (VAR)							←------ 1st dose ------→					2nd dose				
Hepatitis A[10] (HepA)							←------ 2-dose series, See footnote 10 ------→									
Meningococcal[11] (Hib-MenCY ≥ 6 weeks; MenACWY-D ≥9 mos; MenACWY-CRM ≥ 2 mos)					See footnote 11									1st dose		Booster
Tetanus, diphtheria, & acellular pertussis[12] (Tdap: ≥7 yrs)														(Tdap)		
Human papillomavirus[13] (2vHPV: females only; 4vHPV, 9vHPV: males and females)														(3-dose series)		
Meningococcal B[11]															See footnote 11	
Pneumococcal polysaccharide[5] (PPSV23)												See footnote 5				

Legend:
- Range of recommended ages for all children
- Range of recommended ages for catch-up immunization
- Range of recommended ages for certain high-risk groups
- Range of recommended ages for non-high-risk groups that may receive vaccine, subject to individual clinical decision making
- No recommendation

This schedule includes recommendations in effect as of January 1, 2016. Any dose not administered at the recommended age should be administered at a subsequent visit, when indicated and feasible. The use of a combination vaccine generally is preferred over separate injections of its equivalent component vaccines. Vaccination providers should consult the relevant Advisory Committee on Immunization Practices (ACIP) statement for detailed recommendations, available online at http://www.cdc.gov/vaccines/hcp/acip-recs/index.html. Clinically significant adverse events that follow vaccination should be reported to the Vaccine Adverse Event Reporting System (VAERS) online (http://www.vaers.hhs.gov) or by telephone (800-822-7967). Suspected cases of vaccine-preventable diseases should be reported to the state or local health department. Additional information, including precautions and contraindications for vaccination, is available from CDC online (http://www.cdc.gov/vaccines/recs/vac-admin/contraindications.htm) or by telephone (800-CDC-INFO [800-232-4636]).

This schedule is approved by the Advisory Committee on Immunization Practices (http://www.cdc.gov/vaccines/acip), the American Academy of Pediatrics (http://www.aap.org), the American Academy of Family Physicians (http://www.aafp.org), and the American College of Obstetricians and Gynecologists (http://www.acog.org).

NOTE: The above recommendations must be read along with the footnotes of this schedule.

FIGURE 2. Catch-up immunization schedule for persons aged 4 months through 18 years who start late or who are more than 1 month behind —United States, 2016.

The figure below provides catch-up schedules and minimum intervals between doses for children whose vaccinations have been delayed. A vaccine series does not need to be restarted, regardless of the time that has elapsed between doses. Use the section appropriate for the child's age. Always use this table in conjunction with Figure 1 and the footnotes that follow.

Vaccine	Minimum Age for Dose 1	Minimum Interval Between Doses			
		Dose 1 to Dose 2	Dose 2 to Dose 3	Dose 3 to Dose 4	Dose 4 to Dose 5
Children age 4 months through 6 years					
Hepatitis B[1]	Birth	4 weeks	8 weeks *and* at least 16 weeks after first dose. Minimum age for the final dose is 24 weeks.		
Rotavirus[2]	6 weeks	4 weeks	4 weeks[2]		
Diphtheria, tetanus, and acellular pertussis[3]	6 weeks	4 weeks	4 weeks	6 months	6 months[3]
Haemophilus influenzae type b[4]	6 weeks	4 weeks if first dose was administered before the 1st birthday. 8 weeks (as final dose) if first dose was administered at age 12 through 14 months. No further doses needed if first dose was administered at age 15 months or older.	4 weeks[4] if current age is younger than 12 months **and** first dose was administered at younger than age 7 months, **and** at least 1 previous dose was PRP-T (ActHib, Pentacel) or unknown. 8 weeks *and* age 12 through 59 months (as final dose)[4] • if current age is younger than 12 months **and** first dose was administered at age 7 through 11 months (wait until at least 12 months old); OR • if current age is 12 through 59 months **and** first dose was administered before the 1st birthday, **and** second dose administered at younger than 15 months; OR • if both doses were PRP-OMP (PedvaxHIB; Comvax) **and** were administered before the 1st birthday (wait until at least 12 months old). No further doses needed if previous dose was administered at age 15 months or older.	8 weeks (as final dose) This dose only necessary for children age 12 through 59 months who received 3 doses before the 1st birthday.	
Pneumococcal[5]	6 weeks	4 weeks if first dose administered before the 1st birthday. 8 weeks (as final dose for healthy children) if first dose was administered at the 1st birthday or after. No further doses needed for healthy children if first dose administered at age 24 months or older.	4 weeks if current age is younger than 12 months and previous dose given at <7months old. 8 weeks (as final dose for healthy children) if previous dose given between 7-11 months (wait until at least 12 months old); OR if current age is 12 months or older and at least 1 dose was given before age 12 months. No further doses needed for healthy children if previous dose administered at age 24 months or older.	8 weeks (as final dose) This dose only necessary for children aged 12 through 59 months who received 3 doses before age 12 months or for children at high risk who received 3 doses at any age.	
Inactivated poliovirus[6]	6 weeks	4 weeks[6]	4 weeks[6]	6 months[6] (minimum age 4 years for final dose).	
Measles, mumps, rubella[8]	12 months	4 weeks			
Varicella[9]	12 months	3 months			
Hepatitis A[10]	12 months	6 months			
Meningococcal[11] (Hib-MenCY ≥ 6 weeks; MenACWY-D ≥9 mos; MenACWY-CRM ≥ 2 mos)	6 weeks	8 weeks[11]	See footnote 11	See footnote 11	
Children and adolescents age 7 through 18 years					
Meningococcal[11] (Hib-MenCY ≥ 6 weeks; MenACWY-D ≥9 mos; MenACWY-CRM ≥ 2 mos)	Not Applicable (N/A)	8 weeks[11]			
Tetanus, diphtheria; tetanus, diphtheria, and acellular pertussis[12]	7 years[12]	4 weeks	4 weeks if first dose of DTaP/DT was administered before the 1st birthday. 6 months (as final dose) if first dose of DTaP/DT or Tdap/Td was administered at or after the 1st birthday.	6 months if first dose of DTaP/DT was administered before the 1st birthday.	
Human papillomavirus[13]	9 years	Routine dosing intervals are recommended.[13]			
Hepatitis A[10]	N/A	6 months			
Hepatitis B[1]	N/A	4 weeks	8 weeks **and** at least 16 weeks after first dose.		
Inactivated poliovirus[6]	N/A	4 weeks	4 weeks[6]	6 months[6]	
Measles, mumps, rubella[8]	N/A	4 weeks			
Varicella[9]	N/A	3 months if younger than age 13 years. 4 weeks if age 13 years or older.			

NOTE: The above recommendations must be read along with the footnotes of this schedule.

Footnotes — Recommended immunization schedule for persons aged 0 through 18 years—United States, 2016

For further guidance on the use of the vaccines mentioned below, see: http://www.cdc.gov/vaccines/hcp/acip-recs/index.html.
For vaccine recommendations for persons 19 years of age and older, see the Adult Immunization Schedule.

Additional information
- For contraindications and precautions to use of a vaccine and for additional information regarding that vaccine, vaccination providers should consult the relevant ACIP statement available online at http://www.cdc.gov/vaccines/hcp/acip-recs/index.html.
- For purposes of calculating intervals between doses, 4 weeks = 28 days. Intervals of 4 months or greater are determined by calendar months.
- Vaccine doses administered 4 days or less before the minimum interval are considered valid. Doses of any vaccine administered ≥5 days earlier than the minimum interval or minimum age should not be counted as valid doses and should be repeated as age-appropriate. The repeat dose should be spaced after the invalid dose by the recommended minimum interval. For further details, see *MMWR, General Recommendations on Immunization and Reports* / Vol. 60 / No. 2; Table 1. *Recommended and minimum ages and intervals between vaccine doses* available online at http://www.cdc.gov/mmwr/pdf/rr/rr6002.pdf.
- Information on travel vaccine requirements and recommendations is available at http://wwwnc.cdc.gov/travel/destinations/list.
- For vaccination of persons with primary and secondary immunodeficiencies, see Table 13, *"Vaccination of persons with primary and secondary immunodeficiencies,"* in *General Recommendations on Immunization* (ACIP), available at http://www.cdc.gov/mmwr/pdf/rr/rr6002.pdf.; and American Academy of Pediatrics. "Immunization in Special Clinical Circumstances," in Kimberlin DW, Brady MT, Jackson MA, Long SS eds. *Red Book: 2015 report of the Committee on Infectious Diseases. 30th ed.* Elk Grove Village, IL: American Academy of Pediatrics.

1. **Hepatitis B (HepB) vaccine. (Minimum age: birth)**
   Routine vaccination:
   At birth:
   - Administer monovalent HepB vaccine to all newborns before hospital discharge.
   - For infants born to hepatitis B surface antigen (HBsAg)-positive mothers, administer HepB vaccine and 0.5 mL of hepatitis B immune globulin (HBIG) within 12 hours of birth. These infants should be tested for HBsAg and antibody to HBsAg (anti-HBs) at age 9 through 18 months (preferably at the next well-child visit) or 1 to 2 months after completion of the HepB series if the series was delayed; CDC recently recommended testing occur at age 9 through 12 months; see http://www.cdc.gov/mmwr/preview/mmwrhtml/mm6439a6.htm.
   - If mother's HBsAg status is unknown, within 12 hours of birth administer HepB vaccine regardless of birth weight. For infants weighing less than 2,000 grams, administer HBIG in addition to HepB vaccine within 12 hours of birth. Determine mother's HBsAg status as soon as possible and, if mother is HBsAg-positive, also administer HBIG for infants weighing 2,000 grams or more as soon as possible, but no later than age 7 days.
   Doses following the birth dose:
   - The second dose should be administered at age 1 or 2 months. Monovalent HepB vaccine should be used for doses administered before age 6 weeks.
   - Infants who did not receive a birth dose should receive 3 doses of a HepB-containing vaccine on a schedule of 0, 1 to 2 months, and 6 months starting as soon as feasible. See Figure 2.
   - Administer the second dose 1 to 2 months after the first dose (minimum interval of 4 weeks), administer the third dose at least 8 weeks after the second dose AND at least 16 weeks after the **first** dose. The final (third or fourth) dose in the HepB vaccine series should be administered **no earlier than age 24 weeks**.
   - Administration of a total of 4 doses of HepB vaccine is permitted when a combination vaccine containing HepB is administered after the birth dose.
   Catch-up vaccination:
   - Unvaccinated persons should complete a 3-dose series.
   - A 2-dose series (doses separated by at least 4 months) of adult formulation Recombivax HB is licensed for use in children aged 11 through 15 years.
   - For other catch-up guidance, see Figure 2.

2. **Rotavirus (RV) vaccines. (Minimum age: 6 weeks for both RV1 [Rotarix] and RV5 [RotaTeq])**
   Routine vaccination:
   Administer a series of RV vaccine to all infants as follows:
   1. If Rotarix is used, administer a 2-dose series at 2 and 4 months of age.
   2. If RotaTeq is used, administer a 3-dose series at ages 2, 4, and 6 months.
   3. If any dose in the series was RotaTeq or vaccine product is unknown for any dose in the series, a total of 3 doses of RV vaccine should be administered.
   Catch-up vaccination:
   - The maximum age for the first dose in the series is 14 weeks, 6 days; vaccination should not be initiated for infants aged 15 weeks, 0 days or older.
   - The maximum age for the final dose in the series is 8 months, 0 days.
   - For other catch-up guidance, see Figure 2.

3. **Diphtheria and tetanus toxoids and acellular pertussis (DTaP) vaccine. (Minimum age: 6 weeks.**
   Exception: DTaP-IPV [Kinrix, Quadracel]: 4 years)
   Routine vaccination:
   - Administer a 5-dose series of DTaP vaccine at ages 2, 4, 6, 15 through 18 months, and 4 through 6 years. The fourth dose may be administered as early as age 12 months, provided at least 6 months have elapsed since the third dose.
   - Inadvertent administration of 4th DTaP dose early: If the fourth dose of DTaP was administered at least 4 months, but less than 6 months, after the third dose of DTaP, it need not be repeated.

3. **Diphtheria and tetanus toxoids and acellular pertussis (DTaP) vaccine (cont'd)**
   Catch-up vaccination:
   - The fifth dose of DTaP vaccine is not necessary if the fourth dose was administered at age 4 years or older.
   - For other catch-up guidance, see Figure 2.

4. ***Haemophilus influenzae* type b (Hib) conjugate vaccine. (Minimum age: 6 weeks for PRP-T [AC-THIB, DTaP-IPV/Hib (Pentacel) and Hib-MenCY (MenHibrix)], PRP-OMP [PedvaxHIB or COMVAX], 12 months for PRP-T [Hiberix])**
   Routine vaccination:
   - Administer a 2- or 3-dose Hib vaccine primary series and a booster dose (dose 3 or 4 depending on vaccine used in primary series) at age 12 through 15 months to complete a full Hib vaccine series.
   - The primary series with ActHIB, MenHibrix, or Pentacel consists of 3 doses and should be administered at 2, 4, and 6 months of age. The primary series with PedvaxHib or COMVAX consists of 2 doses and should be administered at 2 and 4 months of age; a dose at age 6 months is not indicated.
   - One booster dose (dose 3 or 4 depending on vaccine used in primary series) of any Hib vaccine should be administered at age 12 through 15 months. An exception is Hiberix vaccine. Hiberix should only be used for the booster (final) dose in children aged 12 months through 4 years who have received at least 1 prior dose of Hib-containing vaccine.
   - For recommendations on the use of MenHibrix in patients at increased risk for meningococcal disease, please refer to the meningococcal vaccine footnotes and also to *MMWR* February 28, 2014 / 63(RR01);1-13, available at http://www.cdc.gov/mmwr/PDF/rr/rr6301.pdf.
   Catch-up vaccination:
   - If dose 1 was administered at ages 12 through 14 months, administer a second (final) dose at least 8 weeks after dose 1, regardless of Hib vaccine used in the primary series.
   - If both doses were PRP-OMP (PedvaxHIB or COMVAX), and were administered before the first birthday, the third (and final) dose should be administered at age 12 through 59 months and at least 8 weeks after the second dose.
   - If the first dose was administered at age 7 through 11 months, administer the second dose at least 4 weeks later and a third (and final) dose at age 12 through 15 months or 8 weeks after second dose, whichever is later.
   - If first dose is administered before the first birthday and second dose administered at younger than 15 months, a third (and final) dose should be administered 8 weeks later.
   - For unvaccinated children aged 15 months or older, administer only 1 dose.
   - For other catch-up guidance, see Figure 2. For catch-up guidance related to MenHibrix, please see the meningococcal vaccine footnotes and also *MMWR* February 28, 2014 / 63(RR01);1-13, available at http://www.cdc.gov/mmwr/PDF/rr/rr6301.pdf.
   Vaccination of persons with high-risk conditions:
   - Children aged 12 through 59 months who are at increased risk for Hib disease, including chemotherapy recipients and those with anatomic or functional asplenia (including sickle cell disease), human immunodeficiency virus (HIV) infection, immunoglobulin deficiency, or early component complement deficiency, who have received either no doses or only 1 dose of Hib vaccine before 12 months of age, should receive 2 additional doses of Hib vaccine 8 weeks apart; children who received 2 or more doses of Hib vaccine before 12 months of age should receive 1 additional dose.
   - For patients younger than 5 years of age undergoing chemotherapy or radiation treatment who received a Hib vaccine dose(s) within 14 days of starting therapy or during therapy, repeat the dose(s) at least 3 months following therapy completion.
   - Recipients of hematopoietic stem cell transplant (HSCT) should be revaccinated with a 3-dose regimen of Hib vaccine starting 6 to 12 months after successful transplant, regardless of vaccination history; doses should be administered at least 4 weeks apart.
   - A single dose of any Hib-containing vaccine should be administered to unimmunized* children and adolescents 15 months of age and older undergoing an elective splenectomy; if possible, vaccine should be administered at least 14 days before procedure.

For further guidance on the use of the vaccines mentioned below, see: http://www.cdc.gov/vaccines/hcp/acip-recs/index.html.

4. *Haemophilus influenzae* type b (Hib) conjugate vaccine (cont'd)
   - Hib vaccine is not routinely recommended for patients 5 years or older. However, 1 dose of Hib vaccine should be administered to unimmunized* persons aged 5 years or older who have anatomic or functional asplenia (including sickle cell disease) and unvaccinated persons 5 through 18 years of age with HIV infection.
     Patients who have not received a primary series and booster dose or at least 1 dose of Hib vaccine after 14 months of age are considered unimmunized.

5. **Pneumococcal vaccines. (Minimum age: 6 weeks for PCV13, 2 years for PPSV23)**
   Routine vaccination with PCV13:
   - Administer a 4-dose series of PCV13 vaccine at ages 2, 4, and 6 months and at age 12 through 15 months.
   - For children aged 14 through 59 months who have received an age-appropriate series of 7-valent PCV (PCV7), administer a single supplemental dose of 13-valent PCV (PCV13).
   Catch-up vaccination with PCV13:
   - Administer 1 dose of PCV13 to all healthy children aged 24 through 59 months who are not completely vaccinated for their age.
   - For other catch-up guidance, see Figure 2.
   Vaccination of persons with high-risk conditions with PCV13 and PPSV23:
   - All recommended PCV13 doses should be administered prior to PPSV23 vaccination if possible.
   - For children 2 through 5 years of age with any of the following conditions: chronic heart disease (particularly cyanotic congenital heart disease and cardiac failure); chronic lung disease (including asthma if treated with high-dose oral corticosteroid therapy); diabetes mellitus; cerebrospinal fluid leak; cochlear implant; sickle cell disease and other hemoglobinopathies; anatomic or functional asplenia; HIV infection; chronic renal failure; nephrotic syndrome; diseases associated with treatment with immunosuppressive drugs or radiation therapy, including malignant neoplasms, leukemias, lymphomas, and Hodgkin disease; solid organ transplantation; or congenital immunodeficiency:
     1. Administer 1 dose of PCV13 if any incomplete schedule of 3 doses of PCV (PCV7 and/or PCV13) were received previously.
     2. Administer 2 doses of PCV13 at least 8 weeks apart if unvaccinated or any incomplete schedule of fewer than 3 doses of PCV (PCV7 and/or PCV13) were received previously.
     3. Administer 1 supplemental dose of PCV13 if 4 doses of PCV7 or other age-appropriate complete PCV7 series was received previously.
     4. The minimum interval between doses of PCV (PCV7 or PCV13) is 8 weeks.
     5. For children with no history of PPSV23 vaccination, administer PPSV23 at least 8 weeks after the most recent dose of PCV13.
   - For children aged 6 through 18 years who have cerebrospinal fluid leak; cochlear implant; sickle cell disease and other hemoglobinopathies; anatomic or functional asplenia; congenital or acquired immunodeficiencies; HIV infection; chronic renal failure; nephrotic syndrome; diseases associated with treatment with immunosuppressive drugs or radiation therapy, including malignant neoplasms, leukemias, lymphomas, and Hodgkin disease; generalized malignancy; solid organ transplantation; or multiple myeloma:
     1. If neither PCV13 nor PPSV23 has been received previously, administer 1 dose of PCV13 now and 1 dose of PPSV23 at least 8 weeks later.
     2. If PCV13 has been received previously but PPSV23 has not, administer 1 dose of PPSV23 at least 8 weeks after the most recent dose of PCV13.
     3. If PPSV23 has been received but PCV13 has not, administer 1 dose of PCV13 at least 8 weeks after the most recent dose of PPSV23.
   - For children 6 through 18 years with chronic heart disease (particularly cyanotic congenital heart disease and cardiac failure), chronic lung disease (including asthma if treated with high-dose oral corticosteroid therapy), diabetes mellitus, alcoholism, or chronic liver disease, who have not received PPSV23, administer 1 dose of PPSV23. If PCV13 has been received previously, then PPSV23 should be administered at least 8 weeks after any prior PCV13 dose.
   - A single revaccination with PPSV23 should be administered 5 years after the first dose to children with sickle cell disease or other hemoglobinopathies; anatomic or functional asplenia; congenital or acquired immunodeficiencies; HIV infection; chronic renal failure; nephrotic syndrome; diseases associated with treatment with immunosuppressive drugs or radiation therapy, including malignant neoplasms, leukemias, lymphomas, and Hodgkin disease; generalized malignancy; solid organ transplantation; or multiple myeloma.

6. **Inactivated poliovirus vaccine (IPV). (Minimum age: 6 weeks)**
   Routine vaccination:
   - Administer a 4-dose series of IPV at ages 2, 4, 6 through 18 months, and 4 through 6 years. The final dose in the series should be administered on or after the fourth birthday and at least 6 months after the previous dose.
   Catch-up vaccination:
   - In the first 6 months of life, minimum age and minimum intervals are only recommended if the person is at risk of imminent exposure to circulating poliovirus (i.e., travel to a polio-endemic region or during an outbreak).
   - If 4 or more doses are administered before age 4 years, an additional dose should be administered at age 4 through 6 years and at least 6 months after the previous dose.
   - A fourth dose is not necessary if the third dose was administered at age 4 years or older and at least 6 months after the previous dose.

6. **Inactivated poliovirus vaccine (IPV). (Minimum age: 6 weeks) (cont'd)**
   - If both OPV and IPV were administered as part of a series, a total of 4 doses should be administered, regardless of the child's current age. If only OPV were administered, and all doses were given prior to 4 years of age, one dose of IPV should be given at 4 years or older, at least 4 weeks after the last OPV dose.
   - IPV is not routinely recommended for U.S. residents aged 18 years or older.
   - For other catch-up guidance, see Figure 2.

7. **Influenza vaccines. (Minimum age: 6 months for inactivated influenza vaccine [IIV], 2 years for live, attenuated influenza vaccine [LAIV])**
   Routine vaccination:
   - Administer influenza vaccine annually to all children beginning at age 6 months. For most healthy, nonpregnant persons aged 2 through 49 years, either LAIV or IIV may be used. However, LAIV should NOT be administered to some persons, including 1) persons who have experienced severe allergic reactions to LAIV, any of its components, or to a previous dose of any other influenza vaccine; 2) children 2 through 17 years receiving aspirin or aspirin-containing products; 3) persons who are allergic to eggs; 4) pregnant women; 5) immunosuppressed persons; 6) children 2 through 4 years of age with asthma or who had wheezing in the past 12 months; or 7) persons who have taken influenza antiviral medications in the previous 48 hours. For all other contraindications and precautions to use of LAIV, see *MMWR* August 7, 2015 / 64(30):818-25 available at http://www.cdc.gov/mmwr/pdf/wk/mm6430.pdf.
   For children aged 6 months through 8 years:
   - For the 2015-16 season, administer 2 doses (separated by at least 4 weeks) to children who are receiving influenza vaccine for the first time. Some children in this age group who have been vaccinated previously will also need 2 doses. For additional guidance, follow dosing guidelines in the 2015-16 ACIP influenza vaccine recommendations, *MMWR* August 7, 2015 / 64(30):818-25, available at http://www.cdc.gov/mmwr/pdf/wk/mm6430.pdf.
   - For the 2016-17 season, follow dosing guidelines in the 2016 ACIP influenza vaccine recommendations.
   For persons aged 9 years and older:
   - Administer 1 dose.

8. **Measles, mumps, and rubella (MMR) vaccine. (Minimum age: 12 months for routine vaccination)**
   Routine vaccination:
   - Administer a 2-dose series of MMR vaccine at ages 12 through 15 months and 4 through 6 years. The second dose may be administered before age 4 years, provided at least 4 weeks have elapsed since the first dose.
   - Administer 1 dose of MMR vaccine to infants aged 6 through 11 months before departure from the United States for international travel. These children should be revaccinated with 2 doses of MMR vaccine, the first at age 12 through 15 months (12 months if the child remains in an area where disease risk is high), and the second dose at least 4 weeks later.
   - Administer 2 doses of MMR vaccine to children aged 12 months and older before departure from the United States for international travel. The first dose should be administered on or after age 12 months and the second dose at least 4 weeks later.
   Catch-up vaccination:
   - Ensure that all school-aged children and adolescents have had 2 doses of MMR vaccine; the minimum interval between the 2 doses is 4 weeks.

9. **Varicella (VAR) vaccine. (Minimum age: 12 months)**
   Routine vaccination:
   - Administer a 2-dose series of VAR vaccine at ages 12 through 15 months and 4 through 6 years. The second dose may be administered before age 4 years, provided at least 3 months have elapsed since the first dose. If the second dose was administered at least 4 weeks after the first dose, it can be accepted as valid.
   Catch-up vaccination:
   - Ensure that all persons aged 7 through 18 years without evidence of immunity (see *MMWR* 2007 / 56 [No. RR-4], available at http://www.cdc.gov/mmwr/pdf/rr/rr5604.pdf) have 2 doses of varicella vaccine. For children aged 7 through 12 years, the recommended minimum interval between doses is 3 months (if the second dose was administered at least 4 weeks after the first dose, it can be accepted as valid); for persons aged 13 years and older, the minimum interval between doses is 4 weeks.

10. **Hepatitis A (HepA) vaccine. (Minimum age: 12 months)**
    Routine vaccination:
    - Initiate the 2-dose HepA vaccine series at 12 through 23 months; separate the 2 doses by 6 to 18 months.
    - Children who have received 1 dose of HepA vaccine before age 24 months should receive a second dose 6 to 18 months after the first dose.
    - For any person aged 2 years and older who has not already received the HepA vaccine series, 2 doses of HepA vaccine separated by 6 to 18 months may be administered if immunity against hepatitis A virus infection is desired.
    Catch-up vaccination:
    - The minimum interval between the 2 doses is 6 months.

For further guidance on the use of the vaccines mentioned below, see: http://www.cdc.gov/vaccines/hcp/acip-recs/index.html.

10. **Hepatitis A (HepA) vaccine (cont'd)**
    Special populations:
    - Administer 2 doses of HepA vaccine at least 6 months apart to previously unvaccinated persons who live in areas where vaccination programs target older children, or who are at increased risk for infection. This includes persons traveling to or working in countries that have high or intermediate endemicity of infection; men having sex with men; users of injection and non-injection illicit drugs; persons who work with HAV-infected primates or with HAV in a research laboratory; persons with clotting-factor disorders; persons with chronic liver disease; and persons who anticipate close personal contact (e.g., household or regular babysitting) with an international adoptee during the first 60 days after arrival in the United States from a country with high or intermediate endemicity. The first dose should be administered as soon as the adoption is planned, ideally 2 or more weeks before the arrival of the adoptee.

11. **Meningococcal vaccines. (Minimum age: 6 weeks for Hib-MenCY [MenHibrix], 9 months for MenACWY-D [Menactra], 2 months for MenACWY-CRM [Menveo], 10 years for serogroup B meningococcal [MenB] vaccines: MenB-4C [Bexsero] and MenB-FHbp [Trumenba])**
    Routine vaccination:
    - Administer a single dose of Menactra or Menveo vaccine at age 11 through 12 years, with a booster dose at age 16 years.
    - Adolescents aged 11 through 18 years with human immunodeficiency virus (HIV) infection should receive a 2-dose primary series of Menactra or Menveo with at least 8 weeks between doses.
    - For children aged 2 months through 18 years with high-risk conditions, see below.
    Catch-up vaccination:
    - Administer Menactra or Menveo vaccine at age 13 through 18 years if not previously vaccinated.
    - If the first dose is administered at age 13 through 15 years, a booster dose should be administered at age 16 through 18 years with a minimum interval of at least 8 weeks between doses.
    - If the first dose is administered at age 16 years or older, a booster dose is not needed.
    - For other catch-up guidance, see Figure 2.
    Clinical discretion:
    - Young adults aged 16 through 23 years (preferred age range is 16 through 18 years) may be vaccinated with either a 2-dose series of Bexsero or a 3-dose series of Trumenba vaccine to provide short-term protection against most strains of serogroup B meningococcal disease. The two MenB vaccines are not interchangeable; the same vaccine product must be used for all doses.
    Vaccination of persons with high-risk conditions and other persons at increased risk of disease:
    Children with anatomic or functional asplenia (including sickle cell disease):
    Meningococcal conjugate ACWY vaccines:
    1. Menveo
       o *Children who initiate vaccination at 8 weeks:* Administer doses at 2, 4, 6, and 12 months of age.
       o *Unvaccinated children who initiate vaccination at 7 through 23 months:* Administer 2 doses, with the second dose at least 12 weeks after the first dose AND after the first birthday.
       o *Children 24 months and older who have not received a complete series:* Administer 2 primary doses at least 8 weeks apart.
    2. MenHibrix
       o *Children who initiate vaccination at 6 weeks:* Administer doses at 2, 4, 6, and 12 through 15 months of age.
       o If the first dose of MenHibrix is given at or after 12 months of age, a total of 2 doses should be given at least 8 weeks apart to ensure protection against serogroups C and Y meningococcal disease.
    3. Menactra
       o *Children 24 months and older who have not received a complete series:* Administer 2 primary doses at least 8 weeks apart. If Menactra is administered to a child with asplenia (including sickle cell disease), do not administer Menactra until 2 years of age and at least 4 weeks after the completion of all PCV13 doses.
    Meningococcal B vaccines:
    1. Bexsero or Trumenba
       o *Persons 10 years or older who have not received a complete series.* Administer a 2-dose series of Bexsero, at least 1 month apart. Or a 3-dose series of Trumenba, with the second dose at least 2 months after the first and the third dose at least 6 months after the first. The two MenB vaccines are not interchangeable; the same vaccine product must be used for all doses.
    Children with persistent complement component deficiency (includes persons with inherited or chronic deficiencies in C3, C5-9, properidin, factor D, factor H, or taking eculizumab (Soliris®):
    Meningococcal conjugate ACWY vaccines:
    1. Menveo
       o *Children who initiate vaccination at 8 weeks:* Administer doses at 2, 4, 6, and 12 months of age.
       o *Unvaccinated children who initiate vaccination at 7 through 23 months:* Administer 2 doses, with the second dose at least 12 weeks after the first dose AND after the first birthday.
       o *Children 24 months and older who have not received a complete series:* Administer 2 primary doses at least 8 weeks apart.
    2. MenHibrix
       o *Children who initiate vaccination 6 weeks:* Administer doses at 2, 4, 6, and 12 through 15 months of age.
       o If the first dose of MenHibrix is given at or after 12 months of age, a total of 2 doses should be given at least 8 weeks apart to ensure protection against serogroups C and Y meningococcal disease.

11. **Meningococcal vaccines (cont'd)**
    3. Menactra
       o *Children 9 through 23 months:* Administer 2 primary doses at least 12 weeks apart.
       o *Children 24 months and older who have not received a complete series:* Administer 2 primary doses at least 8 weeks apart.
    Meningococcal B vaccines:
    1. Bexsero or Trumenba
       o *Persons 10 years or older who have not received a complete series.* Administer a 2-dose series of Bexsero, at least 1 month apart. Or a 3-dose series of Trumenba, with the second dose at least 2 months after the first and the third dose at least 6 months after the first. The two MenB vaccines are not interchangeable; the same vaccine product must be used for all doses.
    For children who travel to or reside in countries in which meningococcal disease is hyperendemic or epidemic, including countries in the African meningitis belt or the Hajj
    - administer an age-appropriate formulation and series of Menactra or Menveo for protection against serogroups A and W meningococcal disease. Prior receipt of MenHibrix is not sufficient for children traveling to the meningitis belt or the Hajj because it does not contain serogroups A or W.
    For children at risk during a community outbreak attributable to a vaccine serogroup
    - administer or complete an age- and formulation-appropriate series of MenHibrix, Menactra, or Menveo, Bexsero or Trumenba.
    For booster doses among persons with high-risk conditions, refer to *MMWR* 2013 / 62(RR02);1-22, available at http://www.cdc.gov/mmwr/preview/mmwrhtml/rr6202a1.htm.

    For other catch-up recommendations for these persons, and complete information on use of meningococcal vaccines, including guidance related to vaccination of persons at increased risk of infection, see *MMWR* March 22, 2013 / 62(RR02);1-22, and *MMWR* October 23, 2015 / 64(41); 1171-1176 available at http://www.cdc.gov/mmwr/pdf/rr/rr6202.pdf, and http://www.cdc.gov/mmwr/pdf/wk/mm6441.pdf.

12. **Tetanus and diphtheria toxoids and acellular pertussis (Tdap) vaccine. (Minimum age: 10 years for both Boostrix and Adacel)**
    Routine vaccination:
    - Administer 1 dose of Tdap vaccine to all adolescents aged 11 through 12 years.
    - Tdap may be administered regardless of the interval since the last tetanus and diphtheria toxoid-containing vaccine.
    - Administer 1 dose of Tdap vaccine to pregnant adolescents during each pregnancy (preferred during 27 through 36 weeks gestation) regardless of time since prior Td or Tdap vaccination.
    Catch-up vaccination:
    - Persons aged 7 years and older who are not fully immunized with DTaP vaccine should receive Tdap vaccine as 1 (preferably the first) dose in the catch-up series; if additional doses are needed, use Td vaccine. For children 7 through 10 years who receive a dose of Tdap as part of the catch-up series, an adolescent Tdap vaccine dose at age 11 through 12 years should NOT be administered. Td should be administered instead 10 years after the Tdap dose.
    - Persons aged 11 through 18 years who have not received Tdap vaccine should receive a dose followed by tetanus and diphtheria toxoids (Td) booster doses every 10 years thereafter.
    - Inadvertent doses of DTaP vaccine:
      - If administered inadvertently to a child aged 7 through 10 years may count as part of the catch-up series. This dose may count as the adolescent Tdap dose, or the child can later receive a Tdap booster dose at age 11 through 12 years.
      - If administered inadvertently to an adolescent aged 11 through 18 years, the dose should be counted as the adolescent Tdap booster.
    - For other catch-up guidance, see Figure 2.

13. **Human papillomavirus (HPV) vaccines. (Minimum age: 9 years for 2vHPV [Cervarix], 4vHPV [Gardasil] and 9vHPV [Gardasil 9])**
    Routine vaccination:
    - Administer a 3-dose series of HPV vaccine on a schedule of 0, 1-2, and 6 months to all adolescents aged 11 through 12 years. 9vHPV, 4vHPV or 2vHPV may be used for females, and only 9vHPV or 4vHPV may be used for males.
    - The vaccine series may be started at age 9 years.
    - Administer the second dose 1 to 2 months after the first dose (minimum interval of 4 weeks); administer the third dose 16 weeks after the second dose (minimum interval of 12 weeks) and 24 weeks after the first dose.
    - Administer HPV vaccine beginning at age 9 years to children and youth with any history of sexual abuse or assault who have not initiated or completed the 3-dose series.
    Catch-up vaccination:
    - Administer the vaccine series to females (2vHPV or 4vHPV or 9vHPV) and males (4vHPV or 9vHPV) at age 13 through 18 years if not previously vaccinated.
    - Use recommended routine dosing intervals (see Routine vaccination above) for vaccine series catch-up.

CS260933-A

Table 5 ADULT IMMUNIZATION

Recommended Adult Immunization Schedule—United States - 2016

Note: These recommendations must be read with the footnotes that follow containing number of doses, intervals between doses, and other important information.

Figure 1. Recommended immunization schedule for adults aged 19 years or older, by vaccine and age group[1]

VACCINE ▼ AGE GROUP ►	19-21 years	22-26 years	27-49 years	50-59 years	60-64 years	≥ 65 years
Influenza[*,2]	1 dose annually					
Tetanus, diphtheria, pertussis (Td/Tdap)[*,3]	Substitute Tdap for Td once, then Td booster every 10 yrs					
Varicella[*,4]	2 doses					
Human papillomavirus (HPV) Female[*,5]	3 doses					
Human papillomavirus (HPV) Male[*,5]	3 doses					
Zoster[6]					1 dose	
Measles, mumps, rubella (MMR)[*,7]	1 or 2 doses depending on indication					
Pneumococcal 13-valent conjugate (PCV13)[*,8]					1 dose	
Pneumococcal 23-valent polysaccharide (PPSV23)[8]			1 or 2 doses depending on indication			1 dose
Hepatitis A[*,9]	2 or 3 doses depending on vaccine					
Hepatitis B[*,10]	3 doses					
Meningococcal 4-valent conjugate (MenACWY) or polysaccharide (MPSV4)[*,11]	1 or more doses depending on indication					
Meningococcal B (MenB)[11]	2 or 3 doses depending on vaccine					
Haemophilus influenzae type b (Hib)[*,12]	1 or 3 doses depending on indication					

*Covered by the Vaccine Injury Compensation Program

▢ Recommended for all persons who meet the age requirement, lack documentation of vaccination, or lack evidence of past infection; zoster vaccine is recommended regardless of past episode of zoster

▢ Recommended for persons with a risk factor (medical, occupational, lifestyle, or other indication)

▢ No recommendation

Report all clinically significant postvaccination reactions to the Vaccine Adverse Event Reporting System (VAERS). Reporting forms and instructions on filing a VAERS report are available at www.vaers.hhs.gov or by telephone, 800-822-7967.

Information on how to file a Vaccine Injury Compensation Program claim is available at www.hrsa.gov/vaccinecompensation or by telephone, 800-338-2382. To file a claim for vaccine injury, contact the U.S. Court of Federal Claims, 717 Madison Place, N.W., Washington, D.C. 20005; telephone, 202-357-6400.

Additional information about the vaccines in this schedule, extent of available data, and contraindications for vaccination is also available at www.cdc.gov/vaccines or from the CDC-INFO Contact Center at 800-CDC-INFO (800-232-4636) in English and Spanish, 8:00 a.m. - 8:00 p.m. Eastern Time, Monday - Friday, excluding holidays.

Use of trade names and commercial sources is for identification only and does not imply endorsement by the U.S. Department of Health and Human Services.

The recommendations in this schedule were approved by the Centers for Disease Control and Prevention's (CDC) Advisory Committee on Immunization Practices (ACIP), the American Academy of Family Physicians (AAFP), the America College of Physicians (ACP), the American College of Obstetricians and Gynecologists (ACOG) and the American College of Nurse-Midwives (ACNM).

Figure 2. Vaccines that might be indicated for adults aged 19 years or older based on medical and other indications[1]

VACCINE ▼ INDICATION ►	Pregnancy	Immuno-compromising conditions (excluding HIV infection)[4,6,7,8,13]	HIV infection CD4+ count (cells/µL)[4,6,7,8,13] < 200	HIV infection CD4+ count (cells/µL)[4,6,7,8,13] ≥ 200	Men who have sex with men (MSM)	Kidney failure, end-stage renal disease, on hemodialysis	Heart disease, chronic lung disease, chronic alcoholism	Asplenia and persistent complement component deficiencies[8,11,12]	Chronic liver disease	Diabetes	Healthcare personnel
Influenza[*,2]	1 dose annually										
Tetanus, diphtheria, pertussis (Td/Tdap)[*,3]	1 dose Tdap each pregnancy	Substitute Tdap for Td once, then Td booster every 10 yrs									
Varicella[*,4]	Contraindicated			2 doses							
Human papillomavirus (HPV) Female[*,5]	3 doses through age 26 yrs				3 doses through age 26 yrs						
Human papillomavirus (HPV) Male[*,5]	3 doses through age 26 yrs				3 doses through age 21 yrs						
Zoster[6]	Contraindicated			1 dose							
Measles, mumps, rubella (MMR)[*,7]	Contraindicated			1 or 2 doses depending on indication							
Pneumococcal 13-valent conjugate (PCV13)[*,8]				1 dose							
Pneumococcal polysaccharide (PPSV23)[8]	1, 2, or 3 doses depending on indication										
Hepatitis A[*,9]	2 or 3 doses depending on vaccine										
Hepatitis B[*,10]	3 doses										
Meningococcal 4-valent conjugate (MenACWY) or polysaccharide (MPSV4)[*,11]	1 or more doses depending on indication										
Meningococcal B (MenB)[11]	2 or 3 doses depending on vaccine										
Haemophilus influenzae type b (Hib)[*,12]	3 doses post-HSCT recipients only			1 dose							

*Covered by the Vaccine Injury Compensation Program

▢ Recommended for all persons who meet the age requirement, lack documentation of vaccination, or lack evidence of past infection; zoster vaccine is recommended regardless of past episode of zoster

▢ Recommended for persons with a risk factor (medical, occupational, lifestyle, or other indication)

▢ No recommendation

▢ Contraindicated

U.S. Department of Health and Human Services
Centers for Disease Control and Prevention

These schedules indicate the recommended age groups and medical indications for which administration of currently licensed vaccines is commonly recommended for adults aged ≥19 years, as of February 2016. For all vaccines being recommended on the Adult Immunization Schedule: a vaccine series does not need to be restarted, regardless of the time that has elapsed between doses. Licensed combination vaccines may be used whenever any components of the combination are indicated and when the vaccine's other components are not contraindicated. For detailed recommendations on all vaccines, including those used primarily for travelers or that are issued during the year, consult the manufacturers' package inserts and the complete statements from the Advisory Committee on Immunization Practices (www.cdc.gov/vaccines/hcp/acip-recs/index.html). Use of trade names and commercial sources is for identification only and does not imply endorsement by the U.S. Department of Health and Human Services.

Footnotes—Recommended Immunization Schedule for Adults Aged 19 Years or Older: United States, 2016

1. Additional information
- Additional guidance for the use of the vaccines described in this supplement is available at www.cdc.gov/vaccines/hcp/acip-recs/index.html.
- Information on vaccination recommendations when vaccination status is unknown and other general immunization information can be found in the General Recommendations on Immunization at www.cdc.gov/mmwr/preview/mmwrhtml/rr6002a1.htm.
- Information on travel vaccine requirements and recommendations (e.g., for hepatitis A and B, meningococcal, and other vaccines) is available at wwwnc.cdc.gov/travel/destinations/list.
- Additional information and resources regarding vaccination of pregnant women can be found at www.cdc.gov/vaccines/adults/rec-vac/pregnant.html.

2. Influenza vaccination
- Annual vaccination against influenza is recommended for all persons aged ≥6 months. A list of currently available influenza vaccines can be found at http://www.cdc.gov/flu/protect/vaccine/vaccines.htm.
- Persons aged ≥6 months, including pregnant women, can receive the inactivated influenza vaccine (IIV). An age-appropriate IIV formulation should be used.
- Intradermal IIV is an option for persons aged 18 through 64 years.
- High-dose IIV is an option for persons aged ≥65 years.
- Live attenuated influenza vaccine (LAIV [FluMist]) is an option for healthy, non-pregnant persons aged 2 through 49 years.
- Recombinant influenza vaccine (RIV [Flublok]) is approved for persons aged ≥18 years.
- RIV, which does not contain any egg protein, may be administered to persons aged ≥18 years with egg allergy of any severity; IIV may be used with additional safety measures for persons with hives-only allergy to eggs.
- Health care personnel who care for severely immunocompromised persons who require care in a protected environment should receive IIV or RIV; health care personnel who receive LAIV should avoid providing care for severely immunosuppressed persons for 7 days after vaccination.

3. Tetanus, diphtheria, and acellular pertussis (Td/Tdap) vaccination
- Administer 1 dose of Tdap vaccine to pregnant women during each pregnancy (preferably during 27–36 weeks' gestation) regardless of interval since prior Td or Tdap vaccination.
- Persons aged ≥11 years who have not received Tdap vaccine or for whom vaccine status is unknown should receive a dose of Tdap followed by tetanus and diphtheria toxoids (Td) booster doses every 10 years thereafter. Tdap can be administered regardless of interval since the most recent tetanus or diphtheria-toxoid-containing vaccine.
- Adults with an unknown or incomplete history of completing a 3-dose primary vaccination series with Td-containing vaccines should begin or complete a primary vaccination series including a Tdap dose.
- For unvaccinated adults, administer the first 2 doses at least 4 weeks apart and the third dose 6–12 months after the second.
- For incompletely vaccinated (i.e., less than 3 doses) adults, administer remaining doses.
- Refer to the ACIP statement for recommendations for administering Td/Tdap as prophylaxis in wound management (see footnote 1).

4. Varicella vaccination
- All adults without evidence of immunity to varicella (as defined below) should receive 2 doses of single-antigen varicella vaccine or a second dose if they have received only 1 dose.
- Vaccination should be emphasized for those who have close contact with persons at high risk for severe disease (e.g., health care personnel and family contacts of persons with immunocompromising conditions) or are at high risk for exposure or transmission (e.g., teachers; child care employees; residents and staff members of institutional settings, including correctional institutions; college students; military personnel; adolescents and adults living in households with children; nonpregnant women of childbearing age; and international travelers).
- Pregnant women should be assessed for evidence of varicella immunity. Women who do not have evidence of immunity should receive the first dose of varicella vaccine upon completion or termination of pregnancy and before discharge from the health care facility. The second dose should be administered 4–8 weeks after the first dose.
- Evidence of immunity to varicella in adults includes any of the following:
  — documentation of 2 doses of varicella vaccine at least 4 weeks apart;
  — U.S.-born before 1980, except health care personnel and pregnant women;
  — history of varicella based on diagnosis or verification of varicella disease by a health care provider;
  — history of herpes zoster based on diagnosis or verification of herpes zoster disease by a health care provider; or
  — laboratory evidence of immunity or laboratory confirmation of disease.

5. Human papillomavirus (HPV) vaccination
- Three HPV vaccines are licensed for use in females (bivalent HPV vaccine [2vHPV], quadrivalent HPV vaccine [4vHPV], and 9-valent HPV vaccine [9vHPV]) and two HPV vaccines are licensed for use in males (4vHPV and 9vHPV).
- For females, 2vHPV, 4vHPV, or 9vHPV is recommended in a 3-dose series for routine vaccination at age 11 or 12 years and for those aged 13 through 26 years, if not previously vaccinated.
- For males, 4vHPV or 9vHPV is recommended in a 3-dose series for routine vaccination at age 11 or 12 years and for those aged 13 through 21 years, if not previously vaccinated. Males aged 22 through 26 years may be vaccinated.
- HPV vaccination is recommended for men who have sex with men through age 26 years who did not get any or all doses when they were younger.
- Vaccination is recommended for immunocompromised persons (including those with HIV infection) through age 26 years who did not get any or all doses when they were younger.
- A complete HPV vaccination series consists of 3 doses. The second dose should be administered 4–8 weeks (minimum interval of 4 weeks) after the first dose; the third dose should be administered 24 weeks after the first dose and 16 weeks after the second dose (minimum interval of 12 weeks).

- HPV vaccines are not recommended for use in pregnant women. However, pregnancy testing is not needed before vaccination. If a woman is found to be pregnant after initiating the vaccination series, no intervention is needed; the remainder of the 3-dose series should be delayed until completion or termination of pregnancy.

6. Zoster vaccination
- A single dose of zoster vaccine is recommended for adults aged ≥60 years regardless of whether they report a prior episode of herpes zoster. Although the vaccine is licensed by the U.S. Food and Drug Administration for use among and can be administered to persons aged ≥50 years, ACIP recommends that vaccination begin at age 60 years.
- Persons aged ≥60 years with chronic medical conditions may be vaccinated unless their condition constitutes a contraindication, such as pregnancy or severe immunodeficiency.

7. Measles, mumps, rubella (MMR) vaccination
- Adults born before 1957 are generally considered immune to measles and mumps. All adults born in 1957 or later should have documentation of 1 or more doses of MMR vaccine unless they have a medical contraindication to the vaccine or laboratory evidence of immunity to each of the three diseases. Documentation of provider-diagnosed disease is not considered acceptable evidence of immunity for measles, mumps, or rubella.
Measles component:
- A routine second dose of MMR vaccine, administered a minimum of 28 days after the first dose, is recommended for adults who:
  — are students in postsecondary educational institutions,
  — work in a health care facility, or
  — plan to travel internationally.
- Persons who received inactivated (killed) measles vaccine or measles vaccine of unknown type during 1963–1967 should be revaccinated with 2 doses of MMR vaccine.
Mumps component:
- A routine second dose of MMR vaccine, administered a minimum of 28 days after the first dose, is recommended for adults who:
  — are students in a postsecondary educational institution,
  — work in a health care facility, or
  — plan to travel internationally.
- Persons vaccinated before 1979 with either killed mumps vaccine or mumps vaccine of unknown type who are at high risk for mumps infection (e.g., persons who are working in a health care facility) should be considered for revaccination with 2 doses of MMR vaccine.
Rubella component:
- For women of childbearing age, regardless of birth year, rubella immunity should be determined. If there is no evidence of immunity, women who are not pregnant should be vaccinated. Pregnant women who do not have evidence of immunity should receive MMR vaccine upon completion or termination of pregnancy and before discharge from the health care facility.
Health care personnel born before 1957:
- For unvaccinated health care personnel born before 1957 who lack laboratory evidence of measles, mumps, and/or rubella immunity or laboratory confirmation of disease, health care facilities should consider vaccinating personnel with 2 doses of MMR vaccine at the appropriate interval for measles and mumps or 1 dose of MMR vaccine for rubella.

8. Pneumococcal vaccination
- General information
  — Adults are recommended to receive 1 dose of 13-valent pneumococcal conjugate vaccine (PCV13) and 1, 2, or 3 doses (depending on indication) of 23-valent pneumococcal polysaccharide vaccine (PPSV23).
  — PCV13 should be administered at least 1 year after PPSV23.
  — PPSV23 should be administered at least 1 year after PCV13, except among adults with immunocompromising conditions, anatomical or functional asplenia, cerebrospinal fluid leak, or cochlear implant, for whom the interval should be at least 8 weeks; the interval between PPSV23 doses should be at least 5 years.
  — No additional dose of PPSV23 is indicated for adults vaccinated with PPSV23 at age ≥65 years.
  — When both PCV13 and PPSV23 are indicated, PCV13 should be administered first; PCV13 and PPSV23 should not be administered during the same visit.
  — When indicated, PCV13 and PPSV23 should be administered to adults whose pneumococcal vaccination history is incomplete or unknown.
- Adults aged ≥65 years (immunocompetent) who:
  — have not received PCV13 or PPSV23: administer PCV13 followed by PPSV23 at least 1 year after PCV13.
  — have not received PCV13 but have received a dose of PPSV23 at age ≥65 years: administer PCV13 at least 1 year after PPSV23.
  — have not received PCV13 but have received 1 or more doses of PPSV23 at age <65 years: administer PCV13 at least 1 year after the most recent dose of PPSV23. Administer a dose of PPSV23 at least 1 year after PCV13 and at least 5 years after the most recent dose of PPSV23.
  — have received PCV13 but not PPSV23 at age <65 years: administer PPSV23 at least 1 year after PCV13.
  — have received PCV13 and 1 or more doses of PPSV23 at age <65 years: administer PPSV23 at least 1 year after PCV13 and at least 5 years after the most recent dose of PPSV23.
- Adults aged ≥19 years with immunocompromising conditions or anatomical or functional asplenia (defined below) who:
  — have not received PCV13 or PPSV23: administer PCV13 followed by PPSV23 at least 8 weeks after PCV13. Administer a second dose of PPSV23 at least 5 years after the first dose of PPSV23.
  — have not received PCV13 but have received 1 dose of PPSV23: administer PCV13 at least 1 year after the PPSV23. Administer a second dose of PPSV23 at least 8 weeks after PCV13 and at least 5 years after the first dose of PPSV23.

(Continued on next page)

Footnotes—Recommended Immunization Schedule for Adults Aged 19 Years or Older: United States, 2016

— have not received PCV13 but have received 2 doses of PPSV23: administer PCV13 at least 1 year after the most recent dose of PPSV23.
— have received PCV13 but not PPSV23: administer PPSV23 at least 8 weeks after PCV13. Administer a second dose of PPSV23 at least 5 years after the first dose of PPSV23.
— have received PCV13 and 1 dose of PPSV23: administer a second dose of PPSV23 at least 8 weeks after PCV13 and at least 5 years after the first dose of PPSV23.
— If the most recent dose of PPSV23 was administered at age <65 years, at age ≥65 years, administer a dose of PPSV23 at least 8 weeks after PCV13 and at least 5 years after the last dose of PPSV23.
— Immunocompromising conditions that are indications for pneumococcal vaccination are: congenital or acquired immunodeficiency (including B- or T-lymphocyte deficiency, complement deficiencies, and phagocytic disorders excluding chronic granulomatous disease), HIV infection, chronic renal failure, nephrotic syndrome, leukemia, lymphoma, Hodgkin disease, generalized malignancy, multiple myeloma, solid organ transplant, and iatrogenic immunosuppression (including long-term systemic corticosteroids and radiation therapy).
— Anatomical or functional asplenia that are indications for pneumococcal vaccination are: sickle cell disease and other hemoglobinopathies, congenital or acquired asplenia, splenic dysfunction, and splenectomy. Administer pneumococcal vaccines at least 2 weeks before immunosuppressive therapy or an elective splenectomy, and as soon as possible to adults who are newly diagnosed with asymptomatic or symptomatic HIV infection.

- Adults aged ≥19 years with cerebrospinal fluid leaks or cochlear implants: administer PCV13 followed by PPSV23 at least 8 weeks after PCV13; no additional dose of PPSV23 is indicated if aged <65 years. If PPSV23 was administered at age <65 years, at age ≥65 years, administer another dose of PPSV23 at least 5 years after the last dose of PPSV23.
- Adults aged 19 through 64 years with chronic heart disease (including congestive heart failure and cardiomyopathies, excluding hypertension), chronic lung disease (including chronic obstructive lung disease, emphysema, and asthma), chronic liver disease (including cirrhosis), alcoholism, or diabetes mellitus, or who smoke cigarettes: administer PPSV23. At age ≥65 years, administer PCV13 at least 1 year after PPSV23, followed by another dose of PPSV23 at least 1 year after PCV13 and at least 5 years after the last dose of PPSV23.
- Routine pneumococcal vaccination is not recommended for American Indian/Alaska Native or other adults unless they have an indication as above; however, public health authorities may consider recommending the use of pneumococcal vaccines for American Indians/Alaska Natives or other adults who live in areas with increased risk for invasive pneumococcal disease.

9. Hepatitis A vaccination

- Vaccinate any person seeking protection from hepatitis A virus (HAV) infection and persons with any of the following indications:
  — men who have sex with men;
  — persons who use injection or noninjection illicit drugs;
  — persons working with HAV-infected primates or with HAV in a research laboratory setting;
  — persons with chronic liver disease and persons who receive clotting factor concentrates;
  — persons traveling to or working in countries that have high or intermediate endemicity of hepatitis A (see footnote 1); and
  — unvaccinated persons who anticipate close personal contact (e.g., household or regular babysitting) with an international adoptee during the first 60 days after arrival in the United States from a country with high or intermediate endemicity of hepatitis A (see footnote 1). The first dose of the 2-dose hepatitis A vaccine series should be administered as soon as adoption is planned, ideally 2 or more weeks before the arrival of the adoptee.
- Single-antigen vaccine formulations should be administered in a 2-dose schedule at either 0 and 6–12 months (Havrix), or 0 and 6–18 months (Vaqta). If the combined hepatitis A and hepatitis B vaccine (Twinrix) is used, administer 3 doses at 0, 1, and 6 months; alternatively, a 4-dose schedule may be used, administered on days 0, 7, and 21–30 followed by a booster dose at 12 months.

10. Hepatitis B vaccination

- Vaccinate any person seeking protection from hepatitis B virus (HBV) infection and persons with any of the following indications:
  — sexually active persons who are not in a long-term, mutually monogamous relationship (e.g., persons with more than 1 sex partner during the previous 6 months); persons seeking evaluation or treatment for a sexually transmitted disease (STD); current or recent injection drug users; and men who have sex with men;
  — health care personnel and public safety workers who are potentially exposed to blood or other infectious body fluids;
  — persons who are aged <60 years with diabetes as soon as feasible after diagnosis; persons with diabetes who are aged ≥60 years at the discretion of the treating clinician based on the likelihood of acquiring HBV infection, including the risk posed by an increased need for assisted blood glucose monitoring in long-term care facilities, the likelihood of experiencing chronic sequelae if infected with HBV, and the likelihood of immune response to vaccination;
  — persons with end-stage renal disease (including patients receiving hemodialysis), persons with HIV infection, and persons with chronic liver disease;
  — household contacts and sex partners of hepatitis B surface antigen–positive persons, clients and staff members of institutions for persons with developmental disabilities, and international travelers to regions with high or intermediate levels of endemic HBV infection (see footnote 1); and
  — all adults in the following settings: STD treatment facilities, HIV testing and treatment facilities, facilities providing drug abuse treatment and prevention services, health care settings targeting services to injection drug users or men who have sex with men, correctional facilities, end-stage renal disease programs and facilities for chronic hemodialysis patients, and institutions and nonresidential day care facilities for persons with developmental disabilities.
- Administer missing doses to complete a 3-dose series of hepatitis B vaccine to those persons not vaccinated or not completely vaccinated. The second dose should be administered at least 1 month after the first dose; the third dose should be administered at least 2 months after the second dose (and at least 4 months after the first dose). If the combined hepatitis A and hepatitis B vaccine (Twinrix) is used, give 3 doses at 0, 1, and 6 months; alternatively, a 4-dose Twinrix schedule may be used, administered on days 0, 7, and 21–30, followed by a booster dose at 12 months.
- Adult patients receiving hemodialysis or with other immunocompromising conditions should receive 1 dose of 40 mcg/mL (Recombivax HB) administered on a 3-dose schedule at 0, 1, and 6 months or 2 doses of 20 mcg/mL (Engerix-B) administered simultaneously on a 4-dose schedule at 0, 1, 2, and 6 months.

11. Meningococcal vaccination

- General information
  — Serogroup A, C, W, and Y meningococcal vaccine is available as a conjugate (MenACWY [Menactra, Menveo]) or a polysaccharide (MPSV4 [Menomune]) vaccine.
  — Serogroup B meningococcal (MenB) vaccine is available as a 2-dose series of MenB-4C vaccine (Bexsero) administered at least 1 month apart or a 3-dose series of MenB-FHbp (Trumenba) vaccine administered at 0, 2, and 6 months; the two MenB vaccines are not interchangeable, i.e., the same MenB vaccine product must be used for all doses.
  — MenACWY vaccine is preferred for adults with serogroup A, C, W, and Y meningococcal vaccine indications who are aged ≤55 years, and for adults aged ≥56 years: 1) who were vaccinated previously with MenACWY vaccine and are recommended for revaccination or 2) for whom multiple doses of vaccine are anticipated; MPSV4 vaccine is preferred for adults aged ≥56 years who have not received MenACWY vaccine previously and who require a single dose only (e.g., persons at risk because of an outbreak).
  — Revaccination with MenACWY vaccine every 5 years is recommended for adults previously vaccinated with MenACWY or MPSV4 vaccine who remain at increased risk for infection (e.g., adults with anatomical or functional asplenia or persistent complement component deficiencies, or microbiologists who are routinely exposed to isolates of *Neisseria meningitidis*).
  — MenB vaccine is approved for use in persons aged 10 through 25 years; however, because there is no theoretical difference in safety for persons aged >25 years compared to those aged 10 through 25 years, MenB vaccine is recommended for routine use in persons aged ≥10 years who are at increased risk for serogroup B meningococcal disease.
  — There is no recommendation for MenB revaccination at this time.
  — MenB vaccine may be administered concomitantly with MenACWY vaccine but at a different anatomic site, if feasible.
  — HIV infection is not an indication for routine vaccination with MenACWY or MenB vaccine; if an HIV-infected person of any age is to be vaccinated, administer 2 doses of MenACWY vaccine at least 2 months apart.
- Adults with anatomical or functional asplenia or persistent complement component deficiencies: administer 2 doses of MenACWY vaccine at least 2 months apart and revaccinate every 5 years. Also administer a series of MenB vaccine.
- Microbiologists who are routinely exposed to isolates of *Neisseria meningitidis*: administer a single dose of MenACWY vaccine; revaccinate with MenACWY vaccine every 5 years if remain at increased risk for infection. Also administer a series of MenB vaccine.
- Persons at risk because of a meningococcal disease outbreak: if the outbreak is attributable to serogroup A, C, W, or Y, administer a single dose of MenACWY vaccine; if the outbreak is attributable to serogroup B, administer a series of MenB vaccine.
- Persons who travel to or live in countries in which meningococcal disease is hyperendemic or epidemic: administer a single dose of MenACWY vaccine and revaccinate with MenACWY vaccine every 5 years if the increased risk for infection remains (see footnote 1); MenB vaccine is not recommended because meningococcal disease in these countries is generally not caused by serogroup B.
- Military recruits: administer a single dose of MenACWY vaccine.
- First-year college students aged ≤21 years who live in residence halls: administer a single dose of MenACWY vaccine if they have not received a dose on or after their 16th birthday.
- Young adults aged 16 through 23 years (preferred age range is 16 through 18 years): may be vaccinated with a series of MenB vaccine to provide short-term protection against most strains of serogroup B meningococcal disease.

12. *Haemophilus influenzae* type b (Hib) vaccination

- One dose of Hib vaccine should be administered to persons who have anatomical or functional asplenia or sickle cell disease or are undergoing elective splenectomy if they have not previously received Hib vaccine. Hib vaccination 14 or more days before splenectomy is suggested.
- Recipients of a hematopoietic stem cell transplant (HSCT) should be vaccinated with a 3-dose regimen 6–12 months after a successful transplant, regardless of vaccination history; at least 4 weeks should separate doses.
- Hib vaccine is not recommended for adults with HIV infection since their risk for Hib infection is low.

13. Immunocompromising conditions

- Inactivated vaccines (e.g., pneumococcal, meningococcal, and inactivated influenza vaccines) generally are acceptable and live vaccines generally should be avoided in persons with immune deficiencies or immunocompromising conditions. Information on specific conditions is available at www.cdc.gov/vaccines/hcp/acip-recs/index.html.

Table 6 SUMMARY OF ADOLESCENT/ADULT IMMUNIZATION RECOMMENDATIONS					
	TETANUS, DIPTHERIA AND ACELLULAR PERTUSSIS (TD/TDAP)	INFLUENZA	PNEUMOCOCCAL POLYSACCHARIDE (PPSV)	MEASLES AND MUMPS	SMALL POX
Indications	All adults Tdap should replace a single dose of Td for adults aged less than 65 years who have not previously received a Tdap dose.	Ages 19–49 for persons with medical/exposure indications Adults 50 y and older Clients with chronic conditions During influenza season for women in 2nd and 3rd trimester of pregnancy Persons traveling to foreign countries Residents of nursing homes, long-term care, assisted-living facilities	Ages 19–64 for persons with medical/exposure indications Adults 65 y and older Alaskan Natives and some Native Americans Residents of nursing homes, long-term care, assisted-living facilities	Adults born after 1957 without proof of vaccine on or after first birthday HIV-infected persons without severe immunosuppression Travelers to foreign countries Persons entering college	First responders
Schedule	Two doses 4–8 wk apart Third dose 6–12 mo Booster at 10 y intervals for life Tdap or Td vaccine used as indicated	Annually each fall	One dose Should receive at age 65 if received at least 5 y previously Administered if vaccination status unknown	One dose Two doses if in college, in health care profession, or traveling to foreign country with 2nd dose one month after 1st	One dose
Contra-indications	Severe allergic reaction to previous dose Encephalopathy not due to another cause within 7 days of DTaP	Allergy to eggs		Severe allergic reaction Known severe immunodeficiency	History of eczema or other skin conditions that disrupt epidermis, pregnancy or breast feeding, or women who wish to conceive 28 days after vaccination Immunosuppression, allergy to small pox vaccine receiving topical ocular steroid medication, moderate-to-severe recurrent illness, being under the age of 18, household contacts with history of eczema
Comments	Precautions: Moderate or severe illness with or without fever			Check pregnancy status of women Should avoid pregnancy for 30 d after vaccination Elevated temperature may be seen for 1–2 weeks Precautions: Recent receipt of antibody-containing blood product Moderate or severe illness with or without fever	Vaccinia can be transmitted from an unhealed vaccination site to other persons by close contact. Wash hands with soapy water immediately after changing bandage; place bandages in sealed plastic bag; cover site with gauze and wear long-sleeved clothing. When performing client care, keep site covered with gauze and a semiper-meable dressing.

Table 6 SUMMARY OF ADOLESCENT/ADULT IMMUNIZATION RECOMMENDATIONS (CONTINUED)						
	RUBELLA	HEPATITIS B	POLIOVIRUS: IPV	VARICELLA	HEPATITIS A	HUMAN PAPILLOMAVIRUS VACCINE (HPV)
Indications	Persons (especially women) without proof of vaccine on or after first birthday Health-care personnel at risk of exposure to rubella and who have contact with pregnant clients	Persons at risk to exposure to blood or blood-containing body fluids Clients and staff at institutions for developmentally disabled Hemodialysis clients Recipients of clotting-factor concentrates Household contacts and sex partners of clients with HBV Some international travelers Injecting drug users Men who have sex with men Heterosexuals with multiple sex partners or recent STD Inmates of longterm correctional facilities All unvaccinated adolescents	Travelers to countries where it is epidemic Unvaccinated adults whose children receive IPV	Persons without proof of disease or vaccination or who are seronegative Susceptible adolescents/ adults living in house holds with children Susceptible healthcare workers Susceptible family contacts of immunocompromised persons Nonpregnant women of childbearing age International travelers High risk persons: teachers of young children, day care employees, residents and staff in institutional settings, college students, inmates and staff of correctional institutions, military personnel	Travelers to countries with high incidence Men who have sex with men Injecting and illegal drug users Persons with chronic liver disease Persons with clotting factor disorders Food handlers	All females age 11/12 to 25
Schedule	One dose	Three doses Second dose 1–2 mo after 1st Third 4–6 mo after 1st	IPV recommended Two doses at 4–8 wk intervals Third dose 2–12 mo after second OPV no longer recommended in U.S.	Two doses separated by 4–8 wk	Two doses separated by 6–12 mo	Three doses Second dose 2 mo after 1st Third dose 6 mo after 2nd
Contra-indications	Allergy to neomycin Pregnancy Receipt of immune globulin or blood/ blood products in previous 3–11 mo	Severe allergic reaction to vaccine	Severe allergic reaction after previous dose	Severe allergic reaction to vaccine Immunosuppressive therapy or immunodeficiency (including HIV infection) Pregnancy	Severe allergic reaction to vaccine	
Comments	Check pregnancy status of women Should avoid pregnancy for 3 mo after vaccination	Precautions: Low birth weight infant Moderate or severe illness with or without fever	Temperature elevation may be seen for 1–2 weeks Precautions: Pregnancy moderate or severe illness with or without fever	Check pregnancy status of women Should avoid pregnancy for 1 mo after vaccination Immune globulin or blood/ blood product in previous 11 mo Moderate or severe illness with or without fever	Swelling and redness at injection site common Precaution: pregnancy	

Table 7 NURSING CONSIDERATIONS FOR THE CHILD RECEIVING IMMUNIZATION		
NAME	ROUTE	NURSING CONSIDERATIONS
DTaP (diphtheria, tetanus, pertussis)	IM anterior or lateral thigh (No IMs in gluteal muscle until after child is walking)	Potential adverse effects include fever within 24–48 hours, swelling, redness, soreness at injection site More serious adverse effects—continuous screaming, convulsions, high fever, loss of consciousness Do not administer if there is past history of serious reaction
MMR (measles, mumps, rubella)	SC anterior or lateral thigh	Potential adverse effects include rash, fever, and arthritis; may occur 10 days to 2 weeks after vaccination May give DTaP, MMR, and IPV at same time if family has history of not keeping appointments for vaccinations
IPV (inactivated polio)	IM	Reactions very rare
HB (hepatitis B)	IM vastus lateralis or deltoid	Should not be given into dorsogluteal site Mild local tenderness at injection site
Tuberculosis test	Intradermal	May be given 4–6 year and 11–16 years if in high prevalence areas Evaluated in 48–72 hours PPD (purified protein derivative) 0.1 ml Tine test (multiple puncture) less accurate
TD (tetanus/ diphtheria booster)	IM anterior or lateral thigh	Repeat every 10 years
Live attenuated rubella	SC anterior or lateral thigh	Give once only to women who are antibody-negative for rubella, and if pregnancy can be prevented for 3 months postvaccination
Live attenuated mumps	SC	Give once Prevention of orchitis (and therefore sterility) in susceptible males

▶ ALLERGEN RESPONSE

A. Assessment

1. Prodromal—reports weakness, apprehension, impending doom, dry/scratchy throat (feeling of "lump in throat"); nausea and vomiting

2. Cutaneous—generalized intense pruritus and urticaria (hives), angioedema (swelling) of lips and eyelids

3. Bronchial—increasing respiratory distress with audible wheezing, rales; diminished breath sounds heard on auscultation

4. Circulatory—hypotension and a rapid, weak, irregular pulse, dysrhythmias, shock, cardiac arrest can occur within minutes

B. Diagnose

1. Hypersensitivity—exaggerated or inappropriate reaction of a previously sensitized immune system resulting in a typical pathological process and tissue damage

2. Anaphylaxis—serious multiple system response (vasogenic shock) to an antigen-antibody reaction upon subsequent exposure (rarely upon first contact) to a substance (allergen) for which the person has developed a severe hypersensitivity

3. Immense amounts of histamine are rapidly dispersed throughout the circulatory system resulting in extensive vasodilation and increased capillary permeability leading to acute hypovolemia and vascular

collapse; there is also severe edema of bronchial tissue resulting in pulmonary obstruction; without treatment, severe hypoxemia and ultimately death will occur

4. Common allergens—drug/chemicals (penicillin, radiopaque dyes, aspirin, bisulfates, vaccines, blood components), toxins (snake, bee, wasp, hornet), and food (berries, chocolate, eggs, shellfish, seafood, nuts)

5. Potential nursing diagnoses
   a. Skin integrity, impaired
   b. Airway clearance, ineffective

C. Plan/Implementation
1. Establish airway (ABC)
2. Administer aqueous epinephrine (adrenaline) 1:1,000—0.1 ml up to 0.5 ml (0.1 mg/kg body weight) SC in arm opposite to side of injection/sting; same dose may be repeated every 15–20 minutes PRN (three times with children)
3. Start IV with large-bore needle for rapid infusion of fluids, if needed; monitor I and O
4. Tourniquet may be applied on extremity proximal to injection of allergen to prevent further absorption
5. Oxygen, suction, and life support as needed
6. Other medications may be used—diphenhydramine as antihistamine, aminophylline for severe bronchospasm, vasopressors for severe shock, corticosteroids for persistent/recurrent symptoms
7. Assess all clients about possible allergic reactions to foods, medications, insects
8. Ensure that clients remain in health setting at least 20–30 minutes after receiving injection
9. Teach client and family how to avoid the identified allergen; ensure/reinforce wearing Medic-Alert items
10. For sensitivity to insect venom, instruct the client and/or family members in the use of the emergency anaphylaxis kit (either epinephrine and syringes or automatic injector), to be kept with the person at all times
11. Hyposensitization/desensitization/immunotherapy—SC administration of gradually increasing dosages of the offending allergen

D. Evaluation
1. Was the reaction to the allergen controlled?
2. Does the family/client know how to provide emergency care?

▶ LATEX ALLERGY

A. Assessment
1. Contact urticaria; lip, mouth
2. Upper airway edema
3. Flushing and generalized edema
4. Rhinitis, conjunctivitis
5. Bronchospasms
6. Anaphylactic shock

B. Diagnose

    1. Caused by repeated exposure to natural latex rubber protein products

    2. High risk populations

        a. Children with neural tube defects

        b. Clients with urogenital abnormalities

        c. Clients with spinal cord injuries

        d. History of multiple surgeries

        e. Health care workers, hairdressers, cleaning staff

        f. Allergies to banana, avocado, chestnut, kiwi, papaya, peaches

C. Plan/Implementation

    1. Screen for latex sensitivity

    2. Provide latex-safe environment

    3. Instruct client to avoid latex products

        a. Gloves

        b. Catheters

        c. Brown ace bandages

        d. Band-Aid dressing

        e. Elastic pressure stocking

        f. Balloons

        g. Condoms

        h. Feminine hygiene pad

    4. Wear Medic-Alert identification

D. Evaluation

    1. Is the client knowledgeable about how to avoid latex?

▶ ATOPIC ALLERGY

A. Assessment

    1. History of offending allergen, pollens (trees, grass, weeds), or environmental substances (dust, animals, feathers)

    2. Upper respiratory symptoms—rhinorrhea (runny nose), sneezing, mucosal edema, and congestion, pharyngeal and conjunctival itching and tearing

    3. Etiology and severity may be determined by skin testing

B. Diagnose

    1. Airway clearance, ineffective

    2. Includes hay fever, rhinitis, asthma

C. Plan/Implementation

    1. Provide symptomatic relief

    2. Teach client how to avoid allergies

D. Evaluation

    1. Is client knowledgeable about how to avoid offending allergen?

    2. Is client able to control symptoms of allergic response?

▶ PHYSICAL ASSESSMENT

A. Purpose

1. Assess client's current health status
2. Interpret physical data
3. Decide on interventions based on data obtained

B. Preparation

1. Gather equipment
   a. Ophthalmoscope
   b. Tuning fork
   c. Cotton swabs
   d. Snellen eye chart
   e. Thermometer
   f. Penlight
   g. Tongue depressor
   h. Ruler/tape measure
   i. Safety pin
   j. Balance scale
   k. Gloves
   l. Nasal speculum
   m. Vaginal speculum
2. Provide for privacy (drape) in quiet, well-lit environment
3. Explain procedure to client
4. Ask client to empty bladder
5. Drape client for privacy
6. Compare findings on one side of body with other side and compare with normal
7. Make use of teaching opportunities (dental care, eye exams, self-exams of breast or testicle)
8. Use piece of equipment for entire assessment, then return to equipment tray

C. Techniques used in order performed, except for abdominal assessment

1. Inspection (visually examined)
   a. Starts with first interaction
   b. Provide good lighting
   c. Determine
      1) Size
      2) Shape
      3) Color
      4) Texture
      5) Symmetry
      6) Position

2. Palpation (touch)

   a. Warm hands

   b. Approach slowly and proceed systematically

   c. Use fingertips for fine touch (pulses, nodes)

   d. Use dorsum of fingers for temperatures

   e. Use palm or ulnar edge of hand for vibration

   f. Start with light palpation, then do deep palpation

   g. Use bimanual palpation (both hands) for deep palpation and to assess movable structure (kidney)—place sensing hand lightly on skin surface, place active hand over sensing hand and apply pressure

   h. Ballottement—push fluid-filled tissue toward palpating hand so object floats against fingertips

   i. Determines

      1) Masses

      2) Pulsation

      3) Organ size

      4) Tenderness or pain

      5) Swelling

      6) Tissue fullness and elasticity

      7) Vibration

      8) Crepitus

      9) Temperature

      10) Texture

      11) Moisture

3. Percussion (tap to produce sound and vibration)

   a. Types

      1) Direct—strike body surface with 1 or 2 fingers

      2) Indirect—strike finger or hand placed over body surface

      3) Blunt—use reflex hammer to check deep tendon reflexes; Use blunt percussion with fist to assess costovertebral angle (CVA) tenderness

   b. Sounds

      1) Resonance—moderate-to-loud, low-pitched (clear, hollow) sound of moderate duration; found with air-filled tissue (normal lung)

      2) Hyperresonance—loud, booming, low-pitched sound of longer duration found with overinflated air-filled tissue (pulmonary emphysema); normal in child due to thin chest wall

      3) Tympany—loud, drumlike, high-pitched or musical sound of moderately long duration found with enclosed, air-filled structures (bowel)

      4) Dull—soft, muffled, moderate-to-high-pitched sound of short duration; found with dense, fluid-filled tissue (liver)

      5) Flat—very soft, high-pitched sound of short duration; found with very dense tissue (bone, muscle)

  c. Determines

   1) Location, size, density of masses

   2) Pain in areas up to depth of 3–5 cm (1–2 inches)

  d. Performed after inspection and palpation, except for abdominal assessment; for abdomen perform inspection, auscultation, percussion, palpation

 4. Auscultation

  a. Equipment

   1) Use diaphragm of stethoscope to listen to high-pitched sounds (lung, bowel, heart); place firmly against skin surface to form tight seal (leave ring)

   2) Use bell to listen to soft, low-pitched sounds (heart murmurs); place lightly on skin surface

  b. Listen over bare skin (not through clothing); moisten body hair to prevent crackling sounds

Table 8 NORMAL VITAL SIGNS			
AGE	NORMAL RESPIRATORY RATE	NORMAL PULSE RATE	NORMAL BLOOD PRESSURE (BP)
Newborn	30–60 per minute	120–140 beats per minute (bpm) May go to 180 when crying	65/41 mm Hg
1–4 years	20–40 per minute	70–110 beats per minute (bpm)	90/60 mm Hg
5–12 years	16–22 per minute	60–95 beats per minute (bpm)	100/60 mm Hg
Adult	12–20 per minute	60–100 beats per minute (bpm)	less than 120/80 mm Hg
Factors influencing respiration: fever, anxiety, drugs, disease			
Factors influencing BP: disease, drugs, anxiety, cardiac output, peripheral resistance, arterial elasticity, blood volume, blood viscosity, age, weight, exercise			
Factors influencing pulse rate and rhythm: drug, pathology, exercise, age, gender, temperature, BP, serum electrolytes			

D. Findings

 1. General survey

  a. General appearance

   1) Apparent age

   2) Sex

   3) Racial and ethnic group

   4) Apparent state of health

   5) Proportionate height and weight

   6) Posture

   7) Gait, movements, range of motion

   8) Suitable clothing

      9) Hygiene

     10) Body and breath odor

     11) Skin color, condition

     12) Presence of assistive device, hearing aid, glasses

  b. General behavior

     1) Signs of distress

     2) Level of consciousness, oriented ×3, mood, speech, thought process appropriate

     3) Level of cooperation, eye contact (culture must be considered)

2. Vital signs (see Table 8)

  a. Temperature (see Table 9)

     1) Infants—performed axillary

     2) Intra-auricular probe allows rapid, noninvasive reading when appropriate

     3) Tympanic membrane sensors—positioning is crucial, ear canal must be straightened

  b. Pulse (rate, rhythm)

  c. Respirations (rate, pattern, depth)

     1) Adult—costal (chest moves), regular, expiration slower than inspiration, rate 12–20 respirations/minute

     2) Neonates—diaphragmatic (abdomen moves), irregular, 30–60 respirations/minute

     3) Breathing patterns

       a) Abdominal respirations—breathing accomplished by abdominal muscles and diaphragm; may be used to increase effectiveness of ventilatory process in certain conditions

       b) Apnea—temporary cessation of breathing

       c) Cheyne-Stokes respiration—periodic breathing characterized by rhythmic waxing and waning of the depth of respirations

       d) Dyspnea—difficult, labored, or painful breathing (considered "normal" at certain times, e.g., after extreme physical exertion)

       e) Hyperpnea—abnormally deep breathing

       f) Hyperventilation—abnormally rapid, deep, and prolonged breathing

         i) Caused by central nervous system disorders, drugs that increase sensitivity of respiratory center or acute anxiety

         ii) Produces respiratory alkalosis due to reduction in CO_2

       g) Hypoventilation—reduced ventilatory efficiency; produces respiratory acidosis due to elevation in CO_2

       h) Kussmaul's respirations (air hunger)—marked increase in depth and rate

       i) Orthopnea—inability to breathe except when trunk is in an upright position

       j) Paradoxical respirations—breathing pattern in which a lung (or portion of a lung) deflates during inspiration (acts opposite to normal)

Table 9 NORMAL BODY TEMPERATURE		
METHOD USED	FAHRENHEIT	CELSIUS
Oral	98.6°	37.0°
Rectal	99.6°	37.6°
Axillary	97.6°	36.5°
Factors influencing reading: elderly client, faulty thermometer, dehydration, environment, infections		

k) Periodic breathing—rate, depth, or tidal volume changes markedly from one interval to the next; pattern of change is periodically reproduced

4) Cyanosis—skin appears blue because of an excessive accumulation of unoxygenated hemoglobin in the blood

5) Stridor—harsh, high-pitched sound associated with airway obstruction near larynx

6) Cough

   a) Normal reflex to remove foreign material from the lungs

   b) Normally absent in newborns

d. Blood pressure

1) Check both arms and compare results (difference 5–10 mm Hg normal)

2) Pulse pressure (normal 30–40 mm Hg)

3) Cover 50% of limb from shoulder to olecranon with cuff; too narrow: abnormally high reading; too wide: abnormally low reading

3. Nutrition status

a. Height, weight; ideal body weight, men—106 lbs for first 5 feet, then add 6 lbs/inch; women—100 for first 5 feet, then add 5 lbs/inch; add 10% for client with larger frame; subtract 10% for client with small frame

4. Skin

a. Check for pallor on buccal mucosa or conjunctivae, cyanosis on nail beds or oral mucosa, jaundice on sclera

b. Scars, bruises, lesions

c. Edema (eyes, sacrum), moisture, hydration

d. Temperature, texture, turgor (pinch skin, tented 3 seconds or less is normal), check over sternum for elderly

5. Hair

a. Hirsutism—excess

b. Alopecia—loss or thinning

6. Nails (indicate respiratory and nutritional status)

a. Color

    b. Shape, contour (normal angle of nail bed less than or equal to 160°, clubbing: nail bed angle greater than or equal to 180° due to prolonged decreased oxygenation)

    c. Texture, thickness

    d. Capillary refill (normal ≤3–second return of color)

7. Head

    a. Size, shape, symmetry

    b. Temporal arteries

    c. Cranial nerve function (see Table 10)

8. Eyes

    a. Ptosis—drooping of upper eyelid

    b. Color of sclerae, conjunctiva

    c. Pupils

       1) Size, shape, equality, reactivity to light and accommodation (PERRLA)

    d. Photophobia—light intolerance

    e. Nystagmus—abnormal, involuntary, rapid eye movements

    f. Strabismus—involuntary drifting of one eye out of alignment with the other eye; "lazy eye"

    g. Corneal reflex

    h. Visual fields (peripheral vision)

    i. Visual acuity—Snellen chart, normal 20/20

    j. Ophthalmoscope exam

       1) Red reflex—red glow from light reflected from retina

       2) Fundus

       3) Optic disk

       4) Macula

    k. Corneal light reflection—same position on each cornea; asymmetrical reflection—strabismus

9. Ears

    a. Pull pinna up and back to examine children's (3 years of age and older) and adult's ears

    b. Pull pinna down and back to examine infants' and young childrens' (younger than 3 years of age) ears

    c. Tympanic membrane—cone of light at 5 o'clock position right ear, 7 o'clock position left ear

    d. Weber test—assesses bone conduction; vibrating tuning fork placed in middle of forehead; normal—hear sound equally in ears

    e. Rinne test—compares bone conduction with air conduction; vibrating tuning fork placed on mastoid process, when client no longer hears sound, positioned in front of ear canal; normal—should still be able to hear sound; air conduction greater than bone conduction by 2:1 ratio (positive Rinne test)

10. Nose and sinuses
    a. Septum midline
    b. Alignment, color, discharge
    c. Palpate and percuss sinuses

11. Mouth and pharynx
    a. Oral mucosa
    b. Teeth (normal 32)
    c. Tongue
    d. Hard and soft palate
    e. Uvula, midline
    f. Tonsils
    g. Gag reflex
    h. Swallow
    i. Taste

12. Neck
    a. Range of motion of cervical spine
    b. Cervical lymph nodes (normal less than or equal to 1 cm round, soft, mobile) nontender
    c. Trachea position
    d. Thyroid gland
    e. Carotid arteries—check for bruit and thrill
    f. Jugular veins

13. Thorax and lungs
    a. Alignment of spine
    b. Anteroposterior to transverse diameter (normal adult 1:2 to 5:7); 1:1 barrel chest

Table 10 CRANIAL NERVE ASSESSMENT			
#/NERVE	FUNCTION	NORMAL FINDINGS	NURSING CONSIDERATIONS
(I) Olfactory	Sense of smell	Able to detect various odors in each nostril	Have client smell a nonirritating substance such as coffee or tobacco with eyes closed Test each nostril separately
(II) Optic	Sense of vision	Clear (acute) vision near and distant	Snellen eye chart for far vision Read newspaper for near vision Ophthalmoscopic exam
(III) Oculomotor	Pupil constriction, raising of eyelids	Pupils equal in size and equally reactive to light	Instruct client to look up, down, inward Observe for symmetry and eye opening Shine penlight into eye as client stares straight ahead Ask client to watch your finger as you move it toward face

Table 10 CRANIAL NERVE ASSESSMENT *(CONTINUED)*			
#/NERVE	**FUNCTION**	**NORMAL FINDINGS**	**NURSING CONSIDERATIONS**
(IV) Trochlear	Downward and inward movement of eyes	Able to move eyes down and inward	(See Oculomotor)
(V) Trigeminal	Motor—jaw movement Sensory—sensation on the face and neck	Able to clench and relax jaw Able to differentiate between various stimuli touched to the face and neck	Test with pin and wisp of cotton over each division on both sides of face Ask client to open jaw, bite down, move jaw laterally against pressure Stroke cornea with wisp of cotton
(VI) Abducens	Lateral movement of the eyes	Able to move eyes in all directions	(See Oculomotor)
(VII) Facial	Motor—facial muscle movement Sensory—taste on the anterior two-thirds of the tongue (sweet and salty)	Able to smile, whistle, wrinkle forehead Able to differentiate tastes among various agents	Observe for facial symmetry after asking client to frown, smile, raise eyebrows, close eyelids against resistance, whistle, blow Place sweet, sour, bitter, and salty substances on tongue
(VIII) Acoustic	Sense of hearing and balance	Hearing intact Balance maintained while walking	Test with watch ticking into ear, rubbing fingers together, Rinne and Weber tests Test posture, standing with eyes closed Otoscopic exam
(IX) Glossopharyngeal	Motor—pharyngeal movement and swallowing Sensory—taste on posterior one-third of tongue (sour and bitter)	Gag reflex intact, able to swallow Able to taste	Place sweet, sour, bitter, and salty substances on tongue Note ability to swallow and handle secretions Stimulate pharyngeal wall to elicit gag reflex
(X) Vagus	Swallowing and speaking	Able to swallow and speak with a smooth voice	Inspect soft palate—instruct to say "ah" Observe uvula for midline position Rate quality of voice
(XI) Spinal accessory	Motor—flexion and rotation of head; shrugging of shoulders	Able to flex and rotate head; able to shrug shoulders	Inspect and palpate sternocleido-mastoid and trapezius muscles for size, contour, tone Ask client to move head side to side against resistance and shrug shoulders against resistance
(XII) Hypoglossal	Motor—tongue movements	Can move tongue side to side and stick it out symmetrically and in midline	Inspect tongue in mouth Ask client to stick out tongue and move it quickly side to side Observe midline, symmetry, and rhythmic movement

c. Respiratory excursion
d. Respirations
e. Tactile fremitus—(vibration produced when client makes sound of "99")

    f. Diaphragmatic excursion—assesses degree and symmetry of diaphragm movement; percuss from areas of resonance to dullness

    g. Breath sounds—bilaterally equal

       1) Normal

          a) Vesicular—soft and low-pitched breezy sounds heard over most of peripheral lung fields

          b) Bronchovesicular—medium pitched, moderately loud sounds heard over the mainstem bronchi

          c) Bronchial—loud, coarse, blowing sound heard over the trachea

       2) Adventitious (abnormal); caused by fluid or inflammation

          a) Rales—crackling or gurgling sounds (also known as crackles) commonly heard on inspiration

          b) Rhonchi—musical sounds or vibrations commonly heard on expiration

          c) Wheezes—squeaky sounds heard during inspiration and expiration associated with narrow airways

          d) Pleural friction rub—grating sound or vibration heard during inspiration and expiration

    h. Vocal resonance

       1) Bronchophony—say "99" and hear more clearly than normal; loud transmission of voice sounds caused by consolidation of lung

       2) Egophony—say "E" and hear "A" due to distortion caused by consolidation of lung

       3) Whispered pectoriloquy—hear whispered sounds clearly due to dense consolidation of lung

    i. Costovertebral angle percussion—kidneys

14. Heart Sounds (corresponds with Figure 1)

    a. Angle of Louis—manubrial sternal junction at second rib

    b. Aortic and pulmonic areas—right and left second intercostal spaces alongside sternum

    c. Erbs' point—third intercostal space just to the left of the sternum

    d. Tricuspid area—fourth or fifth intercostal space to the left

    e. Mitral area—fifth intercostal space at left midclavicular line (apex of heart)

    f. Point of maximal impulse (PMI)

       1) Impulse of the left ventricle felt most strongly

       2) Adult—left fifth intercostal space in the midclavicular line (8–10 cm to the left of the midsternal line)

       3) Infant—lateral to left nipple

    g. S1 and S2

       1) S1 "lubb"—closure of tricuspid and mitral valves; dull quality and low pitch; onset of ventricular systole (contraction)

       2) S2 "dubb"—closure of aortic and pulmonic valves; snapping quality; onset of diastole (relaxation of atria, then ventricles)

h. Murmurs—abnormal sounds caused by turbulence within the heart valve; turbulence within a blood vessel is called a bruit; three basic factors result in murmurs

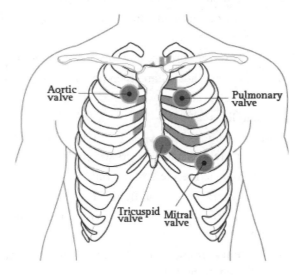

Figure 1 Heart Sounds (intercostal spaces)

   1) High rate of blood flow through either a normal or abnormal valve

   2) Blood flow through a sclerosed or abnormal valve, or into a dilated heart chamber or vessel

   3) Blood flow regurgitated backward through an incompetent valve or septal defect

   i. Pulse deficit—difference between apical and radial rate

   j. Jugular veins—normally distend when the client lies flat, but are not visible when the client's head is raised 30 to 45°

15. Peripheral vascular system

   a. Pulses

      1) Radial—passes medially across the wrist; felt on radial (or thumb) side of the forearm

      2) Ulnar—passes laterally across the wrist; felt on the ulnar (little finger) side of the wrist

      3) Femoral—passes beneath the inguinal ligament (groin area) into the thigh; felt in groin area

      4) Carotid—pulsations can be felt over medial edge of sternocleidomastoid muscle in neck

      5) Pedal (dorsalis pedis: dorsal artery of the foot)—passes laterally over the foot; felt along top of foot

      6) Posterior tibial—felt on inner side of ankle below medial malleous

      7) Popliteal—felt in popliteal fossa, the region at the back of the knee

      8) Temporal—felt lateral to eyes

      9) Apical—left at fifth intercostal space at midclavicular line

16. Breasts and axillae

    a. Size, shape, symmetry

    b. Gynecomastia—breast enlargement in males

    c. Nodes—normal nonpalpable

17. Abdomen

    a. Knees flexed to relax muscles and provide for comfort

    b. Inspect and auscultate, then percuss and palpate

    c. Symmetry, contour

    d. Umbilicus

    e. Bowel sounds; normal high-pitched gurgles heard with the diaphragm of the stethoscope at 5–20-second intervals

        1) Hypoactive– less than 3/minute

        2) Hyperactive—loud, frequent

    f. Aorta, renal, iliac, femoral arteries auscultated with the bell of the stethoscope

    g. Peritoneal friction rub—grating sound varies with respirations; inflammation of liver

    h. Liver and spleen size

    i. Inguinal lymph nodes

    j. Rebound tenderness—inflammation of peritoneum

    k. Kidneys

    l. Abdominal reflexes

18. Neurological system

    a. Deep tendon reflexes (DTRs)—assesses sensory and motor pathways; compare bilaterally; 0 (absent) through 4+ (hyperactive) scale

    b. Cerebellar function—coordination; point-to-point touching, rapid, alternating movements, gait

    c. Mental status (cerebral function)

    d. Cranial nerve function

    e. Motor function

        1) Strength

        2) Tone

    f. Sensory function

        1) Touch, tactile localization

        2) Pain

        3) Pressure

        4) Temperature

        5) Vibration

        6) Proprioception (position sense)

        7) Vision

        8) Hearing

        9) Smell

        10) Taste

19. Musculoskeletal system

    a. Muscle tone and strength

    b. Joint movements; crepitus–grating sound abnormal

20. Genitalia

    a. Provide privacy

    b. Inspect outer structures (labia, urethral meatus, vaginal introitus, anus, penis, scrotum)

    c. Use firm, deliberate touch

    d. Note any abnormalities

        1) Hypospadias—urethral meatus located on the underside of the penile shaft

        2) Epispadias—urethral meatus located on the upper side of the penile shaft

        3) Hemorrhoids—dilated veins in the anal area

    e. Male

        1) Penis—foreskin, glans

        2) Hypospadias—meatus located on underside of penile shaft

        3) Epispadias—meatus located on upper side of penile shaft

        4) Scrotum

        5) Inguinal area

    f. Female

        1) Lithotomy position

        2) Cervix

21. Anus and rectum

    a. Rectal prolapse—protrusion of rectal mucous membrane through anus

    b. Hemorrhoids—dilated veins

    c. Anal sphincter

    d. Male—prostate gland

    e. Female—cervix

    f. Stool—normal color brown; assess for presence of blood

Chapter 9

PSYCHOSOCIAL INTEGRITY

Units

1. **Coping and Adaptation**

2. **Psychosocial Adaptation**

3. **Psychopathology**

4. **Chemical Dependency**

5. **Abuse and Neglect**

COPING AND ADAPTATION | *Unit 1*

▶ MENTAL HEALTH CONCEPTS

A. Assessment

1. Appearance, behavior, or mood
   a. Well groomed, relaxed
   b. Self-confident, self-accepting
2. Speech, thought content, and thought process
   a. Clear, coherent
   b. Reality-based
3. Sensorium
   a. Oriented to person, place, and time
   b. Good memory
   c. Ability to abstract
4. Insight and judgment—accurate self-perception and awareness
5. Family relationships and work habits
   a. Satisfying interpersonal relationships
   b. Ability to trust
   c. Ability to cope effectively with stress
   d. Environmental mastery
6. Level of growth and development

B. Diagnose

1. Potential support systems or stressors
   a. Religious organizations or community support
   b. Family
   c. Socioeconomic resources
   d. Education
   e. Cultural norms
2. Potential risk factors
   a. Family history of mental illness
   b. Medical history—imbalances can cause symptoms resembling emotional illness
3. Satisfaction of basic human needs in order of importance (Maslow) (see Figure 1)
   a. Physical—oxygen, water, food, sleep, sex
   b. Safety—physical, security, order
   c. Love and belonging—affection, companionship, identification
   d. Esteem and recognition—status, success, prestige
   e. Self-actualization—self-fulfillment, creativity

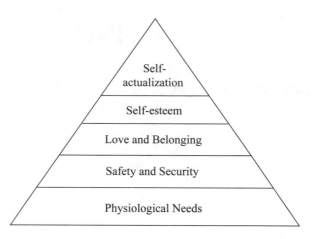

Figure 1 Maslow Hierarchy of Needs

4. Potential nursing diagnoses

    a. Social interaction, impaired

    b. Anxiety

    c. Individual coping, ineffective

    d. Self-esteem disturbance

Table 1 THERAPEUTIC RESPONSES		
RESPONSE	**GOAL/PURPOSE**	**EXAMPLES**
Using silence (nonverbal)	Allows client time to think and reflect; conveys acceptance Allows client to take lead in conversation	Use proper nonverbal communication, remain seated, maintain eye contact, sit quietly and wait
Using general leads or broad openings	Encourages client to talk Indicates interest in client Allows client to choose subject Sets tone for depressed client	"What would you like to talk about? Then what? Go on. . ." "What brought you to the hospital?" "What can you tell me about your family?"
Clarification	Encourages recall and details of particular experience Encourages description of feelings Seeks clarification, pinpoints specifics Makes sure nurse understands client	"Give me an example." "Tell me more." "And how do you feel when you're angry?" "Who are 'they'?"
Reflecting	Paraphrases what client says Reflects what client says, especially feelings conveyed	"It sounds like you're feeling angry." "In other words, you really felt abandoned." "I hear you saying it was hard to come to the hospital."

C. Plan/Implementation

1. Therapeutic communication—listening to and understanding client while promoting clarification and insight (see Tables 1, 2, and 3)

   a. Goals

   1) To understand client's message (verbal and nonverbal)

   2) To facilitate verbalization of feelings

   3) To communicate understanding and acceptance

   4) To identify problems, goals, and objectives

   b. Guidelines

   1) Nonverbal communication constitutes two-thirds of all communication and gives the most accurate reflection of attitude; key point of psychiatric interventions is say nothing, listen

      a) Physical appearance, body movement, posture, gesture, facial expression

      b) Contact—eye contact, physical distance maintained, ability to touch and be touched

   2) The person's feelings and what is verbalized may be incongruent, e.g., client denies feeling sad but appears morose

   3) Implied messages are as important to understand as overt behavior, e.g., continual interruptions may represent loneliness or fear

Table 2 RESPONSES TO AVOID IN THERAPEUTIC COMMUNICATION	
RESPONSE	**EXAMPLES**
Closed-ended questions that can be answered by a "yes" or "no" or other monosyllabic responses; prevents sharing; puts pressure on client	"How many children do you have?" "Who do you live with?" "Are you feeling better today?"
Advice-giving—encourages dependency, may not be right for a particular client	"Why don't you. . . ?" "You really should cut your hair and wear makeup."
Responding to questions that are related to one's qualifications or personal life in an embarrassed or concrete way; keep conversation client-centered	"Yes, I am highly qualified." "You know nurses are not permitted to go out with their clients."
Arguing or responding in a hostile way	"If you do not take your medication, there is really nothing we can do to help you."
Reassuring—client benefits more by exploring own ideas and feelings	"You will start feeling much better any day." "Don't worry, your doctors will do everything necessary for your care."
"Why" questions—can imply disapproval and client may become defensive	"Why didn't you take your medication?"
Judgmental responses—evaluate client from nurse's values	"You were wrong to do that. " "Don't you think your being unfaithful has destroyed your marriage?"

Table 3 TREATMENT MODALITIES FOR MENTAL ILLNESS		
TYPE	ASSUMPTIONS	FOCUS OF TREATMENT
Biological	Emotional problem is an illness Cause may be inherited or chemical in origin	Medications, ECT
Psychoanalytical (individual)	Anxiety results when there is conflict between the id, ego, and superego parts of the personality Defense mechanisms form to ward off anxiety	The therapist helps the client to become aware of unconscious thoughts and feelings; understand anxiety and defenses
Milieu therapy	Providing a therapeutic environment will help increase client's awareness of feelings, increase sense of responsibility, and help him/her return to his/her community	Positive physical and social environment Structured groups and activities One-on-one intervention May be token program, open wards, self-medication
Group therapy	Relationship with others will be recreated among group members and can be worked through; members can also directly help one another	Members meet regularly with a leader to form a stable group Members learn new ways to cope with stress and develop insight into their behavior with others
Family therapy	The problem is a family problem, not an individual one Sick families lack a sense of "I" in each member The tendency is to focus on sick member's behavior as the source of trouble The sick member's symptom serves a function in the family	Therapist treats the whole family Helps members to each develop their own sense of identity Points out function of sick member to the rest of the family
Activity therapy	Important group interactions occur when group members work on a task together or share in recreation	Organized group activities created to promote socialization, increase self-esteem
Play therapy	Children express themselves more easily in play than in verbal communication Choice of colors, toys, and interaction with toys is revealing as reflection of child's situation in the family	Provide materials and toys to facilitate interaction with child, observe play, and help child to resolve problems through play
Behavioral therapy and behavior modification	Psychological problems are the result of learning Deficiencies can be corrected through learning	Operant conditioning—use of rewards to reinforce positive behavior; becomes more important than external reinforcement Desensitization—used to treat phobias; client slowly adjusts to threatening objects

D. Evaluation

1. Is there increased self-knowledge and insight?

2. Has client's self-esteem increased?

3. Has client's interpersonal relationships and work habits improved?

4. Does client demonstrate new and improved coping skills?

5. Does client have an enhanced enjoyment of life?

▶ ANXIETY

A. Assessment

1. Cardiovascular

   a. Increased pulse, blood pressure, and respiration

   b. Palpitations, chest discomfort/pain

   c. Perspiration, flushing, and heat sensations

   d. Cold hands and feet

   e. Headache

2. Gastrointestinal

   a. Nausea, vomiting, and diarrhea

   b. Belching, heartburn, cramps

3. Musculoskeletal

   a. Increased muscle tension and tendon reflexes

   b. Increased generalized fatigue

   c. Tremors, jerking of limbs

   d. Unsteady voice

4. Intellectual

   a. Poor comprehension—may be unable to follow directions

   b. Poor concentration, selective inattention

   c. Focus on detail

   d. Impaired problem solving

   e. Unable to communicate

      1) Thoughts may become random, distorted, disconnected with impaired logic

      2) Rapid, high-pitched speech

5. Social and emotional

   a. Feelings of helplessness and hopelessness

   b. Feelings of increased threat, dread, horror, anger, and rage

   c. Use of defense mechanisms and more primitive coping behaviors

      1) Shouting, arguing, hitting, kicking

      2) Crying, rocking, curling up, and withdrawal

B. Diagnose

1. Definition—feeling of dread or fear in the absence of an external threat or disproportionate to the nature of the threat

2. Predisposing conditions
   a. Prolonged unmet needs of dependency, security, love, and attention
   b. Stress threatening security or self-esteem
   c. Unacceptable thoughts or feelings surfacing to consciousness, e.g., rage, erotic impulses, flashbacks
3. Levels of anxiety
   a. Mild—high degree of alertness, mild uneasiness
   b. Moderate—heart pounds, skin cold and clammy, poor comprehension
   c. Severe—symptoms of moderate anxiety plus hallucinations, delusions
   d. Panic—symptoms of severe anxiety plus inability to see and hear,inability to function; may regress to less appropriate behaviors
4. Ego defense mechanisms—methods, usually unconscious, of managing anxiety by keeping it from awareness; may be adaptive or maladaptive
   a. Denial—failure to acknowledge an intolerable thought, feeling, experience, or reality, e.g., an alcoholic who says he does not have a drinking problem
   b. Displacement—redirection of emotions or feelings to a subject that is more acceptable or less threatening, e.g., yelling at the dog when angry with the boss
   c. Projection—attributing to others one's unacceptable feelings,impulses, thoughts, or wishes, e.g., saying someone you are angry with dislikes you
   d. Undoing—an attempt to erase an unacceptable act, thought, feeling, or desire, e.g., apologizing excessively; obsessive compulsive behavior
   e. Compensation—an attempt to overcome a real or imagined shortcoming, e.g., a small person excels in sports
   f. Substitution—replacing desired, impractical, or unobtainable object with one that is acceptable or attainable, e.g., marrying someone who looks like previous significant other

Table 4 NURSING INTERVENTIONS IN ANXIETY	
GENERAL PRINCIPLES	**NURSING CONSIDERATIONS**
Assess level of anxiety	Use standardized tool for consistency
	Look at body language, speech patterns, facial expressions, defense mechanisms, and behavior used
	Distinguish levels of anxiety
Keep environmental stresses/ stimulation low when anxiety is high	First action
	Need to intervene with severe or panic level
	Brief orientation to unit or procedures
	Written information to read later, when anxiety is lower
	Pleasant, attractive, uncluttered environment
	Provide privacy if presence of other clients is overstimulating
	Provide physical care if necessary
	Avoid offering several alternatives or decisions when anxiety is high

Table 4 NURSING INTERVENTIONS IN ANXIETY *(CONTINUED)*	
GENERAL PRINCIPLES	**NURSING CONSIDERATIONS**
Assist client to cope with anxiety more effectively	Acknowledge anxious behavior; reflect and clarify
	Always remain with client who is moderately or severely anxious
	Assist client to clarify own thoughts and feelings
	Encourage measures to reduce anxiety, e.g., exercise, activities, talking with friends, hobbies
	Assist client to recognize his/her strengths and capabilities realistically
	Provide therapy to develop more effective coping and interpersonal skills, e.g., individual, group
	May need to administer antianxiety medications
Maintain accepting and helpful attitude toward client	Use an unhurried approach
	Acknowledge client's distress and concerns about problem
	Encourage clarification of feelings and thoughts
	Evaluate and manage own anxiety while working with client
	Recognize the value of defense mechanisms and realize that client is attempting to make the anxiety tolerable in the best way possible
	Acknowledge defense but provide reality, e.g., "You do not see that you have a problem with alcohol but your blood level is high."
	Do not attempt to remove a defense mechanism at any time

  g. Introjection—a form of identification in which there is a symbolic taking into oneself the characteristics of another, e.g., blaming oneself when angry with another

  h. Repression—unacceptable thoughts kept from awareness, e.g., inability to remember a traumatic event

  i. Reaction formation—expressing attitude directly opposite to unconscious wish or fear, e.g., being excessively kind to a person who is actually disliked

  j. Regression—return to an earlier developmental phase in the face of stress, e.g., bedwetting, baby-talk

  k. Dissociation—detachment of painful emotional experience from consciousness, e.g., sleepwalking

  l. Suppression—consciously putting a disturbing thought or incident out of awareness, e.g., deciding not to deal with something unpleasant until next day

  m. Sublimation—substituting constructive activity for strong impulses that are not acceptable

5. Potential nursing diagnoses

  a. Individual coping, ineffective

  b. Anxiety

Table 5 ANXIETY DISORDERS		
TYPE	**ASSESSMENT**	**NURSING CONSIDERATIONS**
Phobia	Apprehension, anxiety, helplessness when confronted with phobic situation or feared object Examples of specific fears: Acrophobia—heights Claustrophobia—closed areas Agoraphobia—open spaces	Avoid confrontation and humiliation Do not focus on getting client to stop being afraid Systematic desensitization Relaxation techniques General anxiety measures (see Table 4) May be managed with antidepressants
Obsessive-compulsive disorder (OCD)	Obsession—repetitive, uncontrollable thoughts Compulsion—repetitive, uncontrollable acts, e.g., rituals, rigidity, inflexibility	Accept ritualistic behavior Structure environment Provide for physical needs Offer alternative activities, especially ones using hands Guide decisions, minimize choices Encourage socialization Group therapy Managed with clomipramine, SSRIs Stimulus–response prevention
Functional neurologic disorder	Physical symptoms with no organic basis, unconscious behavior—could include blindness, paralysis, convulsions without loss of consciousness, stocking and glove anesthesia, "la belle indifference"	Diagnostic evaluation Discuss feelings rather than symptoms Promote therapeutic relationship with client Avoid secondary gain

C. Plan/Implementation

1. Goals

   a. Decrease anxiety

   b. Recognize anxiety, e.g., restlessness

   c. Identify precipitants of anxiety

   d. Establish more effective coping mechanisms

   e. Increase self-esteem

2. Institute measures to decrease anxiety (see Table 4)

3. Provide nursing care for anxiety disorders (see Table 5)

4. Administer antianxiety medications as ordered

5. Use realistic, measurable objectives to evaluate effectiveness

6. Medications—benzodiazepines, buspirone, zolpidem, zaleplon, propranolol

D. Evaluation

1. Can client recognize symptoms of anxiety and anxiety-provoking situations?

2. Are client's daily activities less restricted as a result of decreased symptomatic behavior?

3. Are episodes of anxiety decreased as a result of new behaviors?

4. Is the client able to ask for help?

5. Is the client able to talk about feelings?

▶ SITUATIONAL CRISIS

A. Assessment (see Table 6)

1. Stages of crisis

   a. Denial

   b. Increased tension, anxiety

   c. Disorganization, inability to function

   d. Attempts to escape the problem, pretends problem doesn't exist, blames others

   e. Attempts to reorganize

   f. General reorganization

2. Precipitating factors

   a. Developmental stages

      1) Birth, adolescence

      2) Midlife, retirement

   b. Situational factors

      1) Natural disasters

      2) Financial loss

   c. Threats to self-concept

      1) Loss of job

      2) Failure at school

      3) Onset of serious illness

B. Diagnose (see Table 6)

1. Characteristics

   a. Temporary state of disequilibrium precipitated by an event

   b. Self-limiting—usually 4–6 weeks

   c. Crisis can promote growth and new behaviors

2. Potential nursing diagnoses

   a. Individual coping, ineffective

   b. Powerlessness

   c. Complicated grieving

C. Plan/Implementation (see Table 6)

1. Goal-directed, focus on the here and now

2. Focus on client's immediate problems

Table 6 SITUATIONAL/TRAUMATIC CRISES			
	GRIEVING CLIENT	**DYING CLIENT**	**RAPE TRAUMA**

Assessment	Stages of grief
	  a. Shock and disbelief
	  b. Awareness of the pain of loss
	  c. Restitution
	Acute grief period 4–8 wks
	Usual resolution within 1 yr
	Long-term resolution over time
		Stages of dying
		  a. Denial
		  b. Anger
		  c. Bargaining
		  d. Depression
		  e. Acceptance
			Stages of crisis
			  a. Acute reaction lasts 3–4 wk
			  b. Reorganization is long-term
			Common responses to rape
			  a. Self-blame, embarrassment
			  b. Phobias, fear of violence, death,
			     injury
			  c. Anxiety, insomnia
			  d. Wish to escape, move, relocate
			  e. Psychosomatic disturbances

Diagnose	Potential problems
	  a. Family of deceased or separated
	    – Guilt
	    – Anger
	    – Anxiety
	  b. Client undergoing surgery or loss
	    of body part
	    – Anger
	    – Withdrawal
	    – Guilt
	    – Anxiety
	    – Loss of role
		Potential problems
		  a. Avoidance behavior
		  b. Inability to express feelings
		    when in denial
		  c. Feelings of guilt
		  d. Withdrawal
		  e. Lonely, frightened
		  f. Anxiety of client and family
			Potential problems
			  a. Fears, panic reactions,
			    generalized anxiety
			  b. Guilt
			  c. Inability to cope
			Current crisis may reactivate old
			unresolved trauma
			Follow emergency room protocol:
			may include clothing, hair samples,
			NPO
			Be alert for potential internal injuries,
			e.g., hemorrhage

Intervention	Apply crisis theory Focus on the here and now Provide support to family when loved one dies Provide family privacy Encourage verbalization of feelings Facilitate expressions of anger and rage Emphasize strengths Increase ability to cope Support adjustment to illness, loss of body part	Apply crisis theory Support staff having feelings of loss Keep communication open Allow expression of feelings Focus on the here and now Let client know he/she is not alone Provide comforting environment Be attentive to need for privacy Provide physically comforting care, e.g., back rubs Give sense of control and dignity Respect client's wishes	Apply crisis theory Focus on the here and now Write out treatments and appointments for client, as anxiety causes forgetfulness Record all information in chart Give client referrals for legal assistance, supportive psychotherapy, and rape crisis center Follow up regularly until client is improved
Evaluation	Does client express feelings of disbelief, anger, and hurt? Are anxiety and helplessness gradually replaced by a sense of competence? Does client work positively with physical and emotional challenges? Have the bereaved resumed their social activities?	Has an open, honest approach to dying helped all concerned grieve together with less fear and avoidance? Did the client feel less isolated and alone because of openness, daily support, and diligence in spite of prognosis? Were the stages of dying accepted and understood by those around the client?	Is client at precrisis level of functioning? Are there any unresolved emotional responses to the rape trauma experience? Did the client utilize referral services?

3. Explore nurse's and client's understanding of the problem
   a. Define the event (client may truly not know what has precipitated the crisis)
   b. Confirm nurse's perception by reviewing with client
   c. Identify the factors that are affecting problem-solving
   d. Evaluate how realistically client sees the problems or concerns
4. Help client become aware of feelings and validate them
   a. Acknowledge feelings, (e.g., "This must be a painful situation for you.")
   b. Avoid blaming client for problems and concerns
   c. Avoid blaming others, as this prevents insight
   d. Encourage ventilation with nurse to relieve anxiety
   e. Tell client he will feel better, but it may take 1 or 2 months
5. Develop a plan
   a. Encourage client to make as many arrangements as possible (avoid dependence)
   b. Write out information, since comprehension is impaired, (e.g., referrals)
   c. Maximize client's situational supports
6. Find new coping skills and manage feelings
   a. Focus on strengths and present coping skills
   b. Encourage client to form new coping skills and social outlets, reaching out to others
   c. Facilitate future planning
      1) Ask client "What would you like to do?", "Where would you like to go from here?"
      2) Give referrals when needed, family counseling, vocational counseling

D. Evaluation
   1. Has stress decreased?
   2. Is client at precrisis level of functioning?
   3. Does client have a larger repertoire of adaptive coping mechanisms?
   4. Is client able to identify cause and significance of disruption?
   5. Faulty resolution of crisis may occur when individual's behavior compounds the crisis, e.g., breakup of the family in response to a child's problems
   6. Faulty resolution may occur when conflicts re-emerge because new coping skills have not been learned to handle both the old and the new crises at the same time

▶ ACUTE/POST-TRAUMATIC STRESS DISORDER

A. Assessment
   1. Develops after (immediate or delayed) a perceived traumatic event
   2. Timing of exposure to a traumatic event (e.g., combat, rape, murder, fire, other catastrophe)

3. Response to trauma causes intense fear or horror
4. Recurrent or distressing recollections of event (images, thoughts, feelings)
5. Distressing dreams or nightmares
6. Acting or feeling like the trauma is recurring (flashbacks)
7. Hypervigilance and exaggerated startle response
8. Irritability or outbursts of anger
9. Avoidance or numbing

B. Diagnose

1. 9 or more symptoms from the 5 following categories: Intrusion, Negative mood, Dissociative symptoms, Avoidance and Arousal
2. Duration of symptoms is at least one month
3. Syndrome can emerge months to years after traumatizing event
4. Biological changes due to impact of stressor and excessive arousal of sympathetic nervous system

C. Plan/Implementation

1. Help client integrate the traumatic experience
   a. Encourage client to talk about painful stored memories
      1) Have client recall images of traumatic event with as much detail as possible (called flooding); will be done by staff with high level of expertise
      2) Use empathetic responses to the expressed distress (e.g., "That must have been hard for you.")
      3) Remain nonjudgmental about client's shameful or horrific experience
      4) Allow client to grieve over losses
   b. Assist client to challenge existing ideas about event and substitute more realistic thoughts and expectations
      1) Point out irrational thinking to the client
      2) Help client recognize the limits of his/her control over the stressful event

2. Assist client with emotional regulation
   a. Help client label his/her feelings and find ways to express them safely
   b. Teach stress management techniques
   c. Involve client in anger management program
      1) Recognize anger as normal feeling
      2) Teach time-out or other ways of walking away from problematic situations involving anger
      3) Teach nonintrusive communication techniques
         a) Speak in first person
         b) Move away from object (person) of anger
         c) Cognitive restructuring (e.g., using thoughts like "This person cannot make me lose control")
   d. Develop a schedule of regular physical activity with client (e.g., walking, running, weightlifting)

      e. Use empowering strategies such as keeping a journal of disturbed thoughts and feelings in response to flashbacks, nightmares, or other problems

      f. Teach methods to reduce sleep disturbances

          1) Regular bedtime

          2) Use bed for sleeping and lovemaking exclusively; no TV or reading

          3) Do not lie in bed sleepless for more than half an hour; get up and move around and then come back to bed

   3. Enhance the client's support systems

      a. Refer to self-help group

      b. Include family and friends in psycho-educational activities

      c. Explore opportunities for socialization

   4. Educate client regarding the recovery process

      a. Assess for and treat substance abuse

      b. Administer antidepressants

D. Evaluation

   1. Is client performing relaxation techniques?

   2. Is client participating in social situations with family and friends?

   3. Has the client's amount of undisturbed sleep increased?

▶ DEPRESSIVE DISORDERS

A. Assessment

   1. Possible changes in self-esteem/self-confidence

      a. Low self-esteem

      b. Self-deprecation

      c. Feelings of helplessness/hopelessness

      d. Obsessive thoughts and fears

      e. Ruminations and worries

      f. Sense of doom, failure

      g. Regressed behavior–immature, demanding, whines for help

   2. Possible changes in self-care

      a. Unkempt, depressed appearance

      b. Multiple reports of physical discomfort

      c. Prone to injury, accidents, and infections

      d. Lack of energy

      e. Changes in usual sleep pattern

          1) Insomnia

          2) Feels unrested after night's sleep

      f. Weight loss, poor appetite, weight gain

      g. Constipation

      h. Amenorrhea

      i. Lack of sexual desire

3. Possible changes in cognitive/mental functioning
   a. Decreased attention span and concentration
   b. Slowed speech, thought processes, and motor activity
   c. Impaired reality testing (psychotic depression)
   d. Withdrawn
   e. Ambivalent and indecisive behavior
   f. Agitation and psychomotor restlessness
   g. Suicidal ideation
4. Suicide/homicide potential
   a. Has plan and means to carry out plan; actual date established (anniversary, birthdate, etc.)
   b. Identifies others who may become involved in the plan

B. Diagnose
1. Psychodynamics
   a. Depression—response to real or imagined loss
   b. Anger and aggression toward self results from feelings of guilt about negative or ambivalent feelings
   c. Introjection occurs (incorporation of a loved or hated object or person into one's own ego)
2. Types of depression—determined by onset and severity of symptoms
   a. Major depression
   b. Dysthymic disorder
   c. Depression Not Otherwise Specified (NOS)
3. Potential nursing diagnoses
   a. Self-care deficit
   b. Self-esteem disturbance
   c. Individual coping, ineffective
   d. Social interaction, impaired
   e. Violence: self-directed, risk for
   f. Powerlessness
   g. Interrupted family processes

C. Plan/Implementation
1. Be alert for signs of self-destructive behavior
   a. Report all behavior changes to the team, especially increased energy or agitation
   b. In psychotic depression, observe for any signs that voices are commanding client to harm self (e.g., question the client, "What are the voices saying to you?")
2. Meet physical needs
   a. Promote nutrition
      1) Provide pleasant surroundings and companionship during meals
      2) Give more frequent feedings, favorite foods because of decreased appetite, high carbohydrate foods, nutritious drinks
   b. Medicate for constipation PRN and encourage fluids

    c. Promote rest

       1) Medicate for insomnia PRN and watch while client swallows pill

       2) Provide a quiet sleeping arrangement; stay with client if necessary; check on client periodically

    d. Promote self-care as much as possible

3. Decrease anxiety and indecisiveness

    a. Administer antianxiety medications

    b. Listen to and explore feelings

       1) Avoid pep talks; don't disagree with self-deprecation because client will not believe it

       2) Avoid excessive cheeriness and promise of a bright future

       3) Keep encouragement brief; client cannot incorporate compliments

    c. Avoid presenting choices, as client feels too inadequate to make decisions

    d. Be brief and simple, avoid long explanations because of decreased attentiveness and poor concentration

       1) Give a brief orientation

       2) Use simple language and repeat when necessary

    e. Provide a structured, written schedule

4. Support self-esteem

    a. Provide a warm, supportive environment

    b. Be client while client is slowed down and cannot think quickly; demonstrate acceptance to promote client self-acceptance

    c. Provide consistent daily care

       1) One-to-one nursing coverage is ideal

       2) Be consistent and predictable—keep all appointments and make few staff changes (they may be seen as a rejection)

       3) Anticipate staff feelings of ineffectiveness as part of caring for depressed clients and continue a positive approach

    d. Give tasks to relieve guilt and increase self-esteem

       1) Avoid tasks at which the client will fail

       2) Give simple tasks that require minimal concentration

5. Help decrease social withdrawal

    a. Pursue the client who avoids contact because of fear of rejection

       1) Sit with client during long quiet times

       2) Point out when client stays alone excessively

       3) Touch to promote acceptance (note: do *not* touch the psychotic client, as this may be seen as intrusion); be aware of cultural acceptance of touch

    b. Introduce to others when ready

    c. Use other treatment modalities

       1) Group therapy to communicate acceptance and increase self-esteem

       2) Family therapy to prevent scapegoating and explore feelings

       3) Individual therapy to decrease fear of rejection

6. Help with anger and fear of losing control

    a. Channel anger into acceptable outlets, e.g., sports, carpentry

    b. Encourage expressions of anger—small expressions initially; client may become suicidal if anger is expressed before able to do so safely

7. Encourage coping

    a. Imply confidence in client's capabilities

        1) Don't make client dependent

        2) Discuss excessive demands

    b. Give assistance when needed, but work together

8. Administer antidepressant medications

    a. Caution client about adverse effects and time required for medication to become effective

    b. Observe for suicidal tendency as depression lifts, usually at 10 days to 2 weeks after start of medication

9. Assist with electroconvulsive therapy (ECT)—convulsions similar to tonic-clonic seizures are induced to treat depression

    a. Preparation of client (see Table 7)

    b. Procedure

        1) Anesthetist gives short-acting intravenous anesthesia and muscle-relaxing drug, e.g., succinylcholine

        2) Keep oxygen and suction on hand

        3) Position client in supine position with arms at sides during convulsion

    c. Adverse effects and complications

        1) Confusion and memory loss for recent events

        2) Transient headaches, muscle soreness, drowsiness

    d. Post-procedure care

        1) Orient client; client will not remember treatment

        2) Take blood pressure, respirations

        3) Stay with client during period of confusion

        4) Signs of diminished depression appear after 6–12 treatments

10. Alternative/Complementary therapies

    a. Phototherapy

        1) First-line treatment for seasonal affective disorder (SAD)

        2) Minimum 2500 lux of light 30 minutes a day

    b. St. John's wort

        1) Herbal medication

        2) Do not take if major depression, pregnancy, or in children younger than 2 years

        3) Do not take with amphetamines, MAOIs, SSRIs, levodopa, and 5-HT

        4) Avoid tyramine-containing foods, excessive sunlight

        5) Contraindicated in pregnancy and during lactation

    c. Exercise

        1) 30 minutes at least 5 times per week

Table 7 NURSING CONSIDERATIONS FOR ELECTROCONVULSIVE THERAPY (ECT)
1. Prepare client by explaining procedure and telling client about potential temporary memory loss and confusion
2. Informed consent, physical exam, labwork
3. NPO after midnight for an early morning procedure
4. Have client void before ECT
5. Remove dentures, glasses, jewelry
6. Give muscle relaxant and short-acting barbiturate anesthetic to induce brief general anesthesia
7. Given Atropine 30 min before treatment to decrease secretions
8. Have oxygen and suction on hand
9. After procedure, take vital signs, orient client
10. Observe client's reaction and stay with him
11. Observe for sudden improvement and indications of suicidal threats after ECT treatment

D. Evaluation

1. Does the client feel accepted?
2. Is client able to express views without fear of retaliation?
3. Is client able to cope in spite of negative self-view?
4. Are new behaviors evident?
5. Is there an increase in self-esteem?
6. Have potential problems associated with ECT treatments been prevented?

▶ SUICIDE

A. Assessment

1. Symptoms same as in depression
2. Behavioral clues of impending suicide (see Table 8)

Table 8 BEHAVIORAL CLUES OF IMPENDING SUICIDE
1. Any sudden change in client's behavior
2. Becomes energetic after period of severe depression
3. Improved mood 10–14 days after taking antidepressant may mean suicidal plans made
4. Finalizes business or personal affairs
5. Gives away valuable possessions or pets
6. Withdraws from social activities and plans
7. Appears emotionally upset
8. Presence of weapons, razors, pills (means)
9. Has death plan
10. Leaves a note
11. Makes direct or indirect statements (e.g., "I may not be around then.")

    B. Diagnose

       1. Predisposing factors

          a. Male over 50 years old

          b. Age range 15–19 years old

          c. Clients with poor social attachments; isolation

          d. Clients with previous attempts

          e. Clients with personality disorders

          f. Psychotic individuals with command hallucinations to kill themselves

          g. Overwhelming precipitating events

             1) Terminal or degenerative disease, e.g., cancer, kidney disease

             2) Death or loss of loved one through divorce or separation

             3) Financial loss, job loss, school failure

       2. Understanding self-destructive behavior

          a. Attempts to cope fail, leaving the client with low self-esteem and feelings of hopelessness and helplessness

          b. Client feels guilty and overwhelmed in response to precipitating event and may see suicide as relief

          c. Ambivalence about suicide may lead to cry for help or attention

          d. Aggression and rage turned toward self (introjection) or into an attempt to punish others

          e. Most common as depression is lifting

             1) 10–14 days after antidepressant medication begun

             2) New signs of energy or improvement

       3. Potential nursing diagnoses

          a. Violence: self-directed, risk for

          b. Risk for suicide

    C. Plan/Implementation

       1. Implement measures for depression

       2. Be alert for signs of self-destructive behavior (suicide/homicide assessment) (see Table 8)

       3. Remove all potentially dangerous items

       4. Provide strong therapeutic relationship to increase client self-worth

          a. Establish authoritative and credible matter-of-fact manner to increase confidence

          b. Place on one-to-one observation and stay with client to help control self-destructive impulses

          c. Let the client know that the nurse will assist in seeking every possible resource to ease troubles

          d. Relieve client's feelings of embarrassment, e.g., "I see you are upset. You are wise to seek help."

5. Discuss all behavior with team members

    a. Note indirect clues as cry for help, e.g., presence of pills

    b. Observe for sudden increased energy level as indication of possible impending suicide attempt

    c. Note increase in anxiety, insomnia

6. Give client a sense of control other than through suicide

    a. Assist with problem-solving and decision-making

    b. Develop and use a suicidal contract

    c. Avoid excess support, as this encourages dependency and eventual feelings of abandonment

7. Provide family therapy where indicated

    a. Avoid taking client's side as family is not direct cause of suicidal urge

    b. Look for scapegoating or acting out of family destructiveness

8. Intervene quickly and calmly during actual attempts

    a. Remove the harmful objects from the client (e.g., razor, ropes) without inflicting harm on self and/or client

    b. Stay by the client's side and reassure the client that you are there to help

    c. Avoid judgmental remarks or interpretations, e.g., "Why did you do this?"

9. Contract with client

    a. "No suicide," "no harm," or "no self-injury" contracts are made between psychiatric health care professionals and clients who are admitted to a psychiatric unit with depression and/or suicide ideation or self-injurious acting-out

    b. Clients agree to contact staff if they have an impulse to be self-destructive

    c. Client is asked to abide by the signed contract

    d. Client is periodically reminded of the contract

    e. Limit-setting lets client know that self-destructive acts are not permitted

    f. Staff members do anything within power to prevent client self-destruction

D. Evaluation

1. Has self-inflicted injury been avoided?

2. Have self-destructive tendencies decreased?

▶ SITUATIONAL ROLE CHANGES

A. Assessment

1. Death of spouse/significant other

2. Divorce/separation

3. Personal illness/injury

4. Marriage

5. Job loss

6. Retirement

    7. Pregnancy/new baby

    8. Job change/relocation

    9. "Empty nest"/child leaving home

   10. Graduation from high school/college/tech school

   11. Spouse beginning or ending full-time employment

B. Diagnose

    1. Coping strategies—specific skills or actions consciously used to manage effects of stress

    2. Reactions to change can be positive, negative, neutral

    3. Reactions determined by

      a. Client's learned behaviors to cope with change

      b. Significance of event

      c. Client's physical and emotional state at time of change

      d. Client's control over change

      e. Number of changes over lifetime

      f. Positive or negative resolution to previous changes

C. Plan/Implementation

    1. Place changes in time line; rank from least to most severe

    2. Discuss resolution to previous changes; determine what was helpful in the past

    3. Use learned coping strategies

      a. Establish and maintain a routine

      b. Limit or avoid changes

      c. Designate time to focus on adaptation to change

      d. Use time efficiently

      e. Change environment to reduce stress

      f. Regular exercise

      g. Humor

      h. Good nutrition

      i. Rest/sleep

      j. Relaxation techniques

      k. Utilize support system

      l. Work on increasing self-esteem

      m. Pray/meditate

      n. Some cultures use rituals

D. Evaluation

    1. Has client coped with role change effectively?

    2. Have new coping strategies been learned?

▶ STRESS

A. Assessment

1. Headache

2. Sleep problems, fatigue, irritability

3. Restlessness, rapid speech and movement

4. GI upset

5. Tachycardia, palpitations, hot flashes

6. Frequent urination, dry mouth

7. Crying

8. Use of alcohol or drugs

9. Withdrawal from friends and family

B. Diagnose

1. Stressors

   a. Family

   b. Job

   c. Environment

   d. Lifestyle

   e. Body image changes

   f. Situational role change

C. Plan/Implementation

1. Determine what client sees as stressful

2. Identify how stressful these items are to client

3. Determine how client has coped with stressors in the past

4. Provide support—encourage family visits, listen to client's concerns, involve pastoral and social services

5. Provide control—maintain client independence; allow client to make choice concerning timing and sequencing of activities

6. Provide information—answer questions, provide information about procedures, events

7. Recognize client feelings—acknowledge anger

8. Support client's own coping strategies

9. Interventions

   a. Biofeedback—use of electrical instruments to identify somatic changes (e.g., muscle activity, skin surface activity)

   b. Progressive muscle relaxation—tensing then relaxing major muscle groups in sequential steps

   c. Meditation—conscious removal of thoughts filling mind, or filling mind with only one thought

   d. Guided imagery—thinking about peaceful scene involving total relaxation

D. Evaluation

1. Is client able to identify stressors?

2. Has client used appropriate coping strategies to deal with stress?

▶ BURNOUT

A. Assessment

1. Emotional or physical exhaustion
2. Depersonalization, inability to become involved with others
3. Decreased effectiveness
4. Stress-related behavior becomes persistent problem
5. Usual coping strategies ineffective
6. Person feels overwhelmed, helpless
7. At risk for physical or mental illness

B. Diagnose

1. Process in which the person disengages from work in response to excessive or prolonged stress
2. Sources of stress may be in environment, self, or in interactions
3. Determined by the person's ability to adapt

C. Plan/Implementation

1. Provide social support
2. Begin counseling
3. Utilize employee assistance programs

D. Evaluation

1. Is the person demonstrating increased ability to handle day-to-day issues?
2. Is the person re-engaging with persons and the environment?

▶ SUPPORT SYSTEMS

A. Assessment

1. Family—role of each member (authority figure, peacemaker)
2. Spouse/significant other
3. Friends
4. Coworkers
5. Groups, clubs, organizations
6. Pet or inanimate object (security blanket)

B. Diagnose

1. Culture and socioeconomic status influence support systems
2. Social network defines client's self-image and sense of belonging

C. Plan/Implementation

1. Assess developmental stage (adolescence, early adulthood, late adulthood) to plan utilization of support systems
2. Enlist support persons who have been effective in previous, similar, stressful situations

D. Evaluation

1. Has client used support system effectively to deal with change/stressors?
2. Has client maintained a positive self-image?

► SUDDEN INFANT DEATH SYNDROME (SIDS)

A. Assessment

1. Occurs during first year of life, peaks at two to four months
2. Occurs between midnight and 9 AM
3. Increased incidence in winter, peaks in January

B. Diagnose

1. Thought to be brainstem abnormality in neurologic regulation of cardiorespiratory control
2. Third leading cause of death in children from one week to one year of age
3. Higher incidence of SIDS
   a. Infants with documented apparent life-threatening events (ALTEs)
   b. Siblings of infant with SIDS
   c. Preterm infants who have pathological apnea
   d. Preterm infants, especially with low birth weight
   e. African decent infants
   f. Multiple births
   g. Infants of addicted mothers
   h. Infants who sleep on abdomen

C. Plan/Implementation

1. Home apnea monitor
2. Place all healthy infants in supine position to sleep
3. Support parents, family
4. Referral to Sudden Infant Death Foundation

D. Evaluation

1. Has the infant reached one year of age without incident?
2. Does the family cope with the loss of their child?

▶ **COUNSELING TECHNIQUES**

A. Techniques

1. Confrontation—call attention to discrepancies between what the client says (verbal communication) and what the client does (nonverbal communication)

2. Contracting—establish expected behaviors and goals as well as rules and consequences with client that structure nurse/client interactions

3. Focusing—create order, guidelines, and priorities by assisting the client in identifying problems and establishing their relative importance

4. Interpreting—explore with the client possible explanations for feelings

5. Making connections—help the client connect seemingly isolated phenomena by filling in blanks and establishing relationships

6. Modeling—exemplify through actions and verbalizations the behaviors that the client is working toward

7. Providing feedback—give the client constructive information about how the nurse perceives and hears him/her

8. Reframing—look at the issue through a different perspective by using different examples and descriptions

9. Stating observations—describe what is happening in the nurse/client relationship that might have relevance to other things happening in client's life

10. Summarizing—give feedback to client about the general substance of the interview or interpersonal exchange before ending

B. Implementation

1. These techniques aid the nurse in promoting change and growth in clients

2. Nurse should demonstrate behaviors of

    a. Congruence or genuineness

    b. Empathy (the ability to see things from the client's perspective)

    c. Positive regard or respect

▶ **RELIGIOUS AND SPIRITUAL INFLUENCES ON HEALTH**

Not all members of a religion or spiritual path will choose to follow all the traditions.

A. Assessment

1. Wears amulets, charms, clothing, jewelry

2. Carries a talisman (object that has supernatural powers)

3. Makes noise to scare off evil entities

4. Drinks/ingests potions, tonics, or foods

5. Performs or refrains from performing activity at certain times

6. Method of disposal of objects that come into contact with person

7. Performs religious ceremony (e.g., baptism)

8. Avoids doing actions that are harmful to others

9. Avoids behaviors that are not socially sanctioned

10. Emotional investment related to aspects of mind or soul, distinct from body

11. Reflects individual values, beliefs, ethical choices

B. Diagnose

1. Religion provides explanation for illness and misfortune

2. Religion can prevent illness and misfortune

3. Client's spiritual beliefs affect all aspects of life, relationships, sense of right and wrong

4. Religion is the basis for health care behaviors and decisions

5. Religion is a basic human need that must be satisfied for individual's well-being

C. Plan/Implementation

1. Seek assistance from persons knowledgeable about client's religious practices

2. Be aware of your own spirituality and beliefs

3. Be respectful and sensitive to client's religious beliefs

4. Do not impose your own religious beliefs on client or believe that if client finds religion, this will spiritually enrich client

5. Observe client's verbal and nonverbal behavior; may indicate spiritual distress

6. Examples

   a. Roman Catholic—sacrament of the sick

   b. Buddhist—believe in healing through faith

   c. Christian Science—practice spiritual healing

   d. Church of Jesus Christ of Latter Day Saints—anoint with oil, pray, lay on hands

   e. Hinduism—faith healing

   f. Islam—use herbal remedies and faith healing

   g. Jehovah's Witness—mental and spiritual healing

   h. Judaism—prays for sick

   i. Mennonite—prayer and anointing with oil

   j. Seventh-Day Adventist—anointing with oil and prayer

   k. Unitarian/Universalist—use of science to facilitate healing

D. Evaluation

1. Have client's spiritual beliefs been preserved and accommodated?

2. Has client felt free to express spiritual beliefs?

▶ BIPOLAR DISORDER

A. Assessment

1. Disoriented, incoherent
2. Delusions of grandeur, cheerful, euphoria
3. Flight of ideas, easily distractable
4. Inappropriate dress; excessive makeup and jewelry
5. Lacks inhibitions
6. Uses sarcastic, profane, and abusive language
7. Quick-tempered, agitated
8. Talks excessively, jokes, dances, sings; hyperactive
9. Can't stop moving to eat, easily stimulated by environment
10. Decreased appetite
11. Weight loss
12. Insomnia
13. Regressed behavior
14. Sexually indiscreet, hypersexual

B. Diagnose

1. Classifications

   a. Bipolar I: at least one manic episode and one depressive episode or mixed episodes

   b. Bipolar II: lifetime experience of at least one episode of major depression or at leas hone hypomanic episode

   c. Cyclothymic disorder: adults at least 2 years (children 1 year) of both hypomanic and depression periods without fulfilling criteria for and episode of mania, hypo mania or major depression

2. Psychodynamics

   a. Bipolar disorder is an affective disorder

   b. Reality contact is less disturbed than in schizophrenia

   c. Elation or grandiosity can be a defense against underlying depression or feelings of low self-esteem

   d. Testing, manipulative behavior results from poor self-esteem

3. Predisposing factors

   a. Hereditary—genetic

   b. Biochemical

4. Problems

   a. Easily stimulated by surroundings

      1) Hyperactive and anxious

      2) Unable to meet physical needs

   b. Aggressive and hostile due to poor self-esteem

        c. Denial

        d. Testing, manipulative, demanding, disruptive, intrusive behavior

        e. Superficial social relationships

    5. Potential nursing diagnoses

        a. Disturbed thought processes

        b. Self-care deficit

        c. Violence: self-directed or directed at others, risk for

        d. Social interaction, impaired

        e. Interrupted family processes

        f. Self-esteem disturbance

C. Plan/Implementation

    1. Institute measures to deal with hyperactivity/agitation

        a. Simplify the environment and decrease environmental stimuli

            1) Assign to a single room away from activity

            2) Keep noise level low

            3) Soft lighting

        b. Limit people

            1) Anticipate situations that will provoke or overstimulate client, e.g., activities, competitive situations

            2) Remove to quiet areas

        c. Distract and redirect energy

            1) Choose activities for brief attention span, e.g., chores, walks

            2) Choose physical activities using large movements until acute mania subsides, e.g., dance

            3) Provide writing materials for busy work when acute mania subsides, e.g., political suggestions, plans

    2. Provide external controls

        a. Assign one staff person to provide controls

        b. Do not encourage client when telling jokes or performing, e.g., avoid laughing

        c. Accompany client to room when hyperactivity is escalating

        d. Guard vigilantly against suicide as elation subsides and mood evens out

    3. Institute measures to deal with manipulativeness

        a. Set limits, e.g., limit phone calls when excessive

            1) Set firm consistent times for meetings—client often late and unaware of time

            2) Refuse unreasonable demands, e.g., asks for date with the nurse

            3) Explain restrictions on behavior and reasons so client does not feel rejected

        b. Communicate using a firm, unambivalent consistent approach

            1) Use staff consistency in enforcing rules

            2) Remain nonjudgmental, e.g., when client disrobes say, "I cannot allow you to undress here."

          3) Never threaten or make comparisons to others, as it increases hostility and poor coping

     c. Avoid long, complicated discussions

          1) Use short sentences with specific straightforward responses

          2) Avoid giving advice when solicited, e.g., "I notice you want me to take responsibility for your life."

  4. Meet physical needs

     a. Meet nutritional needs

          1) Encourage fluids; offer water every hour because client will not take the time to drink

          2) Give high-calorie finger foods and drinks to be carried while moving, e.g., cupcakes, sandwiches

          3) Serve meals on tray in client's room when too stimulated

     b. Encourage rest

          1) Sedate PRN

          2) Encourage short naps

     c. Supervise bathing routines when client plays with water or is too distracted to clean self

  5. Administer medications—mood-stabilizing medications (lithium, valproic acid, carbamazepine)

  6. Help decrease denial and increase client's awareness of feelings

     a. Encourage expression of real feelings through reflecting

     b. Help client acknowledge the need for help when denying it, e.g., "You say you don't need love, but most people need love. It's okay to feel that."

     c. Function as a role model for client by communicating feelings openly

     d. Help client recognize demanding behavior, e.g., "You seem to want others to notice you."

     e. Encourage client to recognize needs of others

     f. Have client verbalize needs directly, e.g., wishes for attention

D. Evaluation

  1. Are client's needs met?

  2. Does client observe feelings of others as well as self?

  3. Does client realistically see areas of competence?

  4. Is client able to limit destructive and/or impulsive behavior?

  5. Is client able to work cooperatively and honestly with staff?

▶ SCHIZOPHRENIA

A. Assessment

  1. Withdrawal from relationships and from the world

     a. Neologisms, rhyming so that others can't understand communication

     b. Concrete thinking

     c. Social ineptitude—aloof and fails to encourage interpersonal relationships, ambivalence toward others

  2. Inappropriate or flat affect

3. Hypochondriasis and/or depersonalization

4. Suspiciousness—sees world as a hostile, threatening place

5. Poor reality testing—delusions, hallucinations, neurologisms

   a. Hallucinations—false sensory perceptions in the absence of an external stimulus; may be auditory, visual, olfactory, or tactile

   b. Delusions—persistent false beliefs, e.g., client may believe stomach is missing

      1) Grandeur—belief that one is special, e.g., a monarch

      2) Persecutory—belief that one is victim of a plot

      3) Ideas of reference—belief that environmental events are directed toward the self, e.g., client sees people talking and believes they are discussing the client

6. Loose associations

7. Short attention span, decreased ability to comprehend stimuli

8. Regression

9. Inability to meet basic survival needs

   a. Unable to feed oneself (poor nutritional habits)

   b. Poor personal hygiene

   c. Inappropriate dress for the weather/environment

B. Diagnose

1. Specific types of schizophrenia (see Table 1)

Table 1 SCHIZOPHRENIA	
SUB-TYPE	**PRESENTING SYMPTOMS**
Disorganized	Inappropriate behavior such as silly laughing and regression, transient hallucinations; disorganized behavior and speech
Catatonic	Sudden-onset mutism, bizarre mannerisms, remains in stereotyped position with waxy flexibility; may have dangerous periods of agitation and explosive behavior
Paranoid	Late onset in life, characterized by suspicion and ideas of persecution and delusions and hallucinations; may be angry or hostile
Undifferentiated	General symptoms of schizophrenia Symptoms of more than one type of schizophrenia
Residual	No longer exhibits overt psychotic symptoms; difficulty with social relationships

2. Potential nursing diagnoses

   a. Disturbed thought processes

   b. Disturbed sensory perception

   c. Self-care deficit

   d. Violence: directed toward self or others, risk for

   e. Social isolation

C. Plan/Implementation (see Tables 2 and 3)

    1. Maintain client safety

        a. Protect from altered thought processes

            1) Decrease sensory stimuli, remove from areas of tension

            2) Validate reality

            3) Recognize that client is experiencing hallucination

            4) Do not argue with client

            5) Respond to feeling or tone of hallucination or delusion

            6) Be alert to hallucinations that command client to harm self or others

Table 2 NURSING CARE OF CLIENT WHO ACTS WITHDRAWN	
PROBLEM	**INTERVENTIONS**
Lack of trust and feeling of safety and security	Keep interactions brief, especially orientation
	Structure environment
	Be consistent and reliable; notify client of anticipated schedule changes
	Decrease physical contact
	Eye contact during greeting
	Maintain attentiveness with head slightly leaning toward client and nonintrusive attitude
	Allow physical distance
	Accept client's behavior, e.g., silence; maintain matter-of-fact attitude toward behavior
Hallucinations	Maintain accepting attitude
	Do not argue with client about reality of hallucinations
	Comment on feeling, tone of hallucination, e.g., "That must be frightening to you."
	Encourage diversional activities, e.g., playing cards, especially activities in which client can gain a sense of mastery, e.g., artwork
	Encourage discussions of reality-based interests
Lack of attention to personal needs, e.g., nutrition, hygiene	Assess adequacy of hydration, nutrition
	Structure routine for bathing, mealtime
	Offer encouragement or assistance if necessary, e.g., sit with client or feed client if appropriate
	Decrease environmental stimuli at mealtime, e.g., suggest early dinner before dining room crowds
	Positioning and skin care for catatonic client

        b. Protect from erratic and inappropriate behavior

            1) Communicate in calm, authoritative tone

            2) Address client by name

            3) Observe client for early signs of escalating behavior

        c. Administer antipsychotic medications

2. Meet physical needs of severely regressed clients

    a. Poor basic hygiene—may have to be washed initially

    b. Poor nutritional habits—may have to be fed

        1) Ask client to pick up fork; if unable to make decision, then feeding is necessary

        2) When ready, encourage client to eat in dining room with others

    c. May be nonverbal initially; do not force into groups

3. Establish a therapeutic relationship—engage in individual therapy

    a. Institute measures to promote trust

        1) Same as general withdrawal from reality (see Table 2)

        2) Be consistent and reliable in keeping all scheduled appointments

        3) Avoid direct questions (client may feel threatened)

        4) Accept client's indifference, e.g., failure to smile or greet nurse, and avoidance behavior, e.g., hostility or sarcasm

        5) Discuss all staff changes, especially vacations and absences

    b. Encourage client's affect by verbalizing what you observe, e.g., "You seem to think that I don't want to stay." Use client's name in a calm, authoritative tone

    c. Tolerate silences—may have to sit through long silences with client who is too anxious to speak (catatonic)

    d. Accept regression as a normal part of treatment when new stresses are encountered

        1) With delusional regression, respond to associated feeling, not to the delusion, e.g., client claims he has no heart, nursing response: "You must feel empty."

        2) Help pinpoint source of regression, e.g., anxiety about discharge

Table 3 NURSING CARE OF A CLIENT WHO ACTS SUSPICIOUS	
PROBLEM	**INTERVENTIONS**
Mistrust and feeling of rejection	Keep appointments with clients
	Clear, consistent communication
	Allow client physical distance and keep door open when interviewing
	Genuineness and honesty in interactions
	Recognize testing behavior and show persistence of interest in client
Delusions	Allow client to verbalize the delusion in a limited way
	Do not argue with client or try to convince that delusions are not real
	Point out feeling tone of delusion
	Provide activities to divert attention from delusions
	Solitary activities best at first and then may progress to noncompetitive games or activities
	Do not reinforce delusions by validating them
	Focus on potential real concerns of client

4. Engage in family therapy—especially when client is returning to family; understand the problem involves the family; establish a "family client" in need of support

5. Engage in socialization or activity group therapy according to client's ability

   a. Accept nonverbal behavior initially

   b. If client cannot tolerate group, do not force or embarrass

   c. Act as a social role model for client

6. Provide simple activities or tasks to promote positive self-esteem and success

   a. Finger painting and clay are good choices for regressed catatonic client

   b. Encourage attendance at occupational, vocational, and art therapy sessions

   c. Avoid competitive situations with paranoid—solitary activities are better

D. Evaluation

1. Is there increased self-knowledge and insight?

2. Has client's self-esteem increased?

3. Have client's interpersonal relationships and work habits improved?

4. Does the client have new and improved coping skills?

5. Does the client have enhanced enjoyment of life?

▶ PERSONALITY DISORDERS

A. Assessment (see Table 4)

B. Diagnose (see Table 4)

C. Plan/Implementation (see Table 4)

D. Evaluation

1. Is the client able to verbally communicate and express feelings with staff members?

2. Is the client able to establish a trusting relationship with key therapeutic staff members?

Table 4 PERSONALITY DISORDERS			
TYPES	ASSESSMENT	DIAGNOSE	NURSING CONSIDERATIONS
Paranoid	Suspiciousness Hypersensitive, humorless, serious Ideas of reference Cold, blunted affect Quick response with anger or rage	Interprets actions of others as personal threat Uses projection: externalizes own feelings by projecting own desires and traits to others Holds grudges	Establish trust Be honest and nonintrusive Low doses of phenothiazines to manage anxiety Structured social situations Be calm, authoritative, matter of fact
Schizoid	Shy and introverted; rarely has close friends Little verbal interaction Cold and detached	Uses intellectualization: describes emotional experiences in matter-of-fact way Daydreaming may be more gratifying than real life	Same as paranoid
Schizotypal	Seems eccentric and odd Sensitive to rejection and anger Vague, stereotypical, overelaborate speech Suspicious of others Blunted or inappropriate affect	Similar to schizophrenia, fewer and milder psychotic episodes Problems in thinking, perceiving, communicating Common disorder among biological relatives of schizophrenics	Same as paranoid Low-dose neuroleptics may decrease transient psychotic symptoms
Antisocial	Disregard for rights of others Lying, cheating, stealing, promiscuous behaviors Appears charming and intellectual, smooth-talking Unlawful, aggressive and reckless behaviors Lack of guilt, remorse, and conscience Immature and irresponsible, especially in finances	Genetic predisposition Correlates with substance abuse and dependency problems More common in males Rationalizes and denies own behaviors	Firm limit-setting Confront behaviors consistently Enforce consequences Group therapy
Borderline	Seeks brief and intense relationships Blames others for own problems Depression, intense anger, labile mood, posttraumatic symptoms Temper tantrums, physical fights Impulsiveness, manipulative Repetitive self-destructiveness, self-mutilation, suicidal Overspending, promiscuity, compulsive overeating	75% are women and have been sexually abused Problems with identity, self image, thinking, and mood Uses splitting to avoid pain and to protect self Projective identification used to protect the self Biological, environmental, and stress-related factors, including traumatic home environment Abnormalities in serotonin systems Suicidal behaviors occur when blocked, frustrated, or stressed	Help person identify and verbalize feelings and control negative behaviors Use empathy Behavioral contracts to decrease self-mutilation Journal-writing Consistent limit-setting needed Supportive confrontation Enforce unit rules Psychopharmacology used sparingly for anxiety, psychotic states, suicidal ideation, mood swings Group therapy

		Table 4 PERSONALITY DISORDERS *(CONTINUED)*	
TYPES	**ASSESSMENT**	**DIAGNOSE**	**NURSING CONSIDERATIONS**
Narcissistic	Arrogant, appears indifferent to criticism while hiding anger, rage, or emptiness Lacks ability to feel or demonstrate empathy Sense of entitlement Use others to meet their own needs Displays grandiosity	Views others as superior or inferior to self Shallow relationships with others Feelings of others not understood or considered Uses rationalization to blame others Expects special treatment Needs to be admired	Mirror what person sounds like, especially contradictions Supportive confrontation to increase sense of self-responsibility Limit-setting and consistency Focus on the here and now Teach that mistakes are acceptable, imperfections do not decrease worth
Histrionic	Draws attention to self, thrives on being the center of attention Silly, colorful, frivolous, seductive Hurried, restless Temper tantrums and outbursts of anger Overreacts Dissociation used to avoid feelings Somatic reports to avoid responsibility and support dependency	Cannot deal with feelings Shallow, rapidly shifting emotions Easily influenced by others	Positive reinforcement for unselfish or other-centered behaviors Help clarify feelings and facilitate appropriate expression
Dependent	Dependent on others for everyday decisions Passive Problem initiating projects or working independently Anxious or helpless when alone Preoccupied with fear of being alone to care for self	Fears loss of support and approval Lacks self-confidence	Emphasize decision-making to increase self-responsibility Teach assertiveness Assist to clarify feelings, needs, and desires
Anxious–Avoidant	Timid, socially uncomfortable, withdrawn Hypersensitive to criticism Avoids situations where rejection is a possibility Lacks self-confidence	Fears intimate relationships due to fear of ridicule Believes self to be socially inept, unappealing, or inferior	Gradually confront fears Discuss feelings before and after accomplishing a goal Teach assertiveness Increase exposure to small groups
Obsessive–compulsive	Sets high personal standards for self and others Preoccupied with rules, lists, organization, details Overconscientious and inflexible Rigid and stubborn Cold affect, may speak in monotone Indecisive until all facts accumulated Repetitive thoughts and actions	Difficulty expressing warmth Rigid and controlling with others Perfectionism interferes with task fulfillment	Explore feelings Help with decision-making Confront procrastination and intellectualization Teach that mistakes are acceptable

▶ **MANIPULATIVE BEHAVIOR**

A. Assessment

1. Makes unreasonable requests for time, attention, and favors

2. Divides staff against each other—attempts to undermine nurse's role

3. Intimidates others

   a. Uses others' faults to own advantage, e.g., naiveté

   b. Makes others feel guilty

4. Uses seductive and disingenuous approach

   a. Makes personal approach with staff, e.g., acts more like friend than client

   b. Frequently lies and rationalizes

   c. Takes advantage of others for own gain

5. Frequently lies and rationalizes

6. May malinger or behave in helpless manner, e.g., feigns illness to avoid task

B. Diagnose

1. Predisposing conditions

   a. Bipolar disorder

   b. Substance abuse, alcoholism

   c. Antisocial disorders

   d. Adolescent adjustment reactions

2. Potential nursing diagnoses

   a. Impaired social interaction

   b. Social isolation

   c. Violence: self-directed, risk for

   d. Violence: directed at others, risk for

C. Plan/Implementation

1. Goals

   a. Help client set limits on his behavior

   b. Help client learn to see the consequences of his behavior

   c. Help family members understand and deal with client

   d. Promote staff cooperation and consistency in caring for client

2. Use consistent undivided staff approach

   a. Clearly define expectations for client

   b. Adhere to hospital regulations

   c. Hold frequent staff conferences to avoid conflicts and increase staff communication

3. Set limits

   a. Do not allow behaviors that endanger or interfere with the rights or safety of others

   b. Carry out limit-setting, avoid threats and promises

   c. Give alternatives when possible

   d. Remain nonjudgmental

    e. Avoid arguing or allowing client to rationalize behavior

    f. Be brief in discussions

  4. Be constantly alert for potential manipulation

    a. Favors, compliments

    b. Attempts to be personal

    c. Malingering, helplessness

  5. Be alert for signs of destructive behavior

    a. Suicide

    b. Homicide

D. Evaluation

  1. Is staff cohesiveness maintained?

  2. Do the client's actions interfere with the rights of others?

  3. Does client set limits on own behavior?

  4. Has self-injury been avoided?

  5. Has injury to others been avoided?

▶ VIOLENT/AGGRESSIVE BEHAVIOR

A. Assessment

  1. Physical or verbal abuse of staff and/or other clients

  2. Overt anger and passive-aggressive behaviors

  3. Increased anxiety levels, physical signs of tension, change in pace or intensity of speech

B. Diagnose

  1. Assault cycle—triggering phase, escalation phase, verbal aggression phase, crisis phase, recovery phase, postcrisis depression phase

  2. Caused by intrapersonal, familial, interpersonal, and environmental stressors

C. Plan/Implementation (see Table 5)

  1. Consider the source and the target of the anger

  2. Consider displacement of anger in delusions and hallucinations

  3. Assessanger at a safe distance, remain calm, assure that safe escape route is present

  4. Allow client to ventilate without violence, assist client to identify source of anger

  5. Ask client to assess his/her own potential for violence

  6. Contract with the client to use nonviolent methods to control anger

  7. Be prepared to use seclusion if escalation with potential for violence exists

Table 5 NURSING CARE OF A CLIENT WHO ACTS VIOLENT	
PROBLEM	INTERVENTIONS
Increased agitation/anxiety	Recognize signs of impending violence, e.g., increased motor activity, pacing, or sudden stop—"calm before the storm"
	Identify self, speak calmly but firmly, and in normal tone of voice
	Help verbalize feelings
	Use nonthreatening body language, e.g., arms to side, palm outward, keep distance, avoid blocking exit, avoid body contact
	Avoid disagreeing with client or threatening client
	Decrease stimuli—remove threatening objects or people
Violence	Intercede early
	Continue nonthreatening behavior
	If client needs to be restrained to protect self or others, get help (at least four people)
	Move in organized, calm manner, stating that nurse wants to help and that you will not permit client to harm self or others
	Use restraints correctly, e.g., never tie to bedside rail, check circulation frequently

D. Evaluation

1. Client approaches staff and discusses angry impulses without acting-out

2. Violent episodes are minor and controlled

3. Unit safety is maintained

▶ EATING DISORDERS

A. Assessment (see Table 6)

B. Diagnose (see Table 6)

C. Plan/Implementation (see Table 6)

D. Evaluation

1. Have client's physical needs been met?

2. Does client have insight into eating disorder?

Table 6 EATING DISORDERS		
DISORDER	**ASSESSMENT/DIAGNOSE**	**NURSING CONSIDERATIONS**
Anorexia nervosa	Most common in females 12–18 years old Characterized by fear of obesity, dramatic weight loss, distorted body image, very structured food intake Anemia, amenorrhea Cathartics, diuretics, and enemas may be used for purging Excessive exercise Induced vomiting used for purging May have cardiotoxicity secondary to use of ipecac May have electrolyte imbalance	Monitor clinical status (e.g., weight, intake, vital signs) Monitor hydration and electrolytes, especially potassium Behavior modification may help in acute phase Family therapy Support efforts to take responsibility for self Explore issues regarding sexuality Contract with client
Bulimia	Characterized by all of the characteristics of anorexia and binge eating (eating increased amounts of high calorie food in a short period of time) May be of normal weight or overweight Tooth erosion and decay GI bleeding (upper and/or lower) May use vomiting, laxatives, enemas, diuretics or weight-loss medications	May be managed with antidepressants (e.g., SSRI) Nutritional assessment and counseling

▶ **ACUTE ALCOHOL INTOXICATION**

A. Assessment (see Table 1)

B. Diagnose (see Table 1)

C. Plan/Implementation (see Table 1)

Table 1 POTENTIAL ALCOHOL INTOXICATION		
ASSESSMENT	**POTENTIAL NURSING DIAGNOSIS**	**NURSING CONSIDERATIONS**
Drowsiness	Acute confusion	Monitor vital signs frequently
Slurred speech	Risk for injury	Allow client to "sleep it off"
Tremors	Risk for ineffective breathing pattern	Protect airway from aspiration
Impaired thinking/memory loss	Risk for aspiration	Assess need for IV glucose
Nystagmus		Assess for injuries
Diminished reflexes		Assess for signs of withdrawal and chronic alcohol dependence
Nausea/vomiting		
Possible hypoglycemia		Counsel about alcohol use
Increased respiration		Potential problems of alcohol poisoning and CNS depression
Belligerence/grandiosity		
Loss of inhibitions		
Depression		

D. Evaluation

1. Short-term: Has injury been prevented and CNS status maintained?

2. Long-term: Have chronic intoxication and CNS damage been avoided?

▶ **ALCOHOL WITHDRAWAL**

A. Assessment (see Table 2)

B. Diagnose—potential nursing diagnoses

1. Anxiety

2. Injury, risk for

3. Self-care deficit

4. Thought process, altered

C. Plan/Implementation (see Table 2)

Table 2 ALCOHOL WITHDRAWAL		
WITHDRAWAL	**DELIRIUM TREMENS**	**NURSING CONSIDERATIONS**
Tremors	Tremors	Administer (benzodiazepines, chlordiazepoxide, diazepam) sedation as needed
Easily startled	Anxiety	
Insomnia	Panic	Monitor vital signs, particularly pulse, BP, temperature
Anxiety	Disorientation, confusion	
Anorexia	Hallucination	Seizure precautions
Alcoholic hallucinations	Vomiting	Provide quiet, well-lit environment
	Diarrhea	
	Paranoia	Orient client frequently
	Delusional symptoms	Don't leave hallucinating, confused client alone
	Ideas of reference	
	Suicide attempts	Administer anticonvulsants as needed
	Grand mal convulsions (especially first 48 hours after drinking stopped)	Administer thiamine IV or IM as needed
	Potential coma/death	Administer IV glucose as needed 10% mortality rate

D. Evaluation

1. Has injury been avoided (head trauma, aspiration of vomitus)?

2. Have normal serum glucose levels been maintained?

3. Have nutritional deficiencies been treated?

▶ CHRONIC ALCOHOL DEPENDENCE

A. Assessment

1. Persistent incapacitation

2. Cyclic drinking or "binges"

3. Daily drinking with increase in amount

4. Potential chronic central nervous system disorder (see Table 3)

5. Sexual relationships may be disturbed

Table 3 CHRONIC CNS DISORDERS ASSOCIATED WITH ALCOHOLISM			
	ALCOHOLIC CHRONIC BRAIN SYNDROME (DEMENTIA)	WERNICKE'S SYNDROME	KORSAKOFF'S PSYCHOSIS
Symptoms	Fatigue, anxiety, personality changes, depression, confusion Loss of memory of recent events Can progress to dependent, bedridden state	Confusion, diplopia, nystagmus, ataxia Disorientation, apathy	Memory disturbance with confabulation, loss of memory of recent events, learning problem Possible problem with taste and smell, loss of reality testing
Nursing considerations	Balanced diet, abstinence from alcohol	IV or IM thiamine, abstinence from alcohol	Balanced diet, thiamine, abstinence from alcohol

6. Others in family may take over alcoholic's role, e.g., children may take parent's role, resulting in loss of childhood opportunities

7. Children often feel shame and embarrassment

8. High percentage of children develop problems with alcohol themselves

9. Incidence of family violence is increased with alcohol use

B. Diagnose—potential nursing diagnoses

1. Imbalanced nutrition: less than body requirements

2. Chronic low self esteem

3. Social isolation

4. Dysfunctional family processes: alcoholism

C. Plan/Implementation

1. Counseling the alcoholic

a. Identify problems related to drinking—in family relationships, work, medical, and other areas of life

b. Help client to see/admit problem

1) Confront denial with slow persistence

2) Maintain relationship with client

2. Establish control of problem drinking

a. Concrete support to identify potentially troublesome settings that trigger drinking behavior

b. Alcoholics Anonymous—valuable mutual support group

1) Peers share experiences

2) Learn to substitute contact with humans for alcohol

3) Stresses living in the present; stop drinking one day at a time

      c. Disulfiram—drug used to maintain sobriety; based on behavioral therapy

         1) Once sufficient blood level is reached, disulfiram interacts with alcohol to provide severe reaction

         2) Symptoms of disulfiram-alcohol reaction include flushing, coughing, difficulty breathing, nausea, vomiting, pallor, anxiety

         3) Contraindicated in diabetes mellitus, atherosclerotic heart disease, cirrhosis, kidney disease, psychosis

  3. Counsel the spouse of the alcoholic

      a. Initial goal is to help spouse focus on self

      b. Explore life problems from spouse's point of view

      c. Spouse can attempt to help alcoholic once strong enough

      d. Al-Anon: self-help group of spouses and relatives

         1) Learn "loving detachment" from alcoholic

         2) Goal is to try to make one's own life better and not to blame the alcoholic

         3) Provides safe, helpful environment

  4. Counsel children of alcoholic parents

      a. Overcome denial of problem

      b. Establish trusting relationship

      c. Work with parents as well; avoid negative reactions to parents

      d. Referral to Alateen: organization for teenagers of alcoholic parent; self-help, similar to Al-Anon

D. Evaluation

  1. Has client abstained from alcohol?

  2. Has client maintained nutritional status?

  3. Has client reduced his/her social isolation?

▶ NONALCOHOL SUBSTANCE ABUSE

A. Assessment (see Table 4)

B. Diagnose

  1. Drug addiction—a physiological and psychological dependence; increasing doses needed to maintain "high" (tolerance)

  2. Substance abusers have a low frustration tolerance and need for immediate gratification to escape anxiety

  3. Addiction may result from prolonged use of medication for physical or psychological pain

  4. Becomes a problem with some nurses

  5. Potential nursing diagnoses

      a. Ineffective denial/coping

      b. Dysfunctional family processes: substance abuse

      c. Violence: directed toward self or others, risk for

C. Plan/Implementation

1. Observe for signs and symptoms of intoxication or drug use

    a. Examine skin for cuts, needle-marks, abscesses, or bruises

    b. Recognize symptoms of individual drug overdose

        1) Hypotension, decreased respirations with narcotics and sedatives

        2) Agitation with amphetamines and hallucinogens

2. Treat symptoms of overdose

    a. Maintain respiration—airway when needed

    b. IV therapy as necessary

    c. Administer naloxone

        1) Antagonist to narcotics—induces withdrawal, stimulates respirations

        2) Short-acting—symptoms of respiratory depression may return; additional doses may be necessary

    d. Gastric lavage for overdose of sedatives taken orally

    e. Dialysis to eliminate barbiturates from system

3. Observe for signs of withdrawal, e.g., sweating, agitation, panic, hallucinations

    a. Identify drug type

    b. Seizure precautions

    c. Keep airway on hand

    d. Detoxify gradually

        1) Methadone or naltrexone used for long-term maintenance and acute withdrawal (narcotic)

        2) Decreasing doses of drug substitute

4. Treat panic from acute withdrawal and/or marked depression

    a. Hospitalize temporarily for psychotic response

    b. Decrease stimuli, provide calm environment

    c. Protect client from self-destructive behavior

Table 4 NONALCOHOL SUBSTANCE ABUSE			
MEDICATION/DRUG	**SYMPTOMS OF ABUSE**	**SYMPTOMS OF WITHDRAWAL**	**NURSING CONSIDERATIONS**
Barbiturates (downers, barbs, pink ladies, rainbows, yellow jackets) Phenobarbital Nembutal	Respiratory depression Decreased BP and pulse Coma, ataxia, seizures Increasing nystagmus Poor muscle coordination Decreased mental alertness	Anxiety, insomnia Tremors, delirium Convulsions	Maintain airway (intubate, suction) Check LOC and vital signs Start IV with large-gauge needle Give sodium bicarbonate to promote excretion Give activated charcoal, use gastric lavage Hemodialysis
Narcotics Morphine Heroin (horse, junk, smack) Codeine Dilaudid Methadone—for detoxification and maintenance	Marked respiratory depression Hyperpyrexia Seizures, ventricular dysrhythmias Euphoria, then anxiety, sadness, insomnia, sexual indifference Overdose–severe respiratory depression, pinpoint pupils, coma Stupor leading to coma	Watery eyes, runny nose Loss of appetite Irritability, tremors, panic Cramps, nausea Chills and sweating Elevated BP Hallucinations, delusions	Maintain airway (intubate, suction) Control seizures Check LOC and vital signs Start IV, may be given bolus of glucose Have lidocaine and defibrillator available Treat for hyperthermia Give naloxone to reverse respiratory depression Hemodialysis
Stimulants (uppers, pep pills, speed, crystal meth) Cocaine (crack) Amphetamine Benzedrine Dexedrine	Tachycardia, increased BP, tachypnea, anxiety Irritability, insomnia, agitation Seizures, coma, hyperpyrexia, euphoria Nausea, vomiting Hyperactivity, rapid speech Hallucinations Nasal septum perforation (cocaine)	Apathy Long periods of sleep Irritability Depression, disorientation	Maintain airway (intubate, suction) Start IV Use cardiac monitoring Check LOC and vital signs Give activated charcoal, use gastric lavage Monitor for suicidal ideation Keep in calm, quiet environment
Cannabis derivatives (pot, weed, grass, reefer, joint, mary jane) Marijuana Hashish	Fatigue Paranoia, psychosis Euphoria, relaxed inhibitions Increased appetite Disoriented behavior	Insomnia, hyperactivity Decreased appetite	Most effects disappear in 5-8 hr as drug wears off May cause psychosis
Hallucinogens LSD (acid) PCP (angel dust, rocket fuel) Mescaline (buttons, cactus)	Nystagmus, marked confusion, hyperactivity Incoherence, hallucinations, distorted body image Delirium, mania, self-injury Hypertension, hyperthermia Flashbacks, convulsions, coma	None	Maintain airway (intubate, suction) Control seizures Check LOC and vital signs Reduce sensory stimuli Small doses of diazepam Check for trauma, protect from self-injury

      d. Stay with client to reduce anxiety, panic, and confusion

      e. Assure client that hallucinations are from drugs and will subside

      f. Administer medications as indicated to manage symptoms of withdrawal and panic

      g. Monitor vital signs

5. Promote physical health

      a. Identify physical health needs

          1) Rest

          2) Nutrition

          3) Shelter

      b. Complete physical work-up

          1) Heroin addicts need to be followed for liver and cardiac complications, sexually transmitted disease, AIDS

          2) Dental care

6. Administer methadone for maintenance when indicated

      a. Synthetic narcotic—blocks euphoric effects of narcotics

      b. Eliminates craving and withdrawal symptoms

      c. Daily urine collected to monitor for other drug abuse while on methadone

7. Implement measures for antisocial personality disorders/manipulative behaviors

      a. Structured, nonpermissive environment

      b. Milieu therapy—peer pressure to conform

      c. Set limits but remain nonjudgmental

      d. Refer to drug-free programs (Synanon, Phoenix House, Odyssey House) for confrontation and support to remain drug-free

8. Treat underlying emotional problems

      a. Individual therapy—give support and acceptance

      b. Group therapy—to learn new ways of interacting

      c. Promote use of self-help groups

9. Assist client with rehabilitation, e.g., work programs, vocational counseling, family counseling, completion of schooling

D. Evaluation

1. Is client able to abstain from drugs or to be maintained on methadone?

2. Has client's independent functioning resumed?

3. Is treatment ongoing for underlying emotional problems?

4. Has client stopped committing crime to support drug habit (if this was an issue)?

▶ CHILD ABUSE

A. Assessment

1. Inconsistency between type/location of injury (bruises, burns, fractures, especially chip/spiral) with the history of the incident(s)

2. Unexplained physical or thermal injuries

3. Withdraws or is fearful of parents

4. Sexual abuse—genital lacerations, sexually transmitted diseases

5. Emotional neglect, failure to thrive, disturbed sleep, change in behavior at school

B. Diagnose

1. Intentional physical, emotional, and/or sexual misuse/trauma or intentional omission of basic needs (neglect); usually related to diminished/limited ability of parent(s) to cope with, provide for, and/or relate to child

2. Those at high risk include children born prematurely and/or of low birth weight, children under 3 years of age, and children with physical and/or mental disabilities

3. Potential nursing diagnoses
   a. Risk for trauma
   b. Interrupted family processes/impaired parenting

C. Plan/Implementation

1. Provide for physical needs first

2. Mandatory reporting of identified/suspected cases to appropriate agency

3. Nonjudgmental treatment of parents; encourage expression of feelings

4. Provide role modeling and encourage parents to be involved in care

5. Teach growth and development concepts, especially safety, discipline, age-appropriate activities, and human nutrition

6. Provide emotional support for child; play therapy (dolls, drawings, making up stories) may be more appropriate way for child to express feelings

7. Initiate protective placement and/or appropriate referrals for long-term follow-up

8. Documentation should reflect only what nurse saw or was told, not nurse's interpretation or opinion

D. Evaluation

1. Have parents learned appropriate ways to discipline their child?

2. Have the child's physical needs been met?

▶ ELDER ABUSE

A. Assessment

1. Battering, fractures, bruises
2. Over/undermedicated
3. Absence of needed dentures, glasses
4. Poor nutritional status, dehydration
5. Physical evidence of sexual abuse
6. Urine burns, excoriated skin, pressure ulcers
7. Fear, apprehension, withdrawal from usual activities

B. Diagnose

1. Elderly with chronic illness and depletion of financial resources who are dependent on children and grandchildren
2. Population trends of today contribute to decline in amount of people available to care for elderly
3. Potential nursing diagnoses
   a. Compromised family coping
   b. Risk for trauma
   c. Nutrition, less than body requirements

C. Plan/Implementation

1. Provide for safety
2. Provide for physical needs first
3. Report to appropriate agencies (state laws vary)
4. Initiate protective placement and/or appropriate referrals
5. Consider client's rights of self-determination

D. Evaluation

1. Is client safe?
2. Have the client's physical needs been met?
3. Have appropriate referrals been made?

▶ SEXUAL ABUSE

A. Assessment

1. Sexually abused child
   a. Disturbed growth and development
   b. Child becomes protective (parent) of others
   c. Uses defense mechanisms (e.g., denial, dissociation)
   d. Sleep and eating disturbances
   e. Depression and aggression, emotional deadening, amnesia
   f. Poor impulse control
   g. Somatic symptoms (e.g., chronic pain, GI disturbances)
   h. Truancy and running away
   i. Self-destructiveness

2. Adult victims of childhood sexual abuse

    a. Response is similar to delayed postraumatic stress disorder (PTSD)

    b. Nightmares

    c. Unwanted, intrusive memories

    d. Kinesthetic sensations

    e. Flashbacks

    f. Relationship issues, fears of intimacy and abandonment

3. Sexually abused adult

    a. Uses defense mechanisms (e.g., denial, dissociation)

    b. Relationship issues, abusive relationships, fears of intimacy and abandonment

    c. Somatic reports

    d. Homicidal thoughts, violence

    e. Hypervigilance, panic attacks, phobias/agoraphobia

    f. Suicidal thoughts/attempts

    g. Self-mutilation

    h. Compulsive eating/dieting, binging/purging

B. Diagnose

1. Victims from every sociocultural, ethnic, and economic group

2. Within the family (incest) and outside the family

3. Usually involves younger, weaker victim

4. Victim is usually urged and coerced, manipulated through fear

5. Difficult to expose abuse; common for child not to be believed

C. Plan/Implementation

1. Establish trusting relationship

2. Use empathy, active support, compassion, warmth

3. Nonjudgmental approach

4. Group and individual therapy; appropriate referrals

5. Medications as needed (e.g., antianxiety)

6. Report to appropriate agencies

D. Evaluation

1. Does the client demonstrate improved self-esteem?

2. Does the client express self-acceptance and forgiveness of self?

3. Does the client demonstrate adaptive coping to stress?

4. Is the client able to sustain capacity for intimate relationships?

5. Does the client demonstrate reduced anxiety and fear?

▶ DOMESTIC VIOLENCE

A. Assessment

1. Frequent visits to health care provider's office or emergency room for unexplained trauma

2. Client being cued, silenced, or threatened by an accompanying family member

3. Evidence of multiple old injuries, scars, healed fractures seen on x-ray

4. Fearful, evasive, or inconsistent replies and nonverbal behaviors such as flinching when approached or touched

B. Diagnose

1. Family violence is usually accompanied by brainwashing (e.g., victims blame themselves, feel unworthy, and fear that they won't be believed)

2. Long-term results of family violence are depression, suicidal ideation, low self-esteem, and impaired relationships outside the family

3. Women and children are the most common victims, but others include adolescents, men, and parents

C. Plan/Implementation

1. Provide privacy during initial interview to insure that the perpetrator of violence does not remain with client; make a statement, e.g., "This part of the exam is always done in private."

2. Carefully document all injuries using body maps or photographs (with consent)

3. Determine the safety of client by specific questions about weapons in the home, substance abuse, extreme jealousy

4. Develop with client a safety or escape plan

5. Refer the client to community resources such as shelters, hotlines, and support groups

D. Evaluation

1. Is the client focusing on own needs?

2. Is the client developing concrete plan for shelter or legal aid?

INDEX

Thrombosis, 41, 90, 205, 260, 295
Thrombus formation from immobility, 315
Thyroid disorders, 362–364
Thyroid replacement medications, 97
Tic Douloureaux, 157
Tick bites and Lyme disease, 432
Ticlodipine, 90
Tilt tables, 316
Timing for Kaplan resources, 16–17
Timing of NCLEX-RN® exam, 7, 24–25
Timolol maleate, 116
Tine TB skin test, 428, 534, 545
Tinea, 194
Tiotropium, 105
Tissue plasminogen activator, 128
TLSO (thoracolumbosacral orthotic) brace, 325–326
TNA (Total Nutrient Admixture), 383
Tobramycin, 71, 116
Toddlers, 197, 198, 378, 445
    growth and development, 454, 458–459, 532
Toilet training, 386, 459
Tolna flake cream, 79
Tolterodine, 113
Tongue, 77, 160, 294, 367, 554, 555
    glossitis, 138, 294, 369
Tonic neck reflex, 457, 508, 511
Tonic seizures, 258
Tonic-clonic seizures, 258
Tonicity, 37
Tonometry, 145
Tonsillitis (streptococcal), 425
Topical anti-infective medications, 78–79
Topiramate, 58
Topoisomerase antineoplastic medications, 88
Topotecan, 88
TORCH test series, 478
Total anomalous venous return, 285
Total cholesterol test, 206
Toxic hepatitis, 431
Toxic shock syndrome (TSS), 527
Toxoplasmosis and pregnancy, 478
Toys by appropriate age, 457, 459, 460, 461
    play development by age, 453
Trachea, 209, 226, 554, 556
Tracheoesophageal fistula, 173–174
Tracheostomy, 220–221, 235–236
Traction, 262, 348–350
Transfusion of blood, 34–35

Transient ischemic attacks (TIAs), 260, 292
Transplant of kidney, 397–398
Transverse colostomy, 183
Tranylcypromine, 59, 61
Trazodone, 58, 62
Treatment refusal, 401, 403, 405
Trendelenburg, modified, 316
Triage, 447
Tricuspid valve, 556, 557
Tricyclic antidepressants, 60–61
Trifluoperazine adverse effects, 94
Trigeminal cranial nerve (V), 555
Trigeminal neuralgia, 157
Triglycerides test, 206
Trihexyphenidyl, 53, 89
Trimethobenzamide HCl, 66
Trimethoprim/sulfamethoxazole, 75, 77
Triple lumen central catheter, 383
Trisomy 21, 468, 475
Trochlear cranial nerve (IV), 555
Trousseau's sign, 364, 365
Truncus arteriosus, 285
TSH, 296
Tubal ligation, 526
Tuberculosis, 426, 427–429
Tumors, 85–88, 299–308, 527, 528, 529
Tunneled central catheter, 41–42
Turner's sign, 253
Turner's syndrome, 475
Types 1 and 2 diabetes, 163–166

U

Ulcerative colitis, 174–175
Ulcers, 171–173
    medications, 113–114, 132, 133
Ulnar pulse, 557
Ultrasonic flow detection, 208
Ultrasound echocardiogram, 210
Ultrasound of fetus, 477
Ultrasound of kidney, 217
Umbilical cord, 479, 484, 485, 511, 512
Umbilical hernias, 179
Undifferentiated schizophrenia, 592
Undoing against anxiety, 568
Unit conversions, 135
Upper airway obstruction, 235–237
Upper GI series, 214
Ureteral calculi, 388–389
Ureterolithiasis, 388–389
Ureterolithotomy, 389

Ureterosigmoidostomy, 393, 394
Urethra diagnostic tests, 216
Urinalysis, 216
Urinary calculi, 388–389
Urinary catheters, 228–231
Urinary diversions, 393–394
Urinary elimination, 377, 385–386
Urinary incontinence, 488
Urinary malformations, congenital, 387
Urinary retention as surgery complication, 203
Urinary stasis, 315
Urinary system tests, 216–217
Urinary tract infections (UTI), 203, 478
Urinary tract surgeries, 389
Urine culture and sensitivity, 216
Urogenital system.
    See Genitourinary system
Urolithiasis, 388–389
Urticaria (hives), 137, 545
Uterus, 472
    disorders, 527, 528
Uveitis, 147

V

Vagina, 215, 316, 463, 525–526, 559
Vaginitis, 526
Vagotomy, 172
Vagus cranial nerve (X), 555
Valerian, 133
Valproic acid, 57
Valsartan, 79
Valvular heart disease, 288
Vancomycin, 73, 76, 78
Vanillylmandelic acid (VMA) test, 277
Vardenafil, 113, 130
Variances in managed care, 407
Varicella, 424, 426, 478
    immunization, 535, 536, 538, 540, 541, 544
Varicose veins, 291
Vasectomy, 526
Vasodilators, 83, 134
Vasopressin, 296
Vegan diet, 294, 371
Vegetables, 164, 370, 379, 380
Vegetarian diets, 371, 372
Velcro straps as adaptive devices, 319
Venlafaxine, 60, 62
Venous diagnostic tests, 208
Venous peripheral vascular disease, 291